Unanswered Questions in Implant Dentistry

Editor

MOHANAD AL-SABBAGH

DENTAL CLINICS OF NORTH AMERICA

www.dental.theclinics.com

July 2019 • Volume 63 • Number 3

ELSEVIER

1600 John F. Kennedy Boulevard • Suite 1800 • Philadelphia, Pennsylvania, 19103-2899

http://www.dental.theclinics.com

DENTAL CLINICS OF NORTH AMERICA Volume 63, Number 3
July 2019 ISSN 0011-8532, ISBN: 978-0-323-68243-5

Editor: John Vassallo; j.vassallo@elsevier.com
Developmental Editor: Laura Fisher

Dental Clinics of North America (ISSN 0011-8532) is published quarterly by Elsevier Inc., 360 Park Avenue South, New York, NY 10010-1710. Months of issue are January, April, July, and October. Business and Editorial Offices: 1600 John F. Kennedy Boulevard, Suite 1800, Philadelphia, PA 19103-2899. Periodicals postage paid at New York, NY and additional mailing offices. Subscription prices are $304.00 per year (domestic individuals), $603.00 per year (domestic institutions), $100.00 per year (domestic students/residents), $366.00 per year (Canadian individuals), $782.00 per year (Canadian institutions), $424.00 per year (international individuals), $782.00 per year (international institutions), and $200.00 per year (international and Canadian students/residents). International air speed delivery is included in all *Clinics* subscription prices. All prices are subject to change without notice. **POSTMASTER:** Send address changes to *Dental Clinics of North America*, Elsevier Health Sciences Division, Subscription Customer Service, 3251 Riverport Lane, Maryland Heights, MO 63043. **Customer Service (orders, claims, online, change of address): Elsevier Health Sciences Division, Subscription Customer Service, 3251 Riverport Lane, Maryland Heights, MO 63043. Tel: 1-800-654-2452 (U.S. and Canada). Fax: 314-447-8029. E-mail: journalscustomer service-usa@elsevier.com (for print support); journalsonlinesupport-usa@elsevier.com (for online support).**

Reprints. For copies of 100 or more, of articles in this publication, please contact the Commercial Reprints Department, Elsevier Inc., 360 Park Avenue South, New York, NY 10010-1710. Tel.: 212-633-3874; Fax: 212-633-3820; E-mail: reprints@elsevier.com.

The *Dental Clinics of North America* is covered in *MEDLINE/PubMed (Index Medicus), Current Contents/Clinical Medicine, ISI/BIOMED* and *Clinahl.*

Contributors

EDITOR

MOHANAD AL-SABBAGH, DDS, MS
Professor and Chief, Division of Periodontology, Director, Advanced Education Externship Program, Diplomate, American Academy of Periodontology, Department of Oral Health Practice, University of Kentucky College of Dentistry, Chandler Medical Center, Lexington, Kentucky, USA

AUTHORS

FIRAS AL YAFI, DDS
Diplomate, Arab Board of Oral Surgery, Teaching Assistant, Division of Periodontology, Department of Oral Health Practice, University of Kentucky College of Dentistry, Lexington, Kentucky, USA

BASEM ALCHAWAF, DMD, DrMedDent
Assistant Professor, Department of Oral and Maxillofacial Surgery, King Khalid University Hospital and Dental University Hospital, Faculty of Dentistry, King Saud University, Riyadh, Saudi Arabia

FADI AL FARAWATI, DDS, MS, MClinDent, MFDS RCSEd
Assistant Professor, Department of Restorative Sciences, The Dental College of Georgia at Augusta University, Augusta, Georgia, USA

KHALID ALMAS, BDS, MSc, FRACDS, MSc, FDSRCS, DDPHRCS, FICD
Professor, Division of Periodontology, Department of Preventive Dental Sciences, College of Dentistry, Imam Abdulrahman Bin Faisal University, Dammam, Saudi Arabia

NEHAL ALMEHMADI, BDS
Research Assistant, Division of Periodontology, Department of Oral Health Practice, University of Kentucky College of Dentistry, Lexington, Kentucky, USA

MOHANAD AL-SABBAGH, DDS, MS
Professor and Chief, Division of Periodontology, Director, Advanced Education Externship Program, Diplomate, American Academy of Periodontology, Department of Oral Health Practice, University of Kentucky College of Dentistry, Chandler Medical Center, Lexington, Kentucky, USA

FATIMAH AL-SHAIKHLI, BDS, DMD
Research Assistant, Division of Periodontology, Department of Oral Health Practice, University of Kentucky College of Dentistry, Lexington, Kentucky, USA

BRITTANY CAMENISCH, DDS, MS
Private Practice, Richmond, Kentucky, USA; Adjunct Professor, University of Kentucky College of Dentistry, Lexington, Kentucky, USA

DOLPHUS R. DAWSON III, DMD, MS, MPH
Division of Periodontology, Department of Oral Health Practice, University of Kentucky
College of Dentistry, Lexington, Kentucky, USA

ENIF A. DOMINGUEZ, DDS
Assistant Professor, Division of Oral and Maxillofacial Surgery, Department of Oral
Health Science, University of Kentucky College of Dentistry, Albert B. Chandler Hospital,
Lexington, Kentucky, USA

WALIED ELDOMIATY, BDS
Visiting Scholar, Division of Periodontology, Department of Oral Health Practice,
University of Kentucky College of Dentistry, Lexington, Kentucky, USA

AHMED EL-GHANNAM, PhD
Department of Mechanical Engineering and Engineering Science, The University of
North Carolina at Charlotte, Charlotte, North Carolina, USA

CESAR GUERRERO, DDS
Private Practice, Clear Choice Dental Implant Center, Oral and Maxillofacial Surgery,
Houston, Texas, USA; The Woodlands Oral & Facial Surgery Center, The Woodlands,
Texas, USA

AHMED HANAFY, BDS, MSc, PhD
Visiting Lecturer, Department of Periodontology, School of Dental Medicine,
British University in Egypt, Cairo, Egypt

VAUGHAN J. HOEFLER, DDS, MBA
Assistant Professor, Department of Oral Health Practice, Prosthodontist, Division of
Prosthodontics, University of Kentucky College of Dentistry, Albert B. Chandler Hospital,
Lexington, Kentucky, USA

YASSER KHABBAZ, DDS, MS
Consultant Periodontist, Ambulatory Healthcare Services - SEHA, Abu Dhabi,
United Arab Emirates

AMRITPAL S. KULLAR, BDS
Oral Health Practice, University of Kentucky, Lexington, Kentucky, USA

AHMAD KUTKUT, DDS, MS, FICOI, DICOI
Associate Professor, Division of Prosthodontics, University of Kentucky College of
Dentistry, Lexington, Kentucky, USA

CRAIG S. MILLER, DMD, MS
Professor, Oral Health Practice, University of Kentucky, Lexington, Kentucky, USA

PRANAI NAKAPARKSIN, DDS, MSD, FACP, FRCD(C)
Lecturer, Mahidol University, Bangkok, Thailand

NOEL YE NAUNG, BDS, Higher Grad Dip Clin Sc (OMFS), MSc (OMFS), FIAOMS
Visiting Scholar, Division of Oral and Maxillofacial Surgery, Chandler Medical Center,
University of Kentucky College of Dentistry, Lexington, Kentucky, USA

KATJA NELSON, DMD, DrMedDent
Professor and Chair for Translational Implantology, Department of Dental and Craniofacial
Sciences, Clinic of Oral and Maxillofacial Surgery, Freiburg University Hospital, Freiburg
im Breisgau, Germany

GALAL OMAMI, BDS, MSc, MDentSc, FRCD(C), Dip ABOMR
Assistant Professor, Division of Oral Diagnosis, Oral Medicine, Oral Radiology, Department of Oral Health Practice, University of Kentucky College of Dentistry, Lexington, Kentucky, USA

LUCIANA M. SHADDOX, DDS, MS, PhD
Professor, Division of Periodontology, Department of Oral Health Practice, University of Kentucky College of Dentistry, Lexington, Kentucky, USA

EHAB SHEHATA, DDS, MD, MSc (GS), PhD
Assistant Professor, Division of Oral and Maxillofacial Surgery, Department of Oral Health Science, University of Kentucky College of Dentistry, Albert B. Chandler Hospital, Lexington, Kentucky, USA; Associate Professor, Department of Maxillofacial and Plastic Surgery, College of Dentistry, Alexandria University, Alexandria, Egypt

STEPH SMITH, BChD, BChD (Hons), MDent, MChD
Senior Lecturer, Division of Periodontology, Department of Preventive Dental Sciences, College of Dentistry, Imam Abdulrahman Bin Faisal University, Dammam, Saudi Arabia

JOSEPH E. VAN SICKELS, DDS, FACD, FICD, FACS
Professor, Program Director, Division of Oral and Maxillofacial Surgery, Department of Oral Health Science, University of Kentucky College of Dentistry, Albert B. Chandler Hospital, Lexington, Kentucky, USA

PINELOPI XENOUDI, DDS, MS
HS Associate Professor, Division of Periodontology, Department of Orofacial Sciences, University of California, San Francisco, School of Dentistry, San Francisco, California, USA

Contents

topography provides better primary stability and faster osseointegration, allowing for immediate placement or immediate loading. Randomized clinical trials are warranted to compare the response of osseointegration with various implant micro and macro surface topographies in people with various local or systemic risk factors.

The osseointegration and survival of dental implants are linked to primary stability. Good primary stability relies on the mechanical friction between implant surface and surrounding bone with absence of mobility in the osteotomy site immediately after implant placement. Several factors have been found to affect implant primary stability, including bone density, implant design, and surgical technique. Various methods have been used to assess implant primary stability including insertion torque and resonance frequency analysis. This article aims to evaluate the success of osseointegration in the absence of primary stability and to propose recommendations to manage implants that lack primary stability.

Edentulous sites are often characterized by inadequate bone volume for dental implant therapy. Bone augmentation procedures for site development involve longer healing period and are often invasive, costly, and associated with postoperative morbidity. This article discusses alternatives to invasive bone grafting procedures that are often used to develop implant sites. Owing to the broad nature of this topic, it is presented in two articles. In Part I, the use of short and narrow-diameter implants are discussed. Part II reviews the use of tilted as well as fewer implants to support a prosthesis.

Despite improvements in bone preservation following tooth extraction, edentulous sites are often deficient in bone volume for conventional dental implant therapy. Missing bone volume is often recaptured by surgery and grafting. This article discusses noninvasive alternatives to bone grafting. Part I of this topic discussed the use of short and narrow diameter implants. Part II discusses three additional alternatives: the use of tilted implants, the use of four or fewer tilted and axially-loaded implants to support a full-arch fixed-dental-prosthesis (FAFDP), and the use of zygomatic implants to restore the severely-atrophic edentulous maxillae lacking adequate bone for conventional treatment.

Rehabilitation of maxillary atrophy with dental implants is challenging to the clinician despite the wide variety of surgical techniques available. Finding the right indication for a procedure is highly important for the long-term stability of dental implants. With the introduction of the concept of "teeth-in-a-day," clinicians have explored innovative techniques to attain the goal of immediate implant-supported provisional prosthesis. However, costs and comorbidities are limitations to advancing these techniques. This article focuses on algorithms to rehabilitate the atrophic maxilla with the purpose of providing immediate provisional prosthetic teeth regardless of the mandibular dentition.

Implant dentistry has shifted to prosthetically guided implant planning and placement. This shift has influenced the range of available dental materials to restore single crowns and partially and fully edentulous jaws with dental implants. This article presents an overview of the available options to restore dental implants. The qualities that define an ideal restoring material are discussed along with the most commonly used materials with their advantages and limitations. Because clinicians face different clinical scenarios in their practice, the discussion sums up the best techniques and materials that are useful in addressing these nonideal situations.

Cement-retention is a viable option in restoring dental implants. A wide range of dental cements with different properties are commercially available for use in the cementation of implant prostheses. The selection of a dental cement for proper clinical application can be challenging. This article overviews the commercially available dental cements used in cement-retained implant-supported prostheses. Guidelines for cement selection are presented according to abutment and prosthetic material. Cementation techniques to reduce excess cement in peri-implant tissues are also mentioned.

Peri-implant mucositis and peri-implantitis are clinically associated with inflammation of soft tissue around implants; however, peri-implantitis is associated with radiographic bone loss. Recently a new classification scheme—peri-implant health, peri-implant mucositis, peri-implantitis, and peri-implant soft-tissue and hard-tissue deficiencies—was introduced. Although various clinical interventions to treat peri-implant diseases have been suggested, early diagnosis and treatment is the key to successful outcomes. Clinicians can select nonsurgical or surgical techniques according to the clinical parameters present, although surgical intervention seems to be more effective in treating peri-implantitis. The best approach to treat peri-implantitis remains controversial.

The need for keratinized tissue around implants remains a controversial topic. However, reconstruction of keratinized mucosa may be needed to facilitate restorative procedures, improve aesthetics, and control plaque during oral hygiene. Free gingival grafts, connective tissue grafts, allogenic/xenograft materials, and apically positioned flaps have been used to augment soft tissue around implants. Four different timing protocols have been explored with regard to soft-tissue augmentation: before and during implant placement, during the second-stage surgery, or after restoration. The timing and technique of soft-tissue augmentation remain controversial and lack support from literature. Long-term clinical studies to establish clear guidelines are warranted.

DENTAL CLINICS OF NORTH AMERICA

SERIES OF RELATED INTEREST

Atlas of the Oral and Maxillofacial Surgery Clinics
http://www.oralmaxsurgeryatlas.theclinics.com

Oral and Maxillofacial Surgery Clinics
http://www.oralmaxsurgery.theclinics.com

THE CLINICS ARE AVAILABLE ONLINE!
Access your subscription at:
www.theclinics.com

Preface

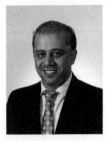

Mohanad Al-Sabbagh, DDS, MS
Editor

Dental implant treatment has become a mainstream reliable method to rehabilitate edentulous and partially edentulous patients. Osseointegration of dental implant is no longer the defining criteria for implant success; the surgical plan should be based on precise prosthetic restoration, accurate treatment planning, and detailed surgical techniques. The ultimate goal of a dental implant is to satisfy the patient's esthetic and functional needs to replace one or more missing teeth in a permanent manner.

The revolution of contemporary implant dentistry includes virtual planning, advanced implant designs and surface modification, and enhanced prosthetic materials. Cone-beam computed tomography (CBCT) and intraoral scanning enable clinicians to digitize the surgical and prosthetic plan, creating a digital workflow to navigate cases that are more complex with ease. In addition, 3D printing and Computer Assisted Design/Computer Assisted Manufacturing technology allow for the rapid production of study casts, surgical guides, and prosthetic temporaries. Nevertheless, with all these novel advancements, research has failed to generate definitive conclusions on many of implant dentist topics, and the decision-making process remains controversial.

The current issue of *Dental Clinics of North America* is an avenue to present evidence-based solutions to unanswered questions in implant dentistry. In the following articles, the authors develop a rational approach to understanding controversial topics in implant dentistry based on literature and the authors' clinical experience. It is our hope to generate a systematic and comprehensive clinical approach for best clinical practices.

The article by Kullar and Miller addresses possible contraindications for placement of dental implants. The authors provide important information on the general precautions of placing dental implants. Available risk factors (local, behavioral, and medical factors) that can contribute to risk of failure are correlated to numerous systematic reviews in the presented article.

The article by Omami and Al Yafi provides insight on the added advantage of CBCT over conventional 2D imaging techniques. CBCTs enhance traditional or virtual implant treatment planning and can decrease the incidence of surgical complications. However, the authors also highlighted the significance in practicing the concept of

Dent Clin N Am 63 (2019) xiii–xv
https://doi.org/10.1016/j.cden.2019.03.001
0011-8532/19/© 2019 Published by Elsevier Inc.

"ALADA" when acquiring images and the overall importance of identifying crucial anatomical landmarks using CBCT.

The article by Al Yafi, Camenisch, and Al-Sabbagh addresses the benefit and accuracy of computer-assisted implant surgery. It also reviews the different steps of digital workflow as well as the deviation between implant virtual plan and implant real position that may occur due to accumulated errors throughout the digital workflow.

The article by Al Yafi, Alchawaf, and Nelson presents the science behind ridge morphology alterations after dental extraction. The article also provides a contemporary review of the different approaches to preserve the alveolar ridge. Furthermore, the article also presents a new classification for single-extraction sockets with correlated treatment approaches.

The article by Naung, Shehata, and Van Sickels presents the rationale for the use of resorbable and nonresorbable membranes in guided bone regeneration for site development. The article assesses the ideal membrane material requirements and different resorbable and nonresorbable membranes commercially available. The authors also conclude that the choice of the membrane will vary according to the choice of bone graft and the nature of the bone defect.

The article by Dawson, El-Ghannam, Van Sickels, and Naung presents the latest concepts in tissue engineering with emphasis on the utilization of mesenchymal stem cells in soft tissue engineering. It also sheds light on maxillofacial bone reconstruction using osteoconductive scaffolds mixed with osteogenic stem and osteoprogenitor cells. The article also emphasizes the role of silica-calcium phosphate composite seeded with human adipose–derived stem cells to enhance bone grafts.

The article by Almas, Smith, and Kutkut presents the available implant microtopographies/macrotopographies to enhance the biologic response. The article discusses the importance of surface characteristics in influencing the rate and quality of early osseointegration and implant stability; these factors are the foundation of immediate placement and/or immediate loading. The authors as well shed light on the importance of identifying implant surface topographies to reduce the risk of peri-implantitis and long-term success of dental implants.

The article by Al-Sabbagh, Eldomiaty, and Khabbaz focuses on the importance of primary stability to achieve successfully osseointegrated dental implants. The article discusses different factors (patient selection, implant design, surgical technique used) that affect primary stability. Moreover, it discusses different methods used to assess primary stability and its importance for immediate loading. The article also provides different recommendations for best practices in circumstances that may lack primary stability.

The articles by Hoefler and Al-Sabbagh address available alternatives to invasive site development, permitting the potential placement of implants in defective sites. Part I discusses the use of short and narrow-diameter dental implants and their rate of success in less than optimum available bone. Part II covers other available alternatives, including the use of tilted implants alone or in combination with tilted and upright implants to support a full-arch fixed dental prosthesis in edentulous ridges.

The article by Dominguez, Guerrero, Shehata, and Van Sickels discusses the use of zygoma implants to rehabilitate severely atrophic maxilla opposing a dentate mandible. The article reviews the high demand of immediate provisional restoration from patients. Zygoma implants can reduce the cost, time, and morbidity associated with regenerative procedures necessary for staged implant placement.

The article by Al Farawati and Nakaparksin discusses the advantages and limitations to commonly used dental implant prosthesis materials (commercially pure titanium, titanium alloys, zirconia, cobalt-chromium alloys, and multiple emerging resin-based materials). They also reviewed the materials of choice to restore dental implants in less than ideal situations. Suggested treatment protocols were also reviewed for each of these complication scenarios.

The article by Almehmadi, Kutkut, and Al-Sabbagh reviews the different characteristics and properties of commercially available luting agents used in the cementation of implant prosthesis. It presents guidelines for cement selection according to abutment and prosthetic material. It also sheds light on using different cementation techniques to reduce excess cement in peri-implant tissues.

The article by Al-Sabbagh and Shaddox tackles one of the most important dilemmas among clinicians: How curable is peri-implantitis? The article presents the origin of disease, new American Academy of Periodontology classification for disease, and clinical manifestations of peri-implant conditions. The authors also have presented rationale of the different clinical interventions to treat peri-implant disease and their efficacy. Furthermore, the article intensely advocates for not only the prevention of peri-implant disease through routine evaluations but also the importance of early diagnosis and treatment of peri-implant diseases with the aim of avoiding any further bone loss.

The article by Al-Sabbagh and colleagues provides information on the importance of keratinized tissue around dental implants and discusses whether it should be considered a prognostic value to assess the success and longevity of dental implants. Furthermore, the article discusses different timing protocols that have been explored with regards to soft tissue augmentation around dental implants.

These richly illustrated articles provide the readers with evidence-based, practical solutions to untangle the most controversial topics in the field of implant dentistry. The reader is provided with the expertise of the authors, which is put into these clinical guidelines. These guidelines provide clinicians with solutions for complicated, or less than ideal, clinical situations. It is the editor's goal to combine the current available literature and clinical experience of the authors into a concise roadmap for everyday clinical use.

Mohanad Al-Sabbagh, DDS, MS
Division of Periodontology
Department of Oral Health Practice
University of Kentucky College of Dentistry
D-438 Chandler Medical Center
800 Rose Street
Lexington, KY 40536-0927, USA

E-mail address:
malsa2@email.uky.edu

Are There Contraindications for Placing Dental Implants?

Amritpal S. Kullar, BDS, Craig S. Miller, DMD, MS*

KEYWORDS

- Contraindication • Risk factors • Dental implants • Implant failure • Implant survival

KEY POINTS

- There are few absolute contraindications to dental implant placement.
- Relative contraindications include cognitive decline, American Society of Anesthesiology Patient Status IV or higher categories, or medical conditions that may jeopardize the life or lifespan of the patient.
- Precautions for placing dental implants should be viewed with respect to the evidence-based exposures that can contribute to risk of failure, including but not limited to local, behavioral, and medical factors.
- Risk for dental implant failure increases in association with (1) past history of periodontal disease, (2) bruxism, (3) smoking, and (4) radiation therapy.

INTRODUCTION

Dental clinicians on a daily basis should be mindful of the indications, precautions, and contraindications of treatment in order to achieve the best patient outcomes. Indications for treatment generally are considered when a patient initially presents with a problem or complaint. After the indication,[1] the precautions and contraindications should be considered as balancing components of the decision-making and informed consent process. Precautions and contraindications involve taking into account the relative seriousness of a particular treatment and when specific treatment would be inadvisable because of the harm or serious adverse outcome that may, or is likely to, occur. A precaution indicates that there is ability to prevent or mitigate the adverse event. In contrast, a contraindication is a more serious situation in which the likelihood and severity of the adverse event outweighs any potential benefit to the patient (**Fig. 1**).

Contraindications are recognized as being either absolute or relative. An absolute contraindication indicates that the procedure could cause a life-threatening event or the risk of the procedure clearly outweighs any possible therapeutic benefit. A relative

Disclosure: The authors have nothing to disclose.
Division of Oral Diagnosis, Oral Medicine, Oral Radiology, MN324 College of Dentistry, University of Kentucky, 800 Rose Street, Lexington, KY 40356-0297, USA
* Corresponding author.
E-mail address: cmiller@uky.edu

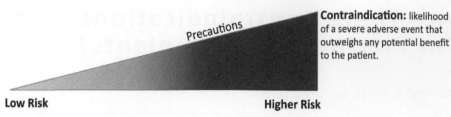

Contraindication: likelihood of a severe adverse event that outweighs any potential benefit to the patient.

Precautions

Low Risk   Higher Risk

Fig. 1. Spectrum of risk when considering placement of a dental implant.

contraindication indicates that caution should be exercised and it is likely that the benefit of the procedure outweighs the risks involved.

Placing a dental implant is an elective procedure that requires consideration for the desires, oral anatomy, potential trauma, and healing capacity of the patient. Hence, indications, precautions, and contraindications are key components of the diagnostic work-up. During the planning phase, health conditions and medical comorbidities are to be respected, and caution should be used before engaging in a procedure or treatment to ensure that the benefits are likely to outweigh the risks.

Expert opinion suggests that there are few situations or medical conditions that create an absolute contraindication for placing a dental implant.[2] Relative contraindications are those situations associated with patients who are categorized with a health condition that may increase the risk of an adverse event, implant failure, or postoperative problem. These patients include those categorized as American Society of Anesthesiology patient status IV or higher (eg, oropharyngeal malignancies, recent cerebrovascular accidents and myocardial infarction, uncontrolled or poorly controlled epilepsy, diabetes mellitus or psychiatric illness, risk of osteoradionecrosis, bleeding disorders, profound immunosuppression, drug and alcohol abuse, active cancer chemotherapy and receiving intravenous antiresorptive medication, or conditions that may jeopardize the life or lifespan of the patient). However, little evidence exists to date to support contraindications to placing a dental implant, but there are contrasting opinions that exist among practitioners.[3–5] Readers are referred to other publications on this topic for additional perspectives.[6–8]

In the context of decision making and dental implants, evidence suggests that 90% to 95% of dental implants are successfully maintained for 10 years[9] and 51.97% to 75.8% survive at 16 to 20 years.[10,11] The most common causes for failure of a dental implant include peri-implantitis, peri-mucositis, failure of osseous integration, placement error, anatomic anomalies, persistent pain, and breakage caused by force applied during function.[8,9,12–14]

In as much as dental implants have a high rate of success and few contraindications for placement,[3] this article focuses on conditions associated with increased risk of dental implant failure, generally defined as cases in which the implant is removed because of disease, pain, or mobility. In this article, our opinions focus on systematic reviews (SRs) of the literature because this is the highest level of evidence. Readers are referred to primary studies on proton pump inhibitors[15,16] and selective serotonin reuptake inhibitors[17] as well as case series regarding chronic pain[18] and neuropathic pain[19–21] following implant placement for additional information on this topic. Readers are cautioned that although SRs provide a high level of evidence for decision making, SRs are not without flaws and some are better than others. Detailing the limitations of SRs is beyond the scope of this article, and the authors do not attempt to analyze the quality of the SR. Readers should be aware that SRs can vary at many levels, including whether investigators of the primary studies or the SR used accurate and consistent definitions of disease or proper inclusion/exclusion criteria; measured publication bias, type, and frequency of treatment provided; or measured the outcome domains (ie, success, survival, failure). For this report, risks for dental implant failure have been categorized into local factors, behavioral factors, and medical factors.

Local

Periodontal disease

Periodontal disease is a global disease[22] that is a diagnostic consideration for patients seeking a dental implant. Both a history and the presence of periodontal disease are well-recognized risk factors for periimplant disease and implant failure.[23,24] The increased risk may be caused by compromised bone level; reduced bone quality; immune dysregulation; or concurrent exposures, such as poor oral hygiene, tobacco use, or persistent periodontal pathogens.[25] At present, there are 10 SRs on periodontal disease and dental implants. Both aggressive and chronic periodontitis have been evaluated in SRs.

There are 2 SRs on the topic of aggressive periodontitis and dental implants (**Table 1**).[23,26] In the Al-Zahrani[26] SR, 9 primary studies involving 72 patients who had a history of aggressive periodontitis were evaluated.[27–35] These patients, in general, received periodontal treatment for several years before implants were placed. There were 4 case reports and 5 longitudinal studies. Patients ranging from 17 to 82 years of age received more than 260 dental implants and were followed for 2 to 36 months. More than 90% of the dental implant survived 24 to 36 months; however, patients with a history of aggressive periodontitis showed greater periimplant crestal bone breakdown than patients without a history of periodontal disease.[35] Hazard ratios were not calculated, and the primary studies were not evaluated for level of evidence or publication bias.

Table 1
Summary data from systemic reviews associated with potential increased risk of dental implant failure

Condition	Number of SRs	Number of Primary Studies	Number of Patients	Number of Implants	Number of Cases	Number of Controls	Duration of Primary Studies	Odds Ratio of Dental Implant Failure
Periodontal disease (aggressive and chronic)[23,24,26,38–43]	10	35	975	14,332[a]	10,481[a]	385[a]	1.2–10 y	NR
Smoking[70–73]	4	110	24,618	104,350[a]	19,836[a]	60,464[a]	8 mo to 20 y	2.92 (95% CI, 1.76–4.83) (P<.001)
Bruxism[80–83]	3	24	2297	7043[a]	1356[a]	3924[a]	1 mo to 15 y	4.72, (95% CI, 2.66–8.36)
Diabetes mellitus[96–103]	8	41	9519	37,782[a]	9606[a]	16,137[a]	4 mo-17 y	0.62, (95% CI, 0.0225–1.705; P = .354)
Osteoporosis[112,113]	2	18	9066	30,381[a]	790[a]	4609[a]	1–22 y	Risk for periimplantitis 1.89, (95% CI, 1.31–2.46; P<.01)
Bisphosphonate[117–121]	5	19	1988	5927[a]	2039[a]	3888[a]	1 mo to 11 y	1.43, P = .156
Radiation[140,144–147]	5	58	2622	10,570[a]	5647[a]	3854[a]	1 mo to 23 y	RR 2.63 (95% CI, 1.93–3.58; P<.001)

Abbreviations: CI, confidence interval; NR, not reported; RR, risk ratio; SRs, systematic reviews.
[a] Not all studies reported the number of implants, cases, or controls.

The Monje and colleagues[23] SR included 6 prospective human studies.[31-34,36,37] Five of the studies were from the Mengal and colleagues author group[32-34,36,37] and 4 studies had been previously evaluated by Al-Zahrani.[26] The 2014 SR provides a more rigorous study design than the Al-Zahrani[26] SR, with the inclusion of meta-analysis and assessments for heterogeneity, quality, and publication bias. Here the survival rates for 264 dental implants in 60 patients with aggressive periodontitis were 83.3% to 100%, with a follow-up period ranging from 12 to 120 months. A meta-analysis yielded an overall failure rate risk ratio (RR) of 4.00 (95% confidence interval [CI], 1.79–8.93; $P<.001$) in patients who had a history of aggressive periodontitis compared with healthy controls. Risk was also increased in patients who had aggressive periodontitis compared with chronic periodontitis (RR, 3.97; 95% CI, 1.68–9.37).

Eight SRs were published between 2008 and 2016 that considered periodontal disease and implant survival.[24,38-43] The most comprehensive data sets were found in the 2014 and 2016 SRs. Here, 22 and 24 primary studies were evaluated, respectively, and 16 primary studies appeared in both data sets. In 12 prospective studies, the investigators evaluated 2825 implants placed in 843 patients with treated periodontitis.[33,44-54] In the 9 retrospective studies,[55-64] 8102 implants were evaluated in 2086 patients. In total, more than 10,000 implants placed in persons who had periodontal disease were compared with 3851 implants placed in 1606 healthy patients over a period of 1.2 to 10 years.[24,38] Evidence from these SRs indicate that there is increased risk of marginal bone loss, periimplantitis, and implant failure (odds ratios [ORs] ranging from 1.7 [CI, 1.23–2.79]; 95% CI, 1.12–8.15) with chronic periodontitis. Survival rates of implants in patients without periodontitis ranged from 91.7% to 100% compared with 71% to 100% for patients with treated periodontitis.[24,38,39] The severity of periodontal disease also contributed to lower implant survival,[24] but duration of disease generally was not assessed in the SRs. Periodic periodontal maintenance program is documented to be associated with improved implant survival.[24] The rationale of increased risk is not well established; however, the literature suggests that adjacent periodontally involved teeth may contribute to the cause through the transfer of periodontal pathogens from adjacent disease sites to the implant site.[25,65]

Although large-scale case-control clinical trials are lacking, the findings from these SRs suggest that dental implants can be used in patients treated for aggressive and chronic periodontitis. However, clinicians need to consider several factors, including the length of time between active periodontal therapy and when an implant should be placed, whether questionable teeth should be extracted before implant placement, and the maintenance program that will be provided regularly to periodontally compromised teeth that are adjacent to the implant. Caveats to consider in the interpretation of these data include that periodontal disease is often associated with confounders (ie, tobacco smoking) and comorbidities (eg, diabetes) and that these factors are not always well controlled for in the SRs published to date. Also, the SRs reviewed generally showed variability in the definitions in periodontitis and implant failure, loading and follow-up period, details regarding the type and frequency of periodontal treatment provided, and outcome criteria, each of which contribute to difficulty in accurate interpretation of the findings.

Behavioral Factors

Smoking

Smoking is a well-recognized risk factor for periodontal diseases that contributes to an anaerobic environment, growth of periodontal pathogens, and detachment of the periodontal ligament.[66,67] Together, these factors can lead to implant failure. It is estimated that 37.8 million (15.5%) adults smoke cigarettes every day,[68] and about 15 of every 100 adults aged 18 years or older in the United States smoke cigarettes.[69] Smoking is considerably higher among American Indians/Alaska Natives (31.8%) and persons of color, and lowest among Asians (9.0%).[68] Smoking is directly correlated with educational status. Although smoking rates decreased from 42.4% in 1965 to 15.7% in 2016, the Healthy People 2020 national objective of 12% has not yet been reached.[68]

There are 4 SRs on smoking and implant failure. These SRs evaluated 113 primary studies and more than 28,000 dental implants over a 20-year period.[70–73] Evidence from these SRs indicates increased risk of implant failure among smokers. The data support that the risk of implant failure, postoperative infections, and marginal bone loss for smokers is at least twice that for nonsmokers.[72] One SR reported 1259 (6.35%) failures of 19,836 dental implants placed in smokers and 1923 failures (3.18%) of 60,464 dental implants placed in nonsmokers.[72] Evidence from this SR indicates that smokers experienced higher rates of implant failure (RR, 2.23; 95% CI, 1.96–2.53).[72] The success rate of dental implants dropped considerably when patients smoked more than 10 cigarettes per day.[74] Overall, the risk of dental implant failure seems to be at least twice as high in smokers as in nonsmokers.

Bruxism

Bruxism, a condition in which the patient clenches and grinds the teeth, is a recognized risk factor for implant fracture and failure as a result of abnormal physical force.[75–79] It is important for clinicians who are planning dental implants to consider that patients who brux often report morning stiffness or tightness in masticatory muscles, and show wear of the dentition. Assessment of these clinical features is critical for the long-term success of dental implants. There are 2 SRs and 1 meta-analysis on bruxism and dental implants that evaluated 38 primary studies over a 15-year period.[80–82] The meta-analysis evaluated 760 implants in patients who showed bruxism and 2989 control (nonbruxism) patients. This analysis reported 49 (6.45%) implant failures that occurred in the patients who showed bruxism compared with 109 (3.65%) implant failures in nonbruxism patients.[82] The findings support about a 2-fold higher risk for those who are bruxers versus nonbruxers.

Medical Factors

Bleeding disorders

Hemorrhage is a potential complication during or after dental implant placement. A surgical procedure can lead to hemorrhage in patients who have a congenital (hemophilia A – factor VIII deficiency; hemophilia B – factor IX deficiency) or acquired bleeding disorder; however, medical consultation with the patient's physician and precise treatment planning before the surgical procedure can minimize adverse outcomes. Most patients taking antiplatelets (low-dose aspirin) or oral anticoagulants (coumadin, Warfarin) should not have their medication discontinued before implant placement.[83–86] However, elective surgery should not be performed if hemostasis is not possible.[3] Patients with International Normalized Ratio (INR; prothrombin ratio = patient prothrombin/control prothrombin) value of higher than 3.5 should be referred to their physicians for improved control and, once controlled, considered for treatment in a setting that will provide for good hemostasis.[87] The INR value should be current (ie, taken between 24 and 72 hours before surgery). Direct oral anticoagulant (DOAC) drugs are newer agents prescribed for persons with deep vein thrombosis, pulmonary embolism, atrial fibrillation, myocardial infarction, and heart valve prosthesis.[88,89] Although there is some controversy regarding whether DOACs should be temporarily discontinued during the surgical placement of a dental implant,[90] accumulating data indicate that DOACs should not be discontinued for this procedure.[89,91,92]

Abnormalities in platelet count and function can also contribute to abnormal bleeding during or after implant surgery. Low platelet levels are associated with leukemia, radiotherapy, idiopathic thrombocytopenia purpura, and myeloablation.[3] The reference value for platelet count is between 150,000 and 400,000 cells/mm³. Abnormal postsurgical hemorrhage may be noticed in mild thrombocytopenia (50,000–100,000 cells/mm³). In case of severe thrombocytopenia, platelet values less than 50,000 cells/mm³ can complicate implant placement or lead to postoperative hemorrhage. In patients with very low platelet values (<20,000 cells/mm³), hemorrhage of mucous membranes often occurs,[93] and these patients require transfusion before invasive dental procedures such as placement of a dental implant.

At present, there are no SRs on the topic of dental implants and failure or contraindications in patients who have bleeding disorders. However, precautions are advised and should be taken with these patients before and during the procedure to prevent bleeding-related adverse events that may occur.

Diabetes mellitus

Diabetes is a well-recognized risk factor for poor wound healing after surgical procedures caused by abnormal glucose blood levels and altered immune response, both of which may contribute to implant failure. Diabetes can also hinder the process of osteointegration.[94] A patient is diagnosed with diabetes if the fasting blood glucose is 126 mg/dL or higher, or the hemoglobin A1c is 6.5% or greater. In the United States, more than 29 million people have diabetes mellitus and 25% of affected persons are unaware of their condition.[95] Approximately 86 million are prediabetic, and 90% of these persons do not know it. Hispanic and Latino people, African Americans, American Indians, Pacific Islanders, and Asian Americans are at higher risk for diabetes than white people.[95]

There are 8 SRs on diabetes that have analyzed 14 to 22 primary studies.[96–103] These SRs evaluated the failure rate of more than 3000 dental implants placed in more than 2000 (type I or type II) diabetic patients. In the Moraschini and colleagues[101] SR, 14 primary studies published between 2000 and 2015 were evaluated. Most involved prospective studies. Overall, this SR analyzed 802 diabetics and 1532 nondiabetic patients between the ages of 15 and 89 years, with a follow-up period of 3 months to 17 years. The investigators did not consider the glycemic control levels, and reported that survival rates of diabetics were similar to those of healthy controls (95.1 vs 97%, 97.2 vs 95%, 92 vs 93.2%, and 97 vs 98.8%) in 4 primary studies[48,104–106] that had a follow-up of more than 1 year; however, 2 studies showed a shorter survival period, which yielded an RR of 4.8 and 2.75 for implant failure in diabetic patients.[107,108] Because of the predominance of favorable outcomes, Moraschini and colleagues[101] reported there was no difference in the rate of implant failure in diabetic patients versus nondiabetic patients. Similar findings are reported by Naujokat and colleagues,[98] who evaluated 22 primary studies in which survival was measured within the first 6 years of placement; however, dental implant failure was observed to be increased in diabetic patients when the observation period was 20 years.

Glycemic control has also been evaluated. Shi and colleagues[99] evaluated the failure rate of 286 dental implants placed in 252 well-controlled diabetics and 301 dental implants placed in poorly controlled patients reported in 7 primary studies. Findings from this meta-analysis showed no difference in the dental implant failure rate among well-controlled versus poorly controlled diabetics (RR, 0.620; 95% CI, 0.0225–1.705; $P = .354$). In contrast, an SR by Monje and colleagues[103] published in 2017 that evaluated 12 primary studies with 2892 implants placed in 1955 subjects with a follow-up period of up to 11 years concluded that the risk of periimplantitis in patients with diabetes mellitus or hyperglycemia is 1.21 to 2.46 times higher than in nondiabetics or persons with normoglycemia.

Bone diseases

The presence of bone disease may be a risk factor for implant disease and failure. The literature to date provides little guidance on dental implant success rates in patients with osteogenesis imperfecta, ankylosing spondylitis, and polyarthritis,[8,14] although SRs are present for osteoporosis. Osteoporosis is a medical condition characterized by low bone mass associated with imbalances in bone metabolism causing the bone to become brittle and fragile because of a decrease in bone volume and quantity. Osteoporosis mainly affects older women (>50 years old).[109,110] Worldwide, more than 200 million women have osteoporosis and it affects approximately 75 million people in the United States, Japan, and Europe according to the International Osteoporosis Foundation.[111] An estimated 14 million people by 2020 will have osteoporosis in the United States.

There are 2 SRs on osteoporosis and dental implants.[112,113] These systematic reviews included 18 studies from 2001 to 2017, and examined more than 20,000 dental implants over a period of 1 to 22 years. Evidence from these SRs indicates that there is no difference in dental implant survival in patients with or without osteoporosis. In these studies, the survival rate is reported to be 96% in the osteoporosis group.[112] Nevertheless, increased periimplant bone loss was observed in patients with osteoporosis.[112]

Antiresorptive medications

Antiresorptive medications are prescribed for several diseases (eg, osteoporosis, Paget disease, hypercalcemia of malignancy, bone metastasis of prostate, lung and breast cancer) that affect bone quality and metabolism.[114] Antiresorptive medications are available as bisphosphonates, receptor activator of nuclear factor kappa-B ligand (RANKL) inhibitors, and antiangiogenic agents (**Box 1**). Antiresorptives are given either orally or intravenously. These agents show various potencies. Bisphosphonates have a high affinity for hydroxyapatite crystals[115] and are used to increase bone strength and reduce the risk for fractures.[116] Bisphosphonates are generally prescribed for osteoporosis as an oral medication or a single annual injection of zoledronic acid. In contrast, the more potent antiresorptive medications (eg, zoledronic acid) are often used intravenously in cancer therapy to limit bone metastases.

The relationship between dental implant survival and bisphosphonate use has been documented in 5 SRs that evaluated more than 4500 dental implants.[117–121] The most comprehensive data sets are found in 2 recent publications.[120,121] Here 14 and 15 primary studies were evaluated. Ten primary studies appeared in both data sets. Data from the de-Freitas and colleagues[121] SR included 8 retrospective studies,[122–129] 1 prospective study,[130] and 6 case series.[131–136] In total, 1330 implants were placed in 528 bisphosphonate users and 2418 implants were placed in 811 healthy patients. The follow-up period was up to 11 years. During this time, 113 dental implants failed in bisphosphonate users (8.5%) and 39 in healthy patients (1.6%).[121] Osteonecrosis was reported to occur in 78 patients (53 in mandible and 23 in maxilla) who used bisphosphonates, with the highest prevalence in those who had combined use of oral and intravenous bisphosphonates.[121]

In 2 SRs, implant survival rates in individuals with a history of bisphosphonate use ranged from 95% to 100% versus 99% in healthy individuals with a follow-up period

---

Box 1
Antiresorptive medications

Bisphosphonates

Non–nitrogen-containing bisphosphonates:
  Etidronate (Didronel)
  Clodronate (Bonefos, Loron)
  Tiludronate (Skelid)

Nitrogen-containing bisphosphonates:
  Pamidronate (APD, Aredia)
  Neridronate (Nerixia)
  Olpadronate
  Aledronate (Fosamax)
  Ibandronate (Boniva)
  Risedronate (Actonel)
  Zoledronate (Zometa, Aclasta)

RANKL inhibitors

Denosumab (Prolia, Xgeva)

Angiogenesis inhibitors

Axitinib (Inlyta)

Bevacizumab (Avastin)

Cabozantinib (Cometriq)

Everolimus (Afinitor, Zortress)

Lenalidomide (Revlimid)

Pazopanib (Votrient)

Ramucirumab (Cyramza)

Regorafenib (Stivarga)

---

of 4 months to 7.4 years.[117,118] In a meta-analysis of 8 primary studies involving 1090 implants in bisphosphonate users and 3472 implants placed in healthy controls, Ata-Ali and colleagues[120] reported only 1 study that offered statistical evidence that bisphosphonates reduce dental implant success, with an overall OR of 1.43 (95% CI, 0.87–2.34; P = .156). Together, these data indicate that patients taking bisphosphonates are not at higher risk of implant failure.[118,120] This finding is consistent with a recent study published by Al-Sabbagh and colleagues[137] who reported no increased risk of implant failure among patient with osteoporosis who took oral bisphosphonates.

There are no SRs available on RANKL inhibitors or antiangiogenic medications as of this date. Accordingly, dental practitioners should be cognizant of the current evidence and review the medical status of each patient before beginning a procedure for dental implant placement in a patient who uses or has received antiresorptive medications.[121] If necessary, the patient's medical practitioner should be consulted.

Radiation therapy

It is estimated that 51,540 new cases of oropharyngeal cancer will be diagnosed in 2018 and an estimated 10,030 lives will be lost because of this disease.[138] Most oropharyngeal cancer diagnoses occur in persons who are at least 60 years of age; however, at least one-quarter of cases occur in persons younger than age 55 years.

Radiation therapy is a common component of the cancer treatment of many of these patients. Radiation therapy is generally administered over a period of 5 to 7 weeks at doses that destroy cancer cells or slow their rate of growth. The high dose of radiotherapy is also damaging to the adjacent tissues and can result in reduced blood supply to bone, bone sclerosis, and reduced ability of osseous regeneration.[139,140] Accordingly, survival of dental implants is potentially affected in the field of irradiation because of hypovascularization and reduced regenerative ability, which can affect the osseointegration process.[141–143]

There are 5 SRs on radiation and implant failure. These SRs evaluated 58 primary studies, and more than 10,000 dental implants over a 23-year period.[140,144–147] Most primary studies were retrospective and only 1 study was a randomized trial. Evidence from these SRs indicate a higher rate of failure (15% to 25%) in irradiated jaw areas compared with nonirradiated areas (5%) over a 60-month period.[140,147] In an analysis based on random effect, the RR of failure was higher (RR, 2.63; 95% CI, 1.93–3.58; $P<.001$) in irradiated patients versus nonirradiated patients.[140] Risk seems to increase when the radiotherapy dose is more than 50 Gy[145]; however, most SRs did not analyze the dose received as a confounder.

The anatomic location is also a consideration. Evidence from a recent SR indicates a higher survival rate of dental implants in irradiated mandible than in irradiated maxilla (OR, 3.67; 95% CI, 2.81–4.79; $P<.0001$).[145] This finding is also reported in the SRs by Shugaa-Addin and colleagues[147] and Schiegnitz and colleagues[146]; however, not all primary studies have reported this finding.[148–150] Hyperbaric oxygen is a consideration when a dental implant is planned for a region that has received greater than 50 Gy; however, consensus is lacking on the need for this treatment.[151] The accumulated evidence from these SRs indicates that irradiated areas in the maxilla or mandible may receive dental implants, but strict evaluation that includes information on the radiation dose received in the site planned for the dental implant, informed consent that includes risks involved, as well as monitoring of the area are needed.[140]

SUMMARY

Although there are no absolute contraindications for placing a dental implant, the factors discussed in this article show increased risk for decreased implant survival when certain factors or comorbidities are present. In situations in which risk is increased, the patient should be informed of the uncertainties and risks, and the practitioner and patient need to understand the requirement for close follow-up and proper periodontal maintenance therapy. It is possible that the factors discussed in this article are additive, thus persons who have periodontal disease, bruxism, and poorly controlled diabetes could be at even higher risk than patients who have only 1 of these exposures. Thus, relative contraindications could relate to the potential additive risk and clinicians should consider these factors carefully when more than 1 exposure is present. Future research should include longitudinal studies and the consideration for additive risk to help expand knowledge on this topic.

REFERENCES

1. Anesthesiologists ASo ASA Physical Status Classification System. Available at: https://www.asahq.org/resources/clinical-information/asa-physical-status-classification-system. Accessed September 2, 2108.
2. Sugerman PB, Barber MT. Patient selection for endosseous dental implants: oral and systemic considerations. Int J Oral Maxillofac Implants 2002;17(2):191–201.

3. Hwang D, Wang HL. Medical contraindications to implant therapy: part I: absolute contraindications. Implant Dent 2006;15(4):353–60.

4. Balshi TJ, Wolfinger GJ. Management of the posterior maxilla in the compromised patient: historical, current, and future perspectives. Periodontol 2000 2003;33:67–81.

5. Hwang D, Wang HL. Medical contraindications to implant therapy: part II: relative contraindications. Implant Dent 2007;16(1):13–23.

6. Scully C, Hobkirk J, Dios PD. Dental endosseous implants in the medically compromised patient. J Oral Rehabil 2007;34(8):590–9.

7. Gomez-de Diego R, Mang-de la Rosa Mdel R, Romero-Perez MJ, et al. Indications and contraindications of dental implants in medically compromised patients: update. Med Oral Patol Oral Cir Bucal 2014;19(5):e483–9.

8. Vissink A, Spijkervet F, Raghoebar GM. The medically compromised patient: are dental implants a feasible option? Oral Dis 2018;24(1–2):253–60.

9. Spiekermann H, Jansen VK, Richter EJ. A 10-year follow-up study of IMZ and TPS implants in the edentulous mandible using bar-retained overdentures. Int J Oral Maxillofac Implants 1995;10(2):231–43.

10. Simonis P, Dufour T, Tenenbaum H. Long-term implant survival and success: a 10-16-year follow-up of non-submerged dental implants. Clin Oral Implants Res 2010;21(7):772–7.

11. Chappuis V, Buser R, Bragger U, et al. Long-term outcomes of dental implants with a titanium plasma-sprayed surface: a 20-year prospective case series study in partially edentulous patients. Clin Implant Dent Relat Res 2013;15(6): 780–90.

12. Chrcanovic BR, Albrektsson T, Wennerberg A. Reasons for failures of oral implants. J Oral Rehabil 2014;41(6):443–76.

13. Chrcanovic BR, Kisch J, Albrektsson T, et al. Factors influencing the fracture of dental implants. Clin Implant Dent Relat Res 2018;20(1):58–67.

14. Diz P, Scully C, Sanz M. Dental implants in the medically compromised patient. J Dent 2013;41(3):195–206.

15. Chrcanovic BR, Kisch J, Albrektsson T, et al. Intake of proton pump inhibitors is associated with an increased risk of dental implant failure. Int J Oral Maxillofac Implants 2017;32(5):1097–102.

16. Wu X, Al-Abedalla K, Abi-Nader S, et al. Proton pump inhibitors and the risk of osseointegrated dental implant failure: a cohort study. Clin Implant Dent Relat Res 2017;19(2):222–32.

17. Chrcanovic BR, Kisch J, Albrektsson T, et al. Is the intake of selective serotonin reuptake inhibitors associated with an increased risk of dental implant failure? Int J Oral Maxillofac Surg 2017;46(6):782–8.

18. Devine M, Taylor S, Renton T. Chronic post-surgical pain following the placement of dental implants in the maxilla: a case series. Eur J Oral Implantol 2016;9. Suppl 1(2):179–86.

19. Politis C, Agbaje J, Van Hevele J, et al. Report of neuropathic pain after dental implant placement: a case series. Int J Oral Maxillofac Implants 2017;32(2): 439–44.

20. Al-Sabbagh M, Okeson JP, Khalaf MW, et al. Persistent pain and neurosensory disturbance after dental implant surgery: pathophysiology, etiology, and diagnosis. Dent Clin North Am 2015;59(1):131–42.

21. Al-Sabbagh M, Okeson JP, Bertoli E, et al. Persistent pain and neurosensory disturbance after dental implant surgery: prevention and treatment. Dent Clin North Am 2015;59(1):143–56.

22. Gross AJ, Paskett KT, Cheever VJ, et al. Periodontitis: a global disease and the primary care provider's role. Postgrad Med J 2017;93(1103):560–5.

23. Monje A, Alcoforado G, Padial-Molina M, et al. Generalized aggressive periodontitis as a risk factor for dental implant failure: a systematic review and meta-analysis. J Periodontol 2014;85(10):1398–407.

24. Sousa V, Mardas N, Farias B, et al. A systematic review of implant outcomes in treated periodontitis patients. Clin Oral Implants Res 2016;27(7):787–844.

25. Mombelli A, Nyman S, Bragger U, et al. Clinical and microbiological changes associated with an altered subgingival environment induced by periodontal pocket reduction. J Clin Periodontol 1995;22(10):780–7.

26. Al-Zahrani MS. Implant therapy in aggressive periodontitis patients: a systematic review and clinical implications. Quintessence Int 2008;39(3):211–5.

27. Malmstrom HS, Fritz ME, Timmis DP, et al. Osseo-integrated implant treatment of a patient with rapidly progressive periodontitis. A case report. J Periodontol 1990;61(5):300–4.

28. Yalcin S, Yalcin F, Gunay Y, et al. Treatment of aggressive periodontitis by osseointegrated dental implants. A case report. J Periodontol 2001;72(3):411–6.

29. Hofer D, Hammerle CH, Lang NP. Comprehensive treatment concept in a young adult patient with severe periodontal disease: a case report. Quintessence Int 2002;33(8):567–78.

30. Wu AY, Chee W. Implant-supported reconstruction in a patient with generalized aggressive periodontitis. J Periodontol 2007;78(4):777–82.

31. De Boever AL, De Boever JA. Early colonization of non-submerged dental implants in patients with a history of advanced aggressive periodontitis. Clin Oral Implants Res 2006;17(1):8–17.

32. Mengel R, Schroder T, Flores-de-Jacoby L. Osseointegrated implants in patients treated for generalized chronic periodontitis and generalized aggressive periodontitis: 3- and 5-year results of a prospective long-term study. J Periodontol 2001;72(8):977–89.

33. Mengel R, Flores-de-Jacoby L. Implants in patients treated for generalized aggressive and chronic periodontitis: a 3-year prospective longitudinal study. J Periodontol 2005;76(4):534–43.

34. Mengel R, Flores-de-Jacoby L. Implants in regenerated bone in patients treated for generalized aggressive periodontitis: a prospective longitudinal study. Int J Periodontics Restorative Dent 2005;25(4):331–41.

35. Hanggi MP, Hanggi DC, Schoolfield JD, et al. Crestal bone changes around titanium implants. Part I: a retrospective radiographic evaluation in humans comparing two non-submerged implant designs with different machined collar lengths. J Periodontol 2005;76(5):791–802.

36. Mengel R, Kreuzer G, Lehmann KM, et al. A telescopic crown concept for the restoration of partially edentulous patients with aggressive generalized periodontitis: a 3-year prospective longitudinal study. Int J Periodontics Restorative Dent 2007;27(3):231–9.

37. Mengel R, Behle M, Flores-de-Jacoby L. Osseointegrated implants in subjects treated for generalized aggressive periodontitis: 10-year results of a prospective, long-term cohort study. J Periodontol 2007;78(12):2229–37.

38. Chrcanovic BR, Albrektsson T, Wennerberg A. Periodontally compromised vs. periodontally healthy patients and dental implants: a systematic review and meta-analysis. J Dent 2014;42(12):1509–27.

39. Ramanauskaite A, Baseviciene N, Wang HL, et al. Effect of history of periodontitis on implant success: meta-analysis and systematic review. Implant Dent 2014;23(6):687–96.

40. Clementini M, Rossetti PH, Penarrocha D, et al. Systemic risk factors for peri-implant bone loss: a systematic review and meta-analysis. Int J Oral Maxillofac Surg 2014;43(3):323–34.

41. Safii SH, Palmer RM, Wilson RF. Risk of implant failure and marginal bone loss in subjects with a history of periodontitis: a systematic review and meta-analysis. Clin Implant Dent Relat Res 2010;12(3):165–74.

42. Ong CT, Ivanovski S, Needleman IG, et al. Systematic review of implant outcomes in treated periodontitis subjects. J Clin Periodontol 2008;35(5):438–62.

43. Schou S. Implant treatment in periodontitis-susceptible patients: a systematic review. J Oral Rehabil 2008;35(Suppl 1):9–22.

44. Watson CJ, Tinsley D, Ogden AR, et al. A 3 to 4 year study of single tooth hydroxylapatite coated endosseous dental implants. Br Dent J 1999;187(2): 90–4.

45. Karoussis IK, Salvi GE, Heitz-Mayfield LJ, et al. Long-term implant prognosis in patients with and without a history of chronic periodontitis: a 10-year prospective cohort study of the ITI Dental Implant System. Clin Oral Implants Res 2003;14(3):329–39.

46. Gatti C, Gatti F, Chiapasco M, et al. Outcome of dental implants in partially edentulous patients with and without a history of periodontitis: a 5-year interim analysis of a cohort study. Eur J Oral Implantol 2008;1(1):45–51.

47. De Boever AL, Quirynen M, Coucke W, et al. Clinical and radiographic study of implant treatment outcome in periodontally susceptible and non-susceptible patients: a prospective long-term study. Clin Oral Implants Res 2009;20(12): 1341–50.

48. Anner R, Grossmann Y, Anner Y, et al. Smoking, diabetes mellitus, periodontitis, and supportive periodontal treatment as factors associated with dental implant survival: a long-term retrospective evaluation of patients followed for up to 10 years. Implant Dent 2010;19(1):57–64.

49. Roccuzzo M, De Angelis N, Bonino L, et al. Ten-year results of a three-arm prospective cohort study on implants in periodontally compromised patients. Part 1: implant loss and radiographic bone loss. Clin Oral Implants Res 2010; 21(5):490–6.

50. Roccuzzo M, Bonino F, Aglietta M, et al. Ten-year results of a three arms prospective cohort study on implants in periodontally compromised patients. Part 2: clinical results. Clin Oral Implants Res 2012;23(4):389–95.

51. Roccuzzo M, Bonino L, Dalmasso P, et al. Long-term results of a three arms prospective cohort study on implants in periodontally compromised patients: 10-year data around sandblasted and acid-etched (SLA) surface. Clin Oral Implants Res 2014;25(10):1105–12.

52. Levin L, Ofec R, Grossmann Y, et al. Periodontal disease as a risk for dental implant failure over time: a long-term historical cohort study. J Clin Periodontol 2011;38(8):732–7.

53. Swierkot K, Lottholz P, Flores-de-Jacoby L, et al. Mucositis, peri-implantitis, implant success, and survival of implants in patients with treated generalized aggressive periodontitis: 3- to 16-year results of a prospective long-term cohort study. J Periodontol 2012;83(10):1213–25.

54. Jiang BQ, Lan J, Huang HY, et al. A clinical study on the effectiveness of implant supported dental restoration in patients with chronic periodontal diseases. Int J Oral Maxillofac Surg 2013;42(2):256–9.

55. Brocard D, Barthet P, Baysse E, et al. A multicenter report on 1,022 consecutively placed ITI implants: a 7-year longitudinal study. Int J Oral Maxillofac Implants 2000;15(5):691–700.

56. Hardt CR, Grondahl K, Lekholm U, et al. Outcome of implant therapy in relation to experienced loss of periodontal bone support: a retrospective 5- year study. Clin Oral Implants Res 2002;13(5):488–94.

57. Evian CI, Emling R, Rosenberg ES, et al. Retrospective analysis of implant survival and the influence of periodontal disease and immediate placement on long-term results. Int J Oral Maxillofac Implants 2004;19(3):393–8.

58. Rosenberg ES, Cho SC, Elian N, et al. A comparison of characteristics of implant failure and survival in periodontally compromised and periodontally healthy patients: a clinical report. Int J Oral Maxillofac Implants 2004;19(6): 873–9.

59. Roos-Jansaker AM, Lindahl C, Renvert H, et al. Nine- to fourteen-year follow-up of implant treatment. Part I: implant loss and associations to various factors. J Clin Periodontol 2006;33(4):283–9.

60. Roos-Jansaker AM, Renvert H, Lindahl C, et al. Nine- to fourteen-year follow-up of implant treatment. Part III: factors associated with peri-implant lesions. J Clin Periodontol 2006;33(4):296–301.

61. Gianserra R, Cavalcanti R, Oreglia F, et al. Outcome of dental implants in patients with and without a history of periodontitis: a 5-year pragmatic multicentre retrospective cohort study of 1727 patients. Eur J Oral Implantol 2010;3(4): 307–14.

62. Matarasso S, Rasperini G, Iorio Siciliano V, et al. A 10-year retrospective analysis of radiographic bone-level changes of implants supporting single-unit crowns in periodontally compromised vs. periodontally healthy patients. Clin Oral Implants Res 2010;21(9):898–903.

63. Aglietta M, Siciliano VI, Rasperini G, et al. A 10-year retrospective analysis of marginal bone-level changes around implants in periodontally healthy and periodontally compromised tobacco smokers. Clin Oral Implants Res 2011;22(1): 47–53.

64. Cho-Yan Lee J, Mattheos N, Nixon KC, et al. Residual periodontal pockets are a risk indicator for peri-implantitis in patients treated for periodontitis. Clin Oral Implants Res 2012;23(3):325–33.

65. Heitz-Mayfield LJ, Lang NP. Comparative biology of chronic and aggressive periodontitis vs. peri-implantitis. Periodontol 2000 2010;53:167–81.

66. Albandar JM, Streckfus CF, Adesanya MR, et al. Cigar, pipe, and cigarette smoking as risk factors for periodontal disease and tooth loss. J Periodontol 2000;71(12):1874–81.

67. Papantonopoulos GH. Effect of periodontal therapy in smokers and nonsmokers with advanced periodontal disease: results after maintenance therapy for a minimum of 5 years. J Periodontol 2004;75(6):839–43.

68. Jamal A, Phillips E, Gentzke AS, et al. Current Cigarette Smoking Among Adults - United States, 2016. MMWR Morb Mortal Wkly Rep 2018;67(2):53–9.

69. Centers for Disease Control and Prevention. Current Cigarette Smoking Among Adults in the United States. Available at: https://www.cdc.gov/tobacco/data_statistics/fact_sheets/adult_data/cig_smoking/index.htm. Accessed August 15, 2018.

70. Chambrone L, Preshaw PM, Ferreira JD, et al. Effects of tobacco smoking on the survival rate of dental implants placed in areas of maxillary sinus floor augmentation: a systematic review. Clin Oral Implants Res 2014;25(4):408–16.

71. Moraschini V, Barboza E. Success of dental implants in smokers and nonsmokers: a systematic review and meta-analysis. Int J Oral Maxillofac Surg 2016;45(2):205–15.

72. Chrcanovic BR, Albrektsson T, Wennerberg A. Smoking and dental implants: a systematic review and meta-analysis. J Dent 2015;43(5):487–98.

73. Alfadda S. Current evidence on dental implants outcomes in smokers and nonsmokers: a systematic review and meta-analysis. J Oral Implantol 2018;44(5):390–9.

74. Koszuta P, Grafka A, Koszuta A, et al. the effect of cigarette smoking on the therapeutic success of dental implants. Iran J Public Health 2016;45(10):1376–7.

75. Simon EW. Are genetic counselors and the social service system for people with intellectual disability reaching rapprochement? J Genet Couns 2012;21(6):777–83.

76. Parel SM, Phillips WR. A risk assessment treatment planning protocol for the four implant immediately loaded maxilla: preliminary findings. J Prosthet Dent 2011;106(6):359–66.

77. Bragger U, Aeschlimann S, Burgin W, et al. Biological and technical complications and failures with fixed partial dentures (FPD) on implants and teeth after four to five years of function. Clin Oral Implants Res 2001;12(1):26–34.

78. Papaspyridakos P, Lal K. Computer-assisted design/computer-assisted manufacturing zirconia implant fixed complete prostheses: clinical results and technical complications up to 4 years of function. Clin Oral Implants Res 2013;24(6):659–65.

79. Balshi TJ. An analysis and management of fractured implants: a clinical report. Int J Oral Maxillofac Implants 1996;11(5):660–6.

80. Zhou Y, Gao J, Luo L, et al. Does bruxism contribute to dental implant failure? A systematic review and meta-analysis. Clin Implant Dent Relat Res 2016;18(2):410–20.

81. Manfredini D, Poggio CE, Lobbezoo F. Is bruxism a risk factor for dental implants? A systematic review of the literature. Clin Implant Dent Relat Res 2014;16(3):460–9.

82. Chrcanovic BR, Albrektsson T, Wennerberg A. Bruxism and dental implants: a meta-analysis. Implant Dent 2015;24(5):505–16.

83. Ardekian L, Gaspar R, Peled M, et al. Does low-dose aspirin therapy complicate oral surgical procedures? J Am Dent Assoc 2000;131(3):331–5.

84. Pototski M, Amenabar JM. Dental management of patients receiving anticoagulation or antiplatelet treatment. J Oral Sci 2007;49(4):253–8.

85. Krishnan B, Shenoy NA, Alexander M. Exodontia and antiplatelet therapy. J Oral Maxillofac Surg 2008;66(10):2063–6.

86. Koskinas KC, Lillis T, Tsirlis A, et al. Dental management of antiplatelet-receiving patients: is uninterrupted antiplatelet therapy safe? Angiology 2012;63(4):245–7.

87. Scully C, Wolff A. Oral surgery in patients on anticoagulant therapy. Oral Surg Oral Med Oral Pathol Oral Radiol Endod 2002;94(1):57–64.

88. Al-Mubarak S, Rass MA, Alsuwyed A, et al. Thromboembolic risk and bleeding in patients maintaining or stopping oral anticoagulant therapy during dental extraction. J Thromb Haemost 2006;4(3):689–91.

89. Wahl MJ, Pinto A, Kilham J, et al. Dental surgery in anticoagulated patients–stop the interruption. Oral Surg Oral Med Oral Pathol Oral Radiol 2015;119(2): 136–57.

90. Bacci C, Berengo M, Favero L, et al. Safety of dental implant surgery in patients undergoing anticoagulation therapy: a prospective case-control study. Clin Oral Implants Res 2011;22(2):151–6.

91. Madrid C, Sanz M. What influence do anticoagulants have on oral implant therapy? A systematic review. Clin Oral Implants Res 2009;20(Suppl 4):96–106.

92. Gomez-Moreno G, Aguilar-Salvatierra A, Fernandez-Cejas E, et al. Dental implant surgery in patients in treatment with the anticoagulant oral rivaroxaban. Clin Oral Implants Res 2016;27(6):730–3.

93. Drews RE. Critical issues in hematology: anemia, thrombocytopenia, coagulopathy, and blood product transfusions in critically ill patients. Clin Chest Med 2003;24(4):607–22.

94. Oates TW, Huynh-Ba G, Vargas A, et al. A critical review of diabetes, glycemic control, and dental implant therapy. Clin Oral Implants Res 2013;24(2):117–27.

95. Centers for Disease Control and Prevention. National Diabetes Statistics Report, 2017: Estimates of Diabetes and Its Burden in the United States. Available at: https://www.cdc.gov/diabetes/pdfs/data/statistics/national-diabetes-statistics-report.pdf. Accessed August 30, 2018.

96. Chen H, Liu N, Xu X, et al. Smoking, radiotherapy, diabetes and osteoporosis as risk factors for dental implant failure: a meta-analysis. PLoS One 2013;8(8): e71955.

97. Chrcanovic BR, Albrektsson T, Wennerberg A. Diabetes and oral implant failure: a systematic review. J Dent Res 2014;93(9):859–67.

98. Naujokat H, Kunzendorf B, Wiltfang J. Dental implants and diabetes mellitus-a systematic review. Int J Implant Dent 2016;2(1):5.

99. Shi Q, Xu J, Huo N, et al. Does a higher glycemic level lead to a higher rate of dental implant failure?: a meta-analysis. J Am Dent Assoc 2016;147(11):875–81.

100. Annibali S, Pranno N, Cristalli MP, et al. Survival analysis of implant in patients with diabetes mellitus: a systematic review. Implant Dent 2016;25(5):663–74.

101. Moraschini V, Barboza ES, Peixoto GA. The impact of diabetes on dental implant failure: a systematic review and meta-analysis. Int J Oral Maxillofac Surg 2016; 45(10):1237–45.

102. Guobis Z, Pacauskiene I, Astramskaite I. General diseases influence on peri-implantitis development: a systematic review. J Oral Maxillofac Res 2016;7(3): e5.

103. Monje A, Catena A, Borgnakke WS. Association between diabetes mellitus/hyperglycaemia and peri-implant diseases: systematic review and meta-analysis. J Clin Periodontol 2017;44(6):636–48.

104. Busenlechner D, Furhauser R, Haas R, et al. Long-term implant success at the Academy for Oral Implantology: 8-year follow-up and risk factor analysis. J Periodontal Implant Sci 2014;44(3):102–8.

105. Morris HF, Ochi S, Winkler S. Implant survival in patients with type 2 diabetes: placement to 36 months. Ann Periodontol 2000;5(1):157–65.

106. Tawil G, Younan R, Azar P, et al. Conventional and advanced implant treatment in the type II diabetic patient: surgical protocol and long-term clinical results. Int J Oral Maxillofac Implants 2008;23(4):744–52.

107. Daubert DM, Weinstein BF, Bordin S, et al. Prevalence and predictive factors for peri-implant disease and implant failure: a cross-sectional analysis. J Periodontol 2015;86(3):337–47.

108. Moy PK, Medina D, Shetty V, et al. Dental implant failure rates and associated risk factors. Int J Oral Maxillofac Implants 2005;20(4):569–77.

109. Tella SH, Gallagher JC. Prevention and treatment of postmenopausal osteoporosis. J Steroid Biochem Mol Biol 2014;142:155–70.

110. Centers for Disease Control and Prevention. National Health and Nutrition Examination Survey: Osteoporosis. Available at: https://www.cdc.gov/nchs/data/nhanes/databriefs/osteoporosis.pdf. Accessed September 1, 2018.

111. Foundation IO Osteoporosis facts and statistics. Available at: https://www.iofbonehealth.org/facts-statistics. Accessed September 1, 2018.

112. de Medeiros F, Kudo GAH, Leme BG, et al. Dental implants in patients with osteoporosis: a systematic review with meta-analysis. Int J Oral Maxillofac Surg 2018;47(4):480–91.

113. Giro G, Chambrone L, Goldstein A, et al. Impact of osteoporosis in dental implants: a systematic review. World J Orthop 2015;6(2):311–5.

114. Drake MT, Clarke BL, Lewiecki EM. The pathophysiology and treatment of osteoporosis. Clin Ther 2015;37(8):1837–50.

115. Rogers MJ, Gordon S, Benford HL, et al. Cellular and molecular mechanisms of action of bisphosphonates. Cancer 2000;88(12 Suppl):2961–78.

116. Kanis JA. Assessment of fracture risk and its application to screening for postmenopausal osteoporosis: synopsis of a WHO report. WHO Study Group. Osteoporos Int 1994;4(6):368–81.

117. Madrid C, Sanz M. What impact do systemically administrated bisphosphonates have on oral implant therapy? A systematic review. Clin Oral Implants Res 2009;20(Suppl 4):87–95.

118. Kumar MN, Honne T. Survival of dental implants in bisphosphonate users versus non-users: a systematic review. Eur J Prosthodont Restor Dent 2012;20(4):159–62.

119. Chadha GK, Ahmadieh A, Kumar S, et al. Osseointegration of dental implants and osteonecrosis of the jaw in patients treated with bisphosphonate therapy: a systematic review. J Oral Implantol 2013;39(4):510–20.

120. Ata-Ali J, Ata-Ali F, Penarrocha-Oltra D, et al. What is the impact of bisphosphonate therapy upon dental implant survival? A systematic review and meta-analysis. Clin Oral Implants Res 2016;27(2):e38–46.

121. de-Freitas NR, Lima LB, de-Moura MB, et al. Bisphosphonate treatment and dental implants: a systematic review. Med Oral Patol Oral Cir Bucal 2016;21(5):e644–51.

122. Fugazzotto PA, Lightfoot WS, Jaffin R, et al. Implant placement with or without simultaneous tooth extraction in patients taking oral bisphosphonates: postoperative healing, early follow-up, and the incidence of complications in two private practices. J Periodontol 2007;78(9):1664–9.

123. Memon S, Weltman RL, Katancik JA. Oral bisphosphonates: early endosseous dental implant success and crestal bone changes. A retrospective study. Int J Oral Maxillofac Implants 2012;27(5):1216–22.

124. Koka S, Babu NM, Norell A. Survival of dental implants in post-menopausal bisphosphonate users. J Prosthodont Res 2010;54(3):108–11.

125. Kwon TG, Lee CO, Park JW, et al. Osteonecrosis associated with dental implants in patients undergoing bisphosphonate treatment. Clin Oral Implants Res 2014;25(5):632–40.

126. Zahid TM, Wang BY, Cohen RE. Influence of bisphosphonates on alveolar bone loss around osseointegrated implants. J Oral Implantol 2011;37(3):335–46.

127. Bell BM, Bell RE. Oral bisphosphonates and dental implants: a retrospective study. J Oral Maxillofac Surg 2008;66(5):1022–4.
128. Grant BT, Amenedo C, Freeman K, et al. Outcomes of placing dental implants in patients taking oral bisphosphonates: a review of 115 cases. J Oral Maxillofac Surg 2008;66(2):223–30.
129. Jacobsen C, Metzler P, Rossle M, et al. Osteopathology induced by bisphosphonates and dental implants: clinical observations. Clin Oral Investig 2013;17(1): 167–75.
130. Siebert T, Jurkovic R, Statelova D, et al. Immediate implant placement in a patient with osteoporosis undergoing bisphosphonate therapy: 1-year preliminary prospective study. J Oral Implantol 2015;41(Spec No):360–5.
131. Shabestari GO, Shayesteh YS, Khojasteh A, et al. Implant placement in patients with oral bisphosphonate therapy: a case series. Clin Implant Dent Relat Res 2010;12(3):175–80.
132. Martin DC, O'Ryan FS, Indresano AT, et al. Characteristics of implant failures in patients with a history of oral bisphosphonate therapy. J Oral Maxillofac Surg 2010;68(3):508–14.
133. Lopez-Cedrun JL, Sanroman JF, Garcia A, et al. Oral bisphosphonate-related osteonecrosis of the jaws in dental implant patients: a case series. Br J Oral Maxillofac Surg 2013;51(8):874–9.
134. Lazarovici TS, Yahalom R, Taicher S, et al. Bisphosphonate-related osteonecrosis of the jaw associated with dental implants. J Oral Maxillofac Surg 2010;68(4): 790–6.
135. Goss A, Bartold M, Sambrook P, et al. The nature and frequency of bisphosphonate-associated osteonecrosis of the jaws in dental implant patients: a South Australian case series. J Oral Maxillofac Surg 2010;68(2):337–43.
136. Tam Y, Kar K, Nowzari H, et al. Osteonecrosis of the jaw after implant surgery in patients treated with bisphosphonates–a presentation of six consecutive cases. Clin Implant Dent Relat Res 2014;16(5):751–61.
137. Al-Sabbagh M, Robinson FG, Romanos G, et al. Osteoporosis and bisphosphonate-related osteonecrosis in a dental school implant patient population. Implant Dent 2015;24(3):328–32.
138. American Cancer Society. Key Statistics for Oral Cavity and Oropharyngeal Cancers. Available at: https://www.cancer.org/cancer/oral-cavity-and-oropharyngeal-cancer/about/key-statistics.html. Accessed October 1, 2018.
139. Verdonck HW, Meijer GJ, Nieman FH, et al. Quantitative computed tomography bone mineral density measurements in irradiated and non-irradiated minipig alveolar bone: an experimental study. Clin Oral Implants Res 2008;19(5):465–8.
140. Smith Nobrega A, Santiago JF Jr, de Faria Almeida DA, et al. Irradiated patients and survival rate of dental implants: a systematic review and meta-analysis. J Prosthet Dent 2016;116(6):858–66.
141. Bolind P, Johansson CB, Johansson P, et al. Retrieved implants from irradiated sites in humans: a histologic/histomorphometric investigation of oral and craniofacial implants. Clin Implant Dent Relat Res 2006;8(3):142–50.
142. Brogniez V, Lejuste P, Pecheur A, et al. Dental prosthetic reconstruction of osseointegrated implants placed in irradiated bone. Int J Oral Maxillofac Implants 1998;13(4):506–12.
143. Mancha de la Plata M, Gias LN, Diez PM, et al. Osseointegrated implant rehabilitation of irradiated oral cancer patients. J Oral Maxillofac Surg 2012;70(5): 1052–63.

144. Javed F, Al-Hezaimi K, Al-Rasheed A, et al. Implant survival rate after oral cancer therapy: a review. Oral Oncol 2010;46(12):854–9.
145. Nooh N. Dental implant survival in irradiated oral cancer patients: a systematic review of the literature. Int J Oral Maxillofac Implants 2013;28(5):1233–42.
146. Schiegnitz E, Al-Nawas B, Kammerer PW, et al. Oral rehabilitation with dental implants in irradiated patients: a meta-analysis on implant survival. Clin Oral Investig 2014;18(3):687–98.
147. Shugaa-Addin B, Al-Shamiri HM, Al-Maweri S, et al. The effect of radiotherapy on survival of dental implants in head and neck cancer patients. J Clin Exp Dent 2016;8(2):e194–200.
148. Andersson G, Andreasson L, Bjelkengren G. Oral implant rehabilitation in irradiated patients without adjunctive hyperbaric oxygen. Int J Oral Maxillofac Implants 1998;13(5):647–54.
149. Granstrom G. Osseointegration in irradiated cancer patients: an analysis with respect to implant failures. J Oral Maxillofac Surg 2005;63(5):579–85.
150. Mericske-Stern R, Perren R, Raveh J. Life table analysis and clinical evaluation of oral implants supporting prostheses after resection of malignant tumors. Int J Oral Maxillofac Implants 1999;14(5):673–80.
151. Schoen PJ, Raghoebar GM, Bouma J, et al. Rehabilitation of oral function in head and neck cancer patients after radiotherapy with implant-retained dentures: effects of hyperbaric oxygen therapy. Oral Oncol 2007;43(4):379–88.

Should Cone Beam Computed Tomography Be Routinely Obtained in Implant Planning?

Galal Omami, BDS, MSc, MDentSc, FRCD(C), Dip ABOMR[a],*,
Firas Al Yafi, DDS[b]

KEYWORDS

- Cone beam CT - Dental implant - Selection criteria - Implant planning

KEY POINTS

- Cone beam CT (CBCT) offers high-quality 3-D images at relatively low radiation doses and costs.
- CBCT should only be used when the question for which the imaging is required cannot be answered adequately by conventional, lower dose dental radiography, applying the As Low As Diagnostically Acceptable (ALADA) principle.
- CBCT imaging allows for 3-D morphometric analysis of the potential implant sites with submillimetric accuracy.
- CBCT allows for identification of anatomic landmarks and pathologies.
- Specialized software can be used for the virtual planning and the fabrication of surgical guides for precise implant placement.

INTRODUCTION

The advent of cone beam CT (CBCT) as a relatively low-dose 3-D dental imaging technology has improved both diagnostic accuracy and implant planning.[1] The 3-D visualization of the alveolar ridge enables clinicians to easily identify anatomic structures and anomalies. CBCT is essential to assess alveolar ridge deficiencies and bone augmentation outcomes. A 3-D evaluation is key in particular techniques, such as zygomatic implants, pterygoid implants, and osteogenic distraction.

CBCT images enable clinicians to discuss the patient-specific clinical scenario while presenting an individualized treatment plan. In this review, the authors discuss the

Disclosure: The authors have nothing to disclose.
[a] Division of Oral Diagnosis, Oral Medicine, Oral Radiology, Department of Oral Health Practice, College of Dentistry, University of Kentucky, 800 Rose Street, MN320, Lexington, KY 40536-0297, USA; [b] Arab Board of Oral Surgery, Division of Periodontology, Department of Oral Health Practice, College of Dentistry, University of Kentucky, 800 Rose Street, Lexington, KY 40536-0297, USA
* Corresponding author.
E-mail address: Galal.Omami@uky.edu

Dent Clin N Am 63 (2019) 363–379
https://doi.org/10.1016/j.cden.2019.02.005
0011-8532/19/© 2019 Elsevier Inc. All rights reserved.

dental.theclinics.com

added value of CBCT in implant dentistry and investigate the question of whether CBCT should be routinely obtained for preoperative implant planning.

CONE BEAM CT RADIATION DOSES

The effective radiation dose associated with CBCT imaging in implant dentistry is varied, ranging from 10 µSv to 271 µSv, depending on the model of CBCT scanner and field of view (FOV) selected.[2–4] CBCT provides an equivalent patient radiation dose of 3 days to 48 days of background radiation or 5 times to 74 times that of a conventional panoramic radiograph[5–7] (**Table 1**). The use of additional personal protection (thyroid collar) and patient positioning modifications (tilting the chin) can substantially reduce the dose by up to 40%.[8] Other methods of reducing patient exposure include decreasing scan time[9,10] or scan arc[11] and increasing voxel size, which decreases the image resolution but does not affect measurement accuracy.[12] Based on a systematic review, it has been suggested that a voxel size of 0.3 to 0.4 mm was adequate to provide CBCT images of acceptable diagnostic quality for implant treatment planning.[13] Many CBCT systems offer ultra–low-dose imaging that has radiation doses comparable to conventional panoramic images, without significant reduction in image quality.[14]

Clinicians should apply the As Low As Diagnostically Acceptable (ALADA) principle in reducing patient exposure during the acquisition of CBCT images. This includes appropriate justification of CBCT use, optimizing exposure parameters, using the smallest FOV necessary for the diagnostic task, and using appropriate personal protective shielding.

CONE BEAM CT VERSUS MULTIDETECTOR CT

In a CBCT machine, the x-ray beam emerges as a divergent cone-shaped or pyramidal beam. Data are acquired as a series of sequential planar projection images (basis images) made with angular differences as the beam rotates around a patient's

Table 1
Effective dose estimates for common dental radiographic examination, cone beam CT, and multidetector CT imaging (estimates for adult patients)

Examination	Effective Dose (µSv)
Four-image posterior bitewings with phosphor storage plate or F-speed film and rectangular collimation	5.0
Panoramic radiograph with digital sensor (charge-coupled device)	3.0–24.3
Cephalometric radiograph with phosphor storage plate	5.1–5.6
Full-mouth radiographs with phosphor storage plate or F-speed film and rectangular collimation	34.9
Full-mouth radiographs with phosphor storage plate or F-speed film and round collimation	170.7
CBCT small FOV	60
CBCT medium FOV	107
CBCT large FOV	151
MDCT mandible	427
MDCT jaws	697
MDCT head	1088

head. Projection data are reconstructed through software algorithms, producing a volumetric data set used to generate primary reconstruction images in 3 orthogonal planes (axial, sagittal, and coronal).

In contrast, the x-ray beam in a multidetector CT (MDCT) scanner emerges as a flat fan beam. Data are acquired as a series of consecutive axial slices of a patient's head obtained from multiple rotations of the x-ray source around the patient. In MDCT, the average density of each voxel is measured in a Hounsfield unit (also known as a CT number); this unit represents the average attenuation coefficient in that voxel. The Hounsfield units that are derived from various CBCT systems, however, are not consistently representative of the actual density values, sometimes even within the same system.[15]

The radiation dose of the CBCT is less than that for an MDCT examination (the dose reduction is between 76.2% and 98.5%).[3,6] Most CBCT systems use x-ray tubes similar to those in panoramic x-ray machines, operating in the range of 2 mA to 14 mA, whereas for MDCT, the tube current may be in excess of 250 mA. CBCT is more reliable for linear measurements than MDCT and less affected by metal artifacts.[16]

PATIENT SELECTION CRITERIA

In addition to a thorough clinical examination, a radiographic assessment is essential to evaluate the potential implant sites. Various conventional and tomographic (cross-sectional) imaging techniques are available for evaluation of the implant site and related anatomical structures. Intraoral periapical images are a valuable tool to estimate the mesiodistal and vertical dimensions of an implant site. Panoramic radiographs are less suited because of inherent distortion. Unlike cross-sectional techniques, however, neither panoramic nor periapical radiographs provide information on the buccolingual width or angulation of the alveolar ridge.

The selection of an appropriate radiograph should be based on the needed diagnostic information while balancing the potential benefits and risks. Evidence-based guidelines for patient selection criteria were published in an American Academy of Oral and Maxillofacial Radiology (AAOMR) position paper.[17] In their guidelines, the initial assessment of a potential dental implant site should be completed using intraoral periapical and/or panoramic radiographs. CBCT is recommended as the imaging modality of choice for presurgical implant planning (**Table 2**).

The use of CBCT for presurgical implant planning provides a morphometric and skeletal analysis of the alveolar ridge, highlighting the proximity to vital anatomic structures. When the clinical examination and conventional radiograph reveals the need for bone augmentation or site development procedure, CBCT should be considered for preoperative and postoperative evaluation (**Figs. 1–3**). In addition, CBCT can be used for an accurate, prosthetically driven implant planning. Intraoral periapical and panoramic radiographs are indicated for postoperative assessment. CBCT imaging, however, may be indicated postoperatively if the implant placement is complicated by local infection or nerve injury (**Fig. 4**).

ANATOMIC CONSIDERATIONS
Alveolar Bone Quality

Assessment of alveolar bone quality takes into consideration overall bone volume and morphology. The cortical thickness, trabecular bone pattern, and bone density (**Figs. 5–7**) are positively correlated with implant primary stability.[18]

Table 2		
Summary of the position statement of the American Academy of Oral and Maxillofacial Radiology on selection criteria of imaging modalities in implant dentistry		
Clinical Situation	**Specific Indication(s)**	**Imaging Modality**
Initial phase		• Panoramic ± periapical radiography
Presurgical phase • Clinical doubt of alveolar bone height, width, and/or shape • Bone density • Anterior esthetic zone • Specific anatomic sites	• Anterior maxilla (nasal floor, incisive fossa) • Posterior maxilla (maxillary sinus, posterior superior alveolar canal) • Anterior mandible (lingual foramen, genial tubercles, incisive canal) • Posterior mandible (inferior alveolar nerve canal, mental foramen, anterior loop, lingual undercut, retromolar foramen) • Zygomatic region (orbital floor, infraorbital foramen, zygomatic bone)	• CBCT + radiographic guide
• Site development	• Sinus floor elevation • Block or particulate bone grafting • Ramus or symphysis grafting • Pathology/impacted in the area of interest • Prior traumatic injury	
• Computer-assisted treatment planning	• Follow manufacturer recommendations	
Postsurgical phase • Postoperative implant integration	• Marginal peri-implant bone height • Bone-implant interface • Postaugmentation assessment • Implant mobility	• Periapical + bitewing radiography • Panoramic radiography in extensive implant therapy
• Postoperative complications	• Altered sensation • Infection (sinusitis)	• CBCT

Nasopalatine Foramen and Canal

The nasopalatine canal (or incisive canal) may show important morphologic and dimensional variations. If the incisive foramen is greater than 10 mm, pathologic conditions should be suspected.[19] Placement of implants in the direct vicinity of the nasopalatine canal have been associated with higher failure rates.[20] Insertion of the implant into the canal may prevent osseointegration or lead to neurosensory damage.

Nasal Cavity and Maxillary Sinus

Atrophy of the maxillary alveolar ridge may pose limitations for implant placement, especially with pneumatization of the maxillary sinuses and the presence of the nasal cavities. CBCT accurately provides a 3-D visualization of the maxillary sinus anatomy. It is possible to assess the thickness of the lateral wall and the presence of the superior alveolar canals in the anterior and lateral antral walls[21] (see **Fig. 7**).

The presence of the maxillary sinus septa is associated with increased risk of schneiderian membrane perforation during sinus augmentation. If perforation occurs, the patient may have an increased risk of sinus infection[22] (**Fig. 8**). In addition, CBCT

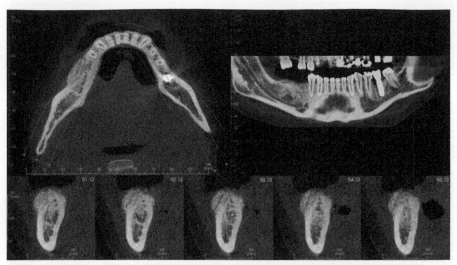

Fig. 1. Comparative sets of axial, reformatted panoramic, and sequential 1-mm–thick cross-sectional CBCT images show consolidation of the graft material to the right mandibular posterior edentulous region. This graft increases the alveolar bone width necessary for implant placement.

can detect conditions that could lead to obstruction of the ostium, which would compromise sinus drainage. These radiographic findings include mucosal thickening and anatomic variations in the antronasal cavity, such as concha bullosa (pneumatized middle turbinate) and Haller cells (infraorbital ethmoidal cells). Sinus lift surgery may be contraindicated when these conditions are detected on the CBCT image (**Fig. 9**).

Lingual Foramen

The lingual canal is a vascular bony channel on the lingual cortical aspect in the midline of the mandible and can be seen in more than 80% of the mandibles[23] (see **Fig. 6**). The anterior region of the mandible has always been considered to be a relative safe zone

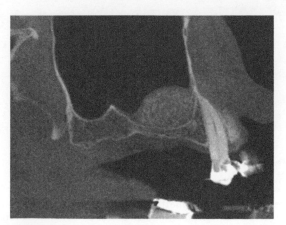

Fig. 2. Parasagittal CBCT image of a partially edentulous maxilla showing homogenous hyperdense sinus-lift graft material with minimal mucosal thickening.

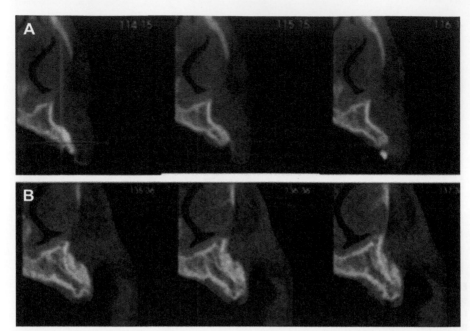

Fig. 3. (*A*) Comparative sets of cross-sectional CBCT images in the anterior maxillary edentulous region show labial cortical concavity. (*B*) Postoperative images show the width gain and bone graft consolidation.

for implant placement. The lingual foramen can be detected on the CBCT, however, to avoid violating the lingual vasculature. This decreases the risk for a potential life-threatening obstruction of the airway caused by hemorrhage into the floor of the mouth.[23,24]

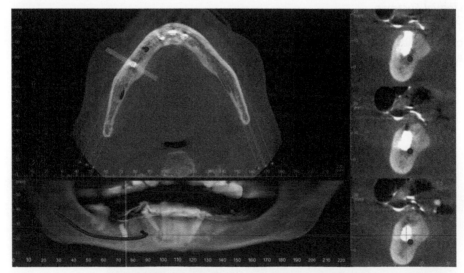

Fig. 4. Comparative sets of axial, reformatted panoramic, and consecutive 1-mm–thick cross-sectional CBCT images of the right mandibular posterior edentulous region demonstrate embarrassment and compression of the mandibular canal by a dental implant. The patient reported postoperative paresthesia of the right lip.

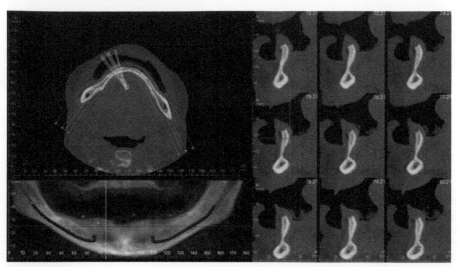

Fig. 5. Comparative sets of axial, reformatted panoramic, and serial 1-mm–thick cross-sectional CBCT images of a completely edentulous mandible. The alveolar ridge in the posterior region shows a constriction between the alveolar process and the basal bone resulting from both a buccal and a lingual concavity, resulting in an hourglass configuration.

Mental Foramen

The mental foramen is a strategically important landmark during implant placement. Presence of 1 or more accessory mental foramina has been reported.[25] The anterior loop of the inferior alveolar nerve, if present, must be identified to avoid nerve injury

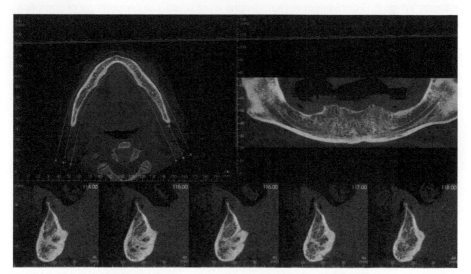

Fig. 6. Comparative sets of axial, reformatted panoramic, and serial 1-mm–thick cross-sectional images of a completely edentulous mandible showing a narrow knife-edge ridge form in the anterior region. Note the thinning of the cortical plates. Note the midline superior and inferior lingual canals exiting through the lingual cortical plate as the corresponding lingual foramen.

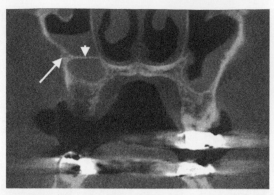

Fig. 7. Coronal CBCT image of the right maxillary posterior edentulous regions showing loss of cortical plates with significant reduction in the trabecular volume. The right maxillary sinus demonstrates a bony septum oriented in a coronal plane (*arrowhead*), with extensive mucosal thickening. Note the posterior superior alveolar canal embedded in the lateral antral wall (*arrow*).

during the implant surgery (**Fig. 10**).[26,27] A 2-mm safety zone should be applied during implant placement.[28]

Mandibular Canal

The mandibular canal (or inferior alveolar canal) can be visualized in most CBCT images; this is important to avoid nerve injury. Bifid mandibular canal, although rare (less than 1%),[29] can pose complications during implant surgery (**Fig. 11**). In 1 study of postimplant neuropathy, a preoperative CBCT was associated with only 10% of the patients. When 2-D conventional radiographs were used, the percentage of complications range from 30% to 50%.[30]

Submandibular Gland Fossa (Lingual Undercut)

A lingual undercut in the posterior mandibular region can be detected in approximately 39% of patients.[31] This is considered an anatomic risk for lingual cortical perforation during implant placement[32] (**Fig. 12**).

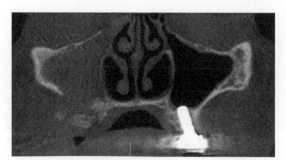

Fig. 8. Coronal CBCT image showing complete radiopacification of the right maxillary sinus associated with thickening of the bony antral walls and dispersion of the bone graft material through the lateral window defect, representing postoperative sinusitis.

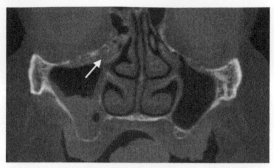

Fig. 9. Coronal CBCT image of a completely edentulous maxilla shows inadequate bone height for implant placement due to bone resorption and sinus pneumatization. The right maxillary sinus shows extensive mucosal thickening associated with obstructed ostium (*arrow*).

COMPUTER-GUIDED IMPLANT PLANNING AND PLACEMENT

Several software programs are available for CBCT analysis and virtual implant planning. Rapid prototyping technology is used to transfer the virtual plan and produce the static surgical guide (**Fig. 13**). Guided implant surgery may improve implant placement accuracy, reduce surgery time, and facilitate minimally invasive flapless approaches.[33,34] An additional application of CBCT in combination with computer-aided design/computer-aided manufacturing technology is to prefabricate the provisional prosthesis.

Facial optical scan can be merged with the CBCT image to evaluate a patient's smile and design the transitional line of implant prosthesis. More recently, CBCT allows the 3-D estimation of a bony defect to mill a customized block graft. Recent advances in dynamic navigation systems have enabled practitioners to precisely place dental implants in real-time surgery. The constant improvements to both static and dynamic systems will allow the full potential of guided surgery.

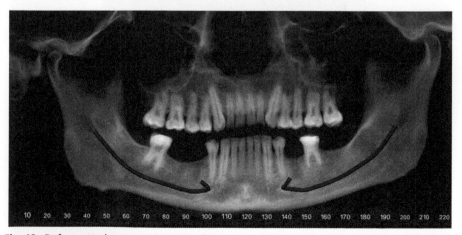

Fig. 10. Reformatted panoramic image demonstrates the anterior loop of the mental nerve, bilaterally. This feature is seen in approximately 10% of the mandibles, posing limitation in implant placement.

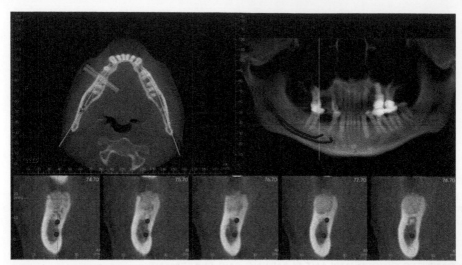

Fig. 11. Comparative sets of axial, reformatted panoramic and serial 1-mm–thick cross-sectional images of the right mandibular posterior edentulous region showing a bifid mandibular canal, presenting potential risk for nerve injury during implant surgery. This feature is demonstrated in less than 1% of the mandibles.

SELECTION GUIDELINES

Many dental professional organizations have developed clinical practice guidelines for the use of CBCT in implant dentistry (**Table 3**). There is an agreement that thorough clinical examination along with 2-D radiographs should be the first step of an implant site assessment. Additionally, there is a consensus on the superiority of CBCT over 2-D radiographs in the diagnosis and planning of complex implant cases. When

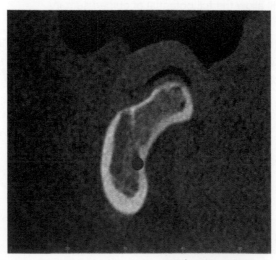

Fig. 12. Cross-sectional CBCT image in the region of the right mandibular molar edentulous region shows resorption of the buccal cortex. The alveolar process and the basal bone depict an S-shaped figure with a marked lingual concavity.

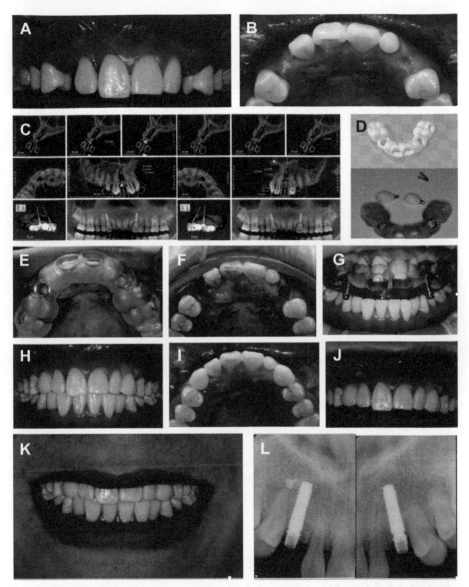

Fig. 13. The digital workflow for guided surgery. (*A, B*) Intraoral frontal and occlusal views of congenitally missed upper cuspids; (*C*) virtual implant planning; (*D*) planning is transferred via the printed implant guide; (*E*) guide in the patient mouth; (*F*) flapless approach; (*G*) fully guided implant placement; (*H–J*) intraoral retracted, occlusal, and frontal views of the prefabricated, immediate restorations; (*K*) patient's smile; and (*L*) PAs showing the implants' angulation and relation to the adjacent teeth.

CBCT is prescribed, the radiation dose should always be optimized, and the whole CBCT data should be reviewed for any incidental findings.

The European Association for Osseointegration[35] recommends cross-sectional imaging for implant placement when information obtained by the clinical assessment and conventional dental radiographs is inadequate. On the other hand, the fifth ITI

Table 3
Summary of the consensus papers on guidelines of cone beam CT in implant dentistry

Title	Organization	Year	Methodology	Recommendations
"2010 Guidelines of the Academy of Osseointegration for the Provision of Dental Implants and Associated Patient Care"[39]	AO	2010	Expert opinion	• Full history and clinical examination should be performed before ordering the CBCT. • Every CBCT requires justification. • Routine CBCT is strongly discouraged. • Large-volume CBCT should not be routinely used. • A comprehensive report, even if not within the maxillofacial region, is needed.
"E.A.O. Guidelines for the Use of Diagnostic Imaging in Implant Dentistry 2011. A Consensus Workshop Organized by the European Association for Osseointegration at the Medical University of Warsaw"[35]	EAO	2011	Expert opinion	• Clinical evaluation and the conventional radiographs may be sufficient for implant placement. • CBCT may be beneficial to 3-D visualize the implant site and anatomic landmarks. • CBCT can aid the prosthetically driven implant placement. • Safety margins should be considered even with the use of CBCT in all cases. • CBCT is beneficial for extensive grafting procedures, sinus grafts, and intraoral autogenous block grafts. • Guided implant surgery should be justified.
"Position Statement of the American Academy of Oral and Maxillofacial Radiology on Selection Criteria for the Use of Radiology Dental Implantology With Emphasis on Cone Beam Computed Tomography"[17]	AAOMR	2012	Research-based expert opinion	• Panoramic and periapical radiographs may be sufficient for initial implant site evaluation. • CBCT is the radiograph of choice for preoperative diagnosis and planning phases. • The CBCT use in implant dentistry can be easily justified. • The smallest FOV should be used and exposure parameters should be optimized. • Periapical and panoramic images are adequate for periodic and postoperative implant follow-ups. • Every CBCT must be interpreted for any incidental findings.

Title	Organization	Year	Type	Findings
"Use of Cone Beam Computed Tomography in Implant Dentistry: The International Congress of Oral Implantologists Consensus Report"[38]	ICOI	2012	Expert opinion	• CBCT use should be justified. • Full history and clinical examination should be performed before ordering the CBCT. • CBCT is the alternative when conventional 2-D radiography may not be sufficient. • The smallest FOV should be used. • Every CBCT must be interpreted for any incidental findings.
"The Use of Cone-Beam Computed Tomography in Dentistry: An Advisory Statement from the American Dental Association Council on Scientific Affairs"[40]	ADA	2012	Expert opinion	• Full history and clinical examination should be performed before ordering the CBCT. • CBCT use should be justified and should not be part of the screening process. • CBCT is an adjunct to conventional dental radiographs. • The radiation dose is optimized (ALADA). • Personal protective methods always should be used. • CBCT-related training should be a prerequisite to order it. • CBCT must be interpreted by a qualified health care provider.
"Guidelines for Clinical Use of CBCT: A Review"[41]	BIR	2014	Review	• 26 publications were included in the review; 11 were particularly for CBCT indications and patient selection criteria. • Only 2 articles had used an evidence-based approach for guideline development and 2 used consensus methods. • The quality of publications was frequently low, as assessed using AGREE II. • There was a general concurrence among the reviewed articles about CBCT clinical indications for dental implant.

(continued on next page)

Table 3
(continued)

Title	Organization	Year	Methodology	Recommendations
"Cone Beam Computed Tomography in Implant Dentistry: A Systematic Review Focusing on Guidelines, Indications, and Radiation Dose Risks"[36]	ITI	2014	A systematic review and consensus	• CBCT indications' range for dental implants includes preoperative assessment for critical anatomy, bone grafting procedure and guided surgery, and, in addition, complications management, especially nerve damage. • The FOV should be limited to the area of interest.
"American Academy of Periodontology Best Evidence Consensus Statement on Selected Oral Applications for Cone-Beam Computed Tomography"[17]	AAP	2017	Expert opinion (best evidence consensus)	• CBCT has a wide range of indications in implant dentistry, including guided implant surgery. • CBCT should be used as an adjunct to 2-D dental radiographs using clinical judgment. • In complex implant cases, CBCT is superior to 2-D radiographs. • CBCT can facilitate patients' education and communication between the dental team. • Every effort should not be preserved to reduce the effective radiation dose.
"Accuracy of Linear Measurements on CBCT Images Related to Presurgical Implant Treatment Planning: A Systematic Review"[13]	ITI	2018	A systematic review and consensus	• CBCT is a valid tool for implant preoperative planning. • 2-mm safety zone role should be applied when CBCT is used for implant planning. • An acceptable diagnostic quality for implant planning can be achieved using voxel size of 0.3–0.4 mm. • CBCT reliability and linear measurement accuracy can be affected by many factors, including radiation exposure, motion artifact, CBCT machine, and software.

Abbreviations: ADA, American Dental Association; AO, Academy of Osseointegration; BIR, British Institute of Radiology; EAO, European Association for Osseointegration.

consensus conference[36] has recommended 3-D imaging in critical anatomic situations, grafting procedures, and guided surgery. The "best evidence review" of the American Academy of Periodontology (AAP),[37] however, emphasized that the benefits of the CBCT should offset the risk. In the International Congress of Oral Implantologists (ICOI) consensus report, the experts stated, "it is virtually impossible to predict which treatment cases would not benefit from having this (CBCT) additional information before obtaining it."[38] Moreover, the AAOMR position paper[17] has suggested CBCT as the imaging modality of choice for implant planning and preoperative preparation.

SUMMARY

CBCT offers high-quality 3-D images at relatively low radiation doses and costs. It provides a 3-D assessment of the dental implant sites and evaluates the proximity to vital anatomic structures with submillimetric accuracy. CBCT should not be routinely used, however, for the initial implant site assessment. The use of CBCT is based on a clinician's professional opinion as to whether or not information from the clinical and conventional radiographic examinations is inadequate and additional 3-D imaging needed to formulate a diagnosis and treatment plan. Radiation dose be should always optimized with a FOV limited to the area of interest.

REFERENCES

1. Sukovic P. Cone beam computed tomography in craniofacial imaging. Orthod Craniofac Res 2003;6(Suppl 1):31–6 [discussion: 179–82].
2. Ludlow JB, Davies-Ludlow LE, Brooks SL, et al. Dosimetry of 3 CBCT devices for oral and maxillofacial radiology: CB mercuray, newtom 3G and i-CAT. Dentomaxillofac Radiol 2006;35:219–26.
3. Schulze D, Heiland M, Thurmann H, et al. Radiation exposure during midfacial imaging using 4- and 16-slice computed tomography, cone beam computed tomography systems and conventional radiography. Dentomaxillofac Radiol 2004; 33:83–6.
4. Scaf G, Lurie AG, Mosier KM, et al. Dosimetry and cost of imaging osseointegrated implants with film-based and computed tomography. Oral Surg Oral Med Oral Pathol Oral Radiol Endod 1997;83:41–8.
5. Pauwels R, Theodorakou C, Walker A, et al. Dose distribution for dental cone beam CT and its implication for defining a dose index. Dentomaxillofac Radiol 2012;41:583–93.
6. Ludlow JB, Ivanovic M. Comparative dosimetry of dental CBCT devices and 64-slice CT for oral and maxillofacial radiology. Oral Surg Oral Med Oral Pathol Oral Radiol Endod 2008;106:106–14.
7. SEDENTEXCT. Radiation protection: cone beam CT for dental and maxillofacial radiology. Evidence Based Guidelines 2011. v2.0 Final. Available at: http://www.sedentexct.eu/files/guidelines_final.pdf. Accessed April, 2018.
8. Aps JK. Cone beam computed tomography in paediatric dentistry: overview of recent literature. Eur Arch Paediatr Dent 2013;14:131–40.
9. Al-Ekrish AA. Effect of exposure time on the accuracy and reliability of cone beam computed tomography in the assessment of dental implant site dimensions in dry skulls. Saudi Dent J 2012;24:127–34.
10. Waltrick KB, Nunes de Abreu Junior MJ, Correa M, et al. Accuracy of linear measurements and visibility of the mandibular canal of cone-beam computed

tomography images with different voxel sizes: an in vitro study. J Periodontol 2013;84:68–77.

11. Neves FS, Vasconcelos TV, Campos PS, et al. Influence of scan mode (180 degrees/360 degrees) of the cone beam computed tomography for preoperative dental implant measurements. Clin Oral Implants Res 2014;25:e155–8.

12. Ganguly R, Ramesh A, Pagni S. The accuracy of linear measurements of maxillary and mandibular edentulous sites in cone-beam computed tomography images with different fields of view and voxel sizes under simulated clinical conditions. Imaging Sci Dent 2016;46:93–101.

13. Fokas G, Vaughn VM, Scarfe WC, et al. Accuracy of linear measurements on CBCT images related to presurgical implant treatment planning: a systematic review. Clin Oral Implants Res 2018;29(Suppl 16):393–415.

14. Ludlow JB, Walker C. Assessment of phantom dosimetry and image quality of i-CAT FLX cone-beam computed tomography. Am J Orthod Dentofacial Orthop 2013;144:802–17.

15. Pauwels R, Jacobs R, Singer SR, et al. CBCT-based bone quality assessment: are hounsfield units applicable? Dentomaxillofac Radiol 2015;44:20140238.

16. Patcas R, Muller L, Ullrich O, et al. Accuracy of cone-beam computed tomography at different resolutions assessed on the bony covering of the mandibular anterior teeth. Am J Orthod Dentofacial Orthop 2012;141:41–50.

17. Tyndall DA, Price JB, Tetradis S, et al. Position statement of the American academy of oral and maxillofacial radiology on selection criteria for the use of radiology in dental implantology with emphasis on cone beam computed tomography. Oral Surg Oral Med Oral Pathol Oral Radiol 2012;113:817–26.

18. de Oliveira RC, Leles CR, Lindh C, et al. Bone tissue microarchitectural characteristics at dental implant sites. Part 1: identification of clinical-related parameters. Clin Oral Implants Res 2012;23:981–6.

19. Swanson KS, Kaugars GE, Gunsolley JC. Nasopalatine duct cyst: an analysis of 334 cases. J Oral Maxillofac Surg 1991;49:268–71.

20. Scher EL. Use of the incisive canal as a recipient site for root form implants: preliminary clinical reports. Implant Dent 1994;3:38–41.

21. Mardinger O, Nissan J, Chaushu G. Sinus floor augmentation with simultaneous implant placement in the severely atrophic maxilla: technical problems and complications. J Periodontol 2007;78:1872–7.

22. Nolan PJ, Freeman K, Kraut RA. Correlation between schneiderian membrane perforation and sinus lift graft outcome: a retrospective evaluation of 359 augmented sinus. J Oral Maxillofac Surg 2014;72:47–52.

23. Tepper G, Hofschneider UB, Gahleitner A, et al. Computed tomographic diagnosis and localization of bone canals in the mandibular interforaminal region for prevention of bleeding complications during implant surgery. Int J Oral Maxillofac Implants 2001;16:68–72.

24. ten Bruggenkate CM, Krekeler G, Kraaijenhagen HA, et al. Hemorrhage of the floor of the mouth resulting from lingual perforation during implant placement: a clinical report. Int J Oral Maxillofac Implants 1993;8:329–34.

25. Toh H, Kodama J, Yanagisako M, et al. Anatomical study of the accessory mental foramen and the distribution of its nerve. Okajimas Folia Anat Jpn 1992;69:85–8.

26. Arzouman MJ, Otis L, Kipnis V, et al. Observations of the anterior loop of the inferior alveolar canal. Int J Oral Maxillofac Implants 1993;8:295–300.

27. Bavitz JB, Harn SD, Hansen CA, et al. An anatomical study of mental neurovascular bundle-implant relationships. Int J Oral Maxillofac Implants 1993;8:563–7.

28. Greenstein G, Tarnow D. The mental foramen and nerve: clinical and anatomical factors related to dental implant placement: a literature review. J Periodontol 2006;77:1933–43.
29. Rouas P, Nancy J, Bar D. Identification of double mandibular canals: literature review and three case reports with CT scans and cone beam CT. Dentomaxillofac Radiol 2007;36:34–8.
30. Renton T, Dawood A, Shah A, et al. Post-implant neuropathy of the trigeminal nerve. A case series. Br Dent J 2012;212:E17.
31. Chan HL, Brooks SL, Fu JH, et al. Cross-sectional analysis of the mandibular lingual concavity using cone beam computed tomography. Clin Oral Implants Res 2011;22:201–6.
32. Watanabe H, Mohammad Abdul M, Kurabayashi T, et al. Mandible size and morphology determined with CT on a premise of dental implant operation. Surg Radiol Anat 2010;32:343–9.
33. D'Haese J, Ackhurst J, Wismeijer D, et al. Current state of the art of computer-guided implant surgery. Periodontol 2000 2017;73:121–33.
34. Tahmaseb A, Wismeijer D, Coucke W, et al. Computer technology applications in surgical implant dentistry: a systematic review. Int J Oral Maxillofac Implants 2014;29(Suppl):25–42.
35. Harris D, Horner K, Grondahl K, et al. E.A.O. guidelines for the use of diagnostic imaging in implant dentistry 2011. A consensus workshop organized by the European Association for Osseointegration at the Medical University of Warsaw. Clin Oral Implants Res 2012;23:1243–53.
36. Bornstein MM, Scarfe WC, Vaughn VM, et al. Cone beam computed tomography in implant dentistry: a systematic review focusing on guidelines, indications, and radiation dose risks. Int J Oral Maxillofac Implants 2014;29(Suppl):55–77.
37. Rios HF, Borgnakke WS, Benavides E. The use of cone-beam computed tomography in management of patients requiring dental implants: an American Academy of Periodontology best evidence review. J Periodontol 2017;88:946–59.
38. Benavides E, Rios HF, Ganz SD, et al. Use of cone beam computed tomography in implant dentistry: the international congress of oral implantologists consensus report. Implant Dent 2012;21:78–86.
39. Academy of Osseointegration. 2010 Guidelines of the Academy of Osseointegration for the provision of dental implants and associated patient care. Int J Oral Maxillofac Implants 2010;25(3):620–7.
40. American Dental Association Council on Scientific Affairs. The use of cone-beam computed tomography in dentistry: an advisory statement from the American Dental Association Council on scientific affairs. J Am Dent Assoc 2012;143:899–902.
41. Horner K, O'Malley L, Taylor K, et al. Guidelines for clinical use of CBCT: a review. Dentomaxillofac Radiol 2015;44:20140225.

Is Digital Guided Implant Surgery Accurate and Reliable?

Firas Al Yafi, DDS[a],*, Brittany Camenisch, DDS, MS[b,c],
Mohanad Al-Sabbagh, DDS, MS[d]

KEYWORDS

- Computer-aided surgery • Implant-guided surgery • Computer-assisted surgery
- Accuracy • Dental implants • Digital workflow • Virtual plan

KEY POINTS

- The benefits of guided implant placement include increased predictability, and decreased surgery time and complication rate.
- Static guides remain the most commonly used guide for computer-assisted implant surgery.
- The digital workflow can be divided into 6 steps. Each step may produce deviations from the virtual plan.
- The accuracy, efficacy, and complication rate of computer-guided implant treatment remain within acceptable clinical limits.
- Proper execution of each digital workflow step must be carefully verified to reduce inaccuracies.

INTRODUCTION

Guided implant surgery simplifies the execution of implant placement procedures and renders optimal clinical outcomes. Digital implant planning allows the accurate diagnosis of an implant site and virtual visualization of the final prosthetic restoration. Additional clinical benefits include reduced surgical time and a lower complication rate leading to increased patient acceptance and satisfaction. However, all the assumed advantages of guided implant surgery over traditional surgeries depend on the precise execution of the virtual implant plan.[1–4]

[a] Arab Board of Oral Surgery, University of Kentucky, College of Dentistry, 4th floor (room D436), Dental Science Bldg, 800 Rose street, Lexington, KY 40536-0297, USA; [b] Private Practice, 519 Hampton Way, Suite 10, Richmond, KY 40475, USA; [c] University of Kentucky, College of Dentistry, 800 Rose Street, Lexington, KY 40536-0297, USA; [d] Division of Periodontology, Advanced Education Externship Program, American Academy of Periodontology, University of Kentucky, College of Dentistry, D-438 Chandler Medical Center, 800 Rose Street, Lexington, KY 40536-0927, USA
* Corresponding author.
E-mail address: firasyafi@uky.edu

Dent Clin N Am 63 (2019) 381–397
https://doi.org/10.1016/j.cden.2019.02.006
0011-8532/19/© 2019 Elsevier Inc. All rights reserved.

dental.theclinics.com

TYPES OF GUIDED SURGERY

Guided implant surgery can generally be classified as dynamic or static. Dynamic guided surgeries involve the use of a computer-aided navigation system to allow for real-time implant surgery. The major advantage to the dynamic design is the ability to intraoperatively adjust the planned implant positioning.[3] Although navigated surgeries are gaining popularity, static guides remain the most commonly used method. This article focuses on static guide–facilitated implant surgeries.

The static guided surgery approach is based on the 3-dimensional (3D) data obtained from cone-beam computed tomography (CBCT) and optical surface scanning, and computer-aided design/computer-aided manufacturing (CAD/CAM) technology for virtual implant planning and guide fabrication. The fabricated surgical guide can be supported by tooth, mucosa, or bone. Additional stabilization and support can be achieved using mini-implants, screws, or pins.[2] Once the guide is fully seated, the planed drilling protocol beings. The drilling protocol can include using the guide for the pilot drill only, or a partially or fully guided drilling protocol. The implant insertion can be executed without the surgical guide or through the guide via a fully guided approach. Proper case selection and planning throughout the digital workflow allow for accurate execution.

THE DIGITAL WORKFLOW

The digital workflow can generally be divided into 6 steps: (1) patient assessment, (2) data collection, (3) data manipulation, (4) virtual implant planning, (5) guide and prosthesis manufacture, and (6) execution of surgery and delivery of an immediate provisional prosthesis (**Fig. 1**). It is worth mentioning that a combination of analog and digital steps may be applied. In addition, different virtual planning implant software may have some variation in the digital workflow.

Step 1: Initial Patient Assessment

During patient assessment, a comprehensive esthetic and functional evaluation should include the following.

Dentition status
Both periodontal and restorative status for the remaining teeth must be assessed. Evaluation of the existing denture must be performed in the case of edentulism.

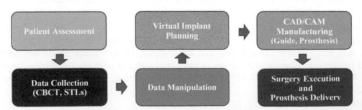

Fig. 1. Digital workflow. The 6 steps of the digital workflow guide clinicians from the initial patient assessment to the execution of the implant surgery. CAD/CAM, computer-aided design/computer-aided manufacturing; CBCT, cone-beam computed tomography; STL, standard tessellation language.

Initial radiographic assessment
The quantity and quality of the bone should be assessed to determine whether grafting or a graftless approach is appropriate; this can be performed on 2-dimensional (2D) radiographs.

Occlusion
Occlusal assessment is essential for acceptable esthetics and function. Adequate mouth opening must be assessed because guided surgery requires extra access, especially in posterior regions.

Aesthetic evaluation and prosthetic consideration
The prosthetic design should ensure appropriate lip support and white/pink display. The prosthetic plan will mandate bone-reduction or augmentation procedures.

Step 2: Data Collection

Data collection includes CBCT acquisition and surface optical scanning. The process of each is reviewed here.

CBCT acquisition
A CBCT is obtained with or without a radiographic guide in dentate patients. A dual-scan technique is the primary method for the edentulous patient (**Fig. 2**); however, direct mucosal scanning techniques are currently being explored.[5]

Limitations to CBCTs include poor soft-tissue contrast and distortion. Distortion can be caused by patient movement[6] and beam-hardening artifacts[7,8] caused by high-density materials such as composite filling, metal restorations, and implants. The distortion affects the quality of the image and hence influences the accuracy of the guided surgery.

Surface optical scanning
Soft-tissue and teeth inaccuracy depicted by CBCT can be compensated by obtaining a surface optical scan, which represents the teeth surface and soft-tissue contour. Hard-tissue and soft-tissue changes must be avoided after the surface scan is captured, otherwise the fit of the surgical guide will be affected. The scan can be created via direct or indirect methods. The patient's impression or stone model is

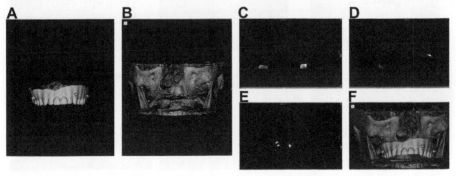

Fig. 2. In the dual-scan technique, fiducial markers are attached to a well-fitting denture; otherwise, a new denture or wax-up should be made. Two separate scans are taken, one of the denture (*A*), and one of the patient with the denture inserted (*B*). Note the superimposition of the 2 scans (*C–F*). The clinician must ensure that the denture is stable and is in the appropriate position, as the intaglio surface of the scanned denture will represent the soft-tissue surface.

scanned using a lab scanner in the indirect method. In the direct method, an intraoral scanner is used to scan the area of interest of the patient's dental arch. Each arch should be scanned individually and then together in occlusion to represent teeth articulation.

The CBCT data are saved in Digital Imaging Communication in Medicine format (DICOM) and the surface optical scan is saved and transferred in a standard tessellation language format (STL). In addition, new CBCTs have the ability to merge facial photographs with the CBCT to obtain an accurate representation of the digital smile.

Step 3: Data Manipulation

Data (the DICOM and STL files) are imported into the digital implant planning software. Data manipulation consists of virtual dissection and orientation of the DICOM file, identification of panoramic curve, tracking of inferior alveolar nerve, and merging the CBCT and surface datasets.

Virtual dissection (segmentation)

CBCT shows both soft and hard tissue, and segmentation of the raw data allows for the differentiation and colorization of anatomic structures and areas of interest. In addition, segmentation reduces the image distortion caused by the metal scattering and motion artifacts. The first step of segmentation is to obtain the appropriate density threshold (also coined as gray-value threshold) to clearly visualize the hard tissues (bone and teeth). Manual setup is the preferred method.[9] Any portion of the scan (known as a voxel) at a selected threshold with the same or larger density will be visible in the selected volume (**Fig. 3**A–C).

CBCT gray values are often not reliable compared with multidetector-row computed tomography.[10–12] Furthermore, different CBCT machines provide variable gray values.[13,14] The selection of the threshold is subjective because it can be affected

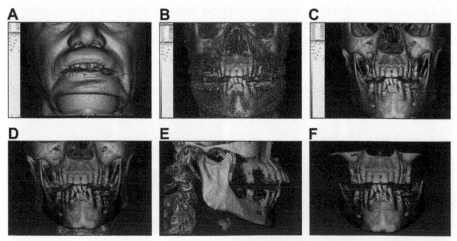

Fig. 3. Segmentation of CBCT volume. The density threshold scale (measured in Hounsfield units) can be adjusted. (*A*) Low-threshold value shows soft tissue. (*B*) Intermediate density threshold between soft tissue and bone. (*C*) Higher-threshold value shows clear bone window. After establishing the proper threshold for bone, the areas of interest can be labeled. (*D, E*) The frontal and lateral view of the segmented maxilla and mandible. (*F*) The segmented 2 jaws after the default volume is turned off.

by the bone irregularities and maturation. Gray-value thresholds can also influence the 3D reconstruction and the fitting of surgical guides.[15]

Orientation and panoramic curve definition
The rendered reconstructed volume has to be correctly oriented into the 3 planes (**Fig. 4**), after which the panoramic arch needs to be defined.

Nerve tracking
The software provides a nerve-tracking tool to detect the inferior alveolar canal by placing dots along its path. Most software programs automatically join the dots and provide a nerve pathway (**Fig. 5**).

Merging of CBCT and surface datasets
The files are merged by selecting identical anatomic landmarks of teeth surfaces or fiducial markers (**Fig. 6**). Misalignment between DICOM and STL data sets can be a possible source of error.

Step 4: Virtual Implant Planning

Once an accurate virtual patient model is obtained, the wax-up of the future prosthesis will allow for the virtual placement of the implants. The surgical guide and prosthesis are designed according to the virtual plan.

The wax-up
The future prosthesis is based on the scanned actual or virtual wax-up (crown-down approach) (**Fig. 7**).

Virtual implant planning
The implant type and size can be chosen from the implant library in the software. Implant position and axis are adjusted according to the available bone. A paralleling tool may be used in the case of multiple implants. Most systems provide an option to set a safety boundary around and between implants (see **Fig. 7**); accordingly, the system will alert the user if these boundaries are violated. In addition, the possibility of a flapless approach or any need for bone augmentation are determined at this time.

Surgical guide design
Once the virtual plan is finalized, the user can design the surgical guide including the type of support (tooth, tissue, bone, or any combination). A minimum of 2 teeth are

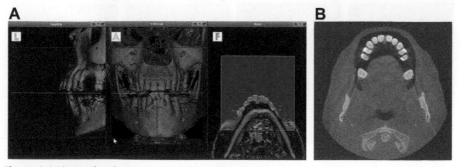

Fig. 4. (*A*) The occlusal plane must be paralleled to the horizontal line in the sagittal view. The patient's midline should be reflected in the coronal view and axial view. (*B*) Panoramic curve definition.

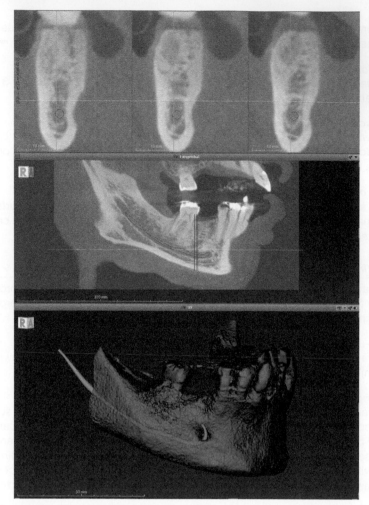

Fig. 5. Nerve tracking allows 3D visualization of the nerve in the posterior mandible.

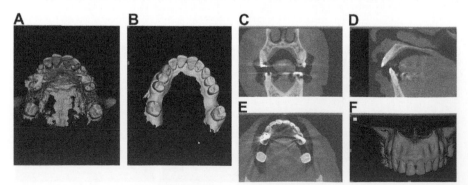

Fig. 6. Files merging. (*A, B*) The segmented DICOM file with selected areas that correspond to those of the STL file in (*B*). (*C–F*) Alignment of the 2 files. Note the homogeneous alignment on different section and views to ensure accurate superimposition.

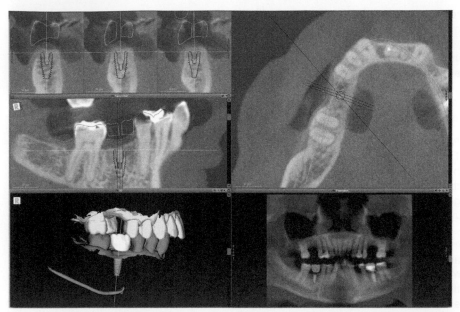

Fig. 7. Virtual implant positioning. The 3D virtual implant placement based on the future prosthesis.

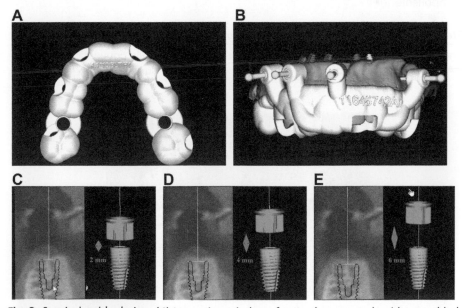

Fig. 8. Surgical guide design. (*A*) Inspection windows for tooth-supported guide are added to allow the confirmation of the intraoperative seating of the guide. (*B*) The position for fixation pins may be incorporated if needed. (*C–E*) Note the different sleeve heights corresponding to the distance from the implant platform.

recommended to support the guide.[16] If additional support is needed, mini-implants may be considered.

The sleeve size (length and diameter) and height (the distance between sleeve and implant platform) may vary among different systems and according to the implant site and plan requirements (**Fig. 8**). In general, decreasing the sleeve height and using a shorter implant may reduce the angular deviation of guided implant placement.[17,18] In addition, this will enable the clinician to perform the guide surgery in cases with limited mouth opening.

Prosthesis design

The wax-up (actual or virtual) can be used as a blueprint to fabricate the custom-made provisional or definitive prosthesis. The restorative space should be assessed during the prosthesis design. Virtual abutments can be inserted to ensure a proper emergence profile and access holes. The fully guided protocol will provide the appropriate implant timing and depth for a prefabricated immediate provisional prosthesis (**Fig. 9**).

The concept of stackable guides was introduced to reduce surgery time and improve the quality of the provisional full-arch prosthesis in implant-retained full-arch cases. A foundation guide can be oriented using the occlusion, or anatomic landmarks and may serve as a bone-reduction guide. The implant guide is stacked onto the foundation guide to perform guided implant placement. Finally, a prefabricated, enhanced provisional prosthesis with premade holes allows for rapid conversion of the provisional (**Fig. 10**).

Surgical and prosthetic report

Following completion of the planning phase, the designed guides and prosthesis are exported into an STL format for fabrication. A detailed report is generated, which includes the drilling protocol with corresponding implants and prosthetic components.

Step 5: Guide and Prosthesis Manufacturing

The fabrication of guide and prosthesis can be carried out via conventional or CAD/ CAM methods. Digital methods for the fabrication of the surgical guide, jaw models,

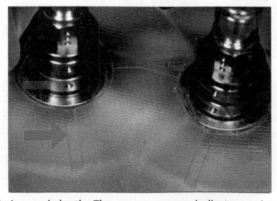

Fig. 9. Implant timing and depth. The orange arrows indicate precise alignment of the implant (the dot on the mount) to the guide indicator (the groove on the guide). The red arrow indicates that the implant is at the appropriate depth; the horizontal line on the implant mount is at the most coronal portion of the guide sleeve.

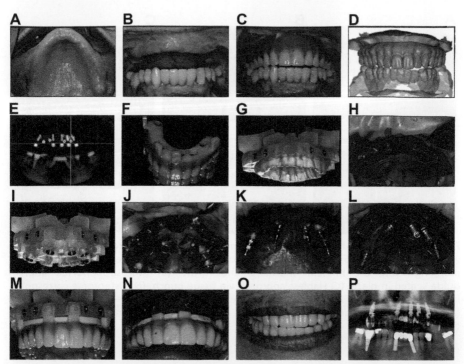

Fig. 10. Digital fully guided surgery of full-arch, screw-retained, fixed immediate provisional restoration. (*A, B*) Intraoral frontal and occlusal views of edentulous maxilla. (*C, D*) Actual and scanned wax-up, which was used as the blueprint for the provisional prosthesis. (*E*) Virtual implant planning. (*F*) Prefabricated monolithic polymethylmethacrylate, stackable provisional prosthesis with premade holes. (*G*) Foundation guide on the stereolithographic model of the jaw. (*H*) Foundation guide is used as a bone-reduction guide and is fixed precisely in position. (*I, J*) Implant guide snaps on the foundation guide. (*K*) Fully guided implant placement. (*L*) Provisional metal abutments screwed on the multiunit abutments. (*M, N*) Provisional prosthesis is seated in place on the foundation guide. Note the blue tissue gasket that is used to isolate the implant plate forms during conversion procedure. (*O*) Patient's smile. (*P*) Postoperative panoramic radiograph.

and the prosthesis include additive (rapid prototyping) or subtractive (milling) techniques. Rapid prototyping involves the use of a 3D printer to cure photosensitive resin in layers to generate the surgical guide and the stereolithographic models of jaws. After the surgical guide is printed, implant system-specific metal sleeves are incorporated.

The CAM milling systems offer many material options to produce the provisional and final prosthesis or abutment.

Step 6: Surgical Execution

Proper fitting and seating of the surgical guide should be verified before surgery. The surgical protocol, which includes the implant size and drilling sequence, is followed. Each guided implant kit is specific to the implant system, and the clinician should be familiar with the components before undertaking the surgery (**Fig. 11**).

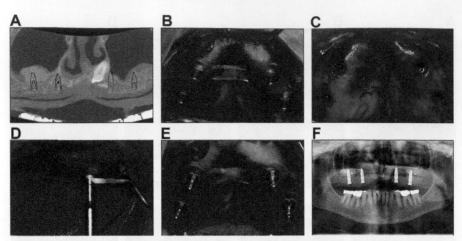

Fig. 11. Fully guided, flapless surgery of a maxillary implants to retain an overdenture with obturator. The patient has a history of cleft lip and palate. (*A*) Virtual implant planning. Note the bilateral maxillary sinus graft. (*B*) Mucosa-supported implant guide seated in place. (*C*) Flapless approach via tissue punch. (*D*) Osteotome corresponding to the same drill size is used through the guide. (*E*) Fully guided implant placement. (*F*) Postoperative panoramic radiograph showing proper implant position and distribution.

Adequate irrigation throughout the surgery is crucial. The surgical guide may prevent sufficient irrigation and therefore induce more heat. Recent in vitro studies[19,20] found that guided surgery generates more heat than the free-handed drilling protocol. However, the additional induced heat was within the acceptable temperature threshold. Jeong and colleagues[21] have found that proper external irrigation in an up-and-down pumping motion may reduce the risk of overheating the bone during the guided drilling protocol. The authors recommend the use of additional irrigation underneath the surgical guide, specifically an irrigation syringe.

ACCURACY OF GUIDED IMPLANT SURGERY

Although guided surgery has become very predictable, deviations will always exist between the virtual plan and execution. Superimposition of preoperative and postoperative CBCT is used to assess the accuracy of the guided implant surgery. The deviation between the planned and the actual implant's positioning in the mouth is assessed through 4 measurements (**Fig. 12**). Model matching using preoperative and postoperative models is an alternative method to assess the accuracy of the guided surgery.[22]

Despite the clinically acceptable deviations of guided surgery, the current level of accuracy does not justify the blind execution of the surgical plan. The 2018 International Team for Implantology consensus paper[1] evaluated the accuracy of static computer-aided implant surgeries. The mean crestal point, apical point, angular, coronal depth, and apical depth deviations were reported to be 1.2 mm, 1.4 mm, 3.5o, 0.2 mm, and 0.5 mm, respectively (**Table 1**). Based on the aforementioned accuracy, a safety margin of 2 mm should always be considered.

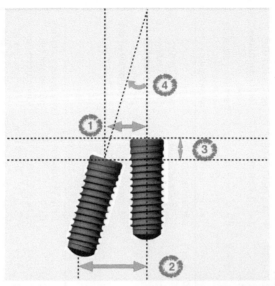

Fig. 12. Deviation measurements. 1, crestal point deviation: the horizontal linear distance between the virtual and actual implants at the center of implant platform. 2, apical point deviation: the horizontal linear distance between the virtual and actual implants at the level of implant apex. 3, depth deviation: the vertical linear distance at between the virtual and actual implants the center of implant platform (however, it can also be measured at the implant apex level). 4, angular deviation: the angle between the long axis of the virtual and actual implants.

SOURCES OF INACCURACY

Each of the aforementioned steps within the digital workflow carry a margin of inaccuracy. Current literature does not provide quantitative data on the deviation of each step. However, overall guided surgery inaccuracy consists of the accumulated deviations throughout. Both patient-related and surgery-related factors affect the accuracy of the computer-aided surgery. Patient-related factors include the type of support and location, whereas surgery-related factors include the skill of the clinician, flap design, and drilling technique.

Patient-Related Factors

Type of support
In general, guided surgeries are more accurate in partially edentulous patients than in fully edentulous patients.[1] Tooth-supported guides are considered the most accurate, followed by mucosa-supported guides (**Box 1**). Bone-supported guides are considered the least accurate.[2,25] Many factors can affect the stability of each of these guides. However, mini-implants, fixation screws, and pins are recommended to further stabilize the guide and enhance the accuracy.[2,23] Three to 4 fixation points were recommended in different studies.[1]

Location
The literature regarding the accuracy of guided surgeries in the maxilla versus mandible remains controversial. There are studies that show no difference.[2,16,32–34] Some studies indicate that guided surgeries in the mandible are more accurate,[6,23,29,35] whereas others indicate greater accuracy of guided surgeries in the maxilla.[36,37]

Table 1
Recent systematic reviews on the accuracy of guided implant surgery

Study Title	Method	Deviation				Conclusion
		Crestal Point	Apex	Angular	Depth	
The accuracy of static computer-aided implant surgery: a systematic review and meta-analysis Tahmaseb et al,[1] 2018	SR and MA 20 CT 2238 implants, 471 patients Fully guided drilling protocol 1883 fully guided implants placed	1.2 mm (1.04–1.44 mm) Partially edentulous: 0.9 mm (0.79–1.00 mm) Edentulous: 1.3 mm (1.09–1.56 mm)	1.4 mm (1.28–1.58 mm) Partially edentulous: 1.2 mm (1.11–1.20 mm) Edentulous: 1.5 mm (1.29–1.62 mm)	3.5° (3.0°–3.96°) Partially edentulous: 3.3° (2.07–4.63) Edentulous: 3.3° (2.71–3.88)	At crestal point 0.2 mm (−0.25 to 0.57 mm) At apex point 0.5 mm (−0.08 to 1.13 mm)	Guided surgery is significantly more accurate in partial edentulism compared with fully edentulous cases The overall accuracy is clinically acceptable
Clinical factors affecting the accuracy of guided implant surgery: a systematic review and meta-analysis Zhou et al,[23] 2018	SR and MA 14 CT, 1513 implants	1.25 mm (1.22–1.29 mm)	1.57 mm (1.53–1.62 mm)	4.1° (3.97°–4.23°)	At crestal point (3 studies, 260 implants) 0.64 mm (0.53–0.74 mm) At apex point (4 studies, 295 implants) 1.24 mm (1.16–1.32 mm)	A totally guided system using fixation screws with a flapless protocol demonstrated the greatest accuracy.
Accuracy of implant placement with computer-guided surgery: a systematic review and meta-analysis comparing cadaver, clinical, and in vitro studies Bover-Ramos et al,[24] 2018	SR: 34 studies, 3033 implants Including: 22 CT, 2244 implants 8 IVS, 543 implants 4 CS, 246 implants (only static guides)	CT 1.10 ± 0.09 mm CS: 1.18 ± 0.12 mm IVS: 0.77 ± 0.15 mm	CT 1.40 ± 0.12 mm CS: 1.52 ± 0.18 mm IVS: 0.17 ± 0.85 mm	CT 3.98° ± 0.33° CS: 2.82° ± 0.40° IVS: 2.39° ± 0.35°	Only 14 studies: CT 0.74 ± 0.103 CS: 0.28 ± 0.049 mm IVS: 0.61 ± 0.149 mm	Fully guided implant placement has lower deviation values compared with half-guided implant placement

Abbreviations: CS, cadaver study; CT, clinical trial; IVS, in vitro study; MA, meta-analysis; SR, systematic review.

> **Box 1**
> **Factors affecting accuracy of mucosal supported guides in edentulous patients**
>
> - Bone density
> - Mucosal thickness
> - Local anesthetics (because of tissue inflation)
> - Smoking (because of increased mucosa thickness)
>
> *Data from* Refs.[26–31]

Surgery-Related Factors

Clinician experience

Current literature is inconsistent on whether experience in guided implant placement plays a role in accuracy.[38–40] Cassetta and Bellardini[41] consider furthering clinicians' experience in conventional implant placement as the gold standard before switching to guided surgery. However, higher levels of accuracy can be obtained by expert surgeons when initially using computer-guided surgery,[41] especially the accuracy of implant depth.[42] Nonetheless, guided surgery has a positive correlation with the reduction of surgical complications.[43]

Flap versus flapless approach

There are advantages and disadvantages to each approach (**Table 2**). Fixation pins[16,33,49] and mucosal resilience[29,32,50] affect the stability and accuracy of the mucosa-supported guides. Fully guided implant placement using the flapless approach with fixation screws is the most accurate approach.[23] Bone-supported guides necessitate extensive flap reflection, which may interfere with the guide positioning; this may be an explanation for the reduced accuracy.[51]

Drilling technique

Eccentric drilling through the sleeve has a substantial effect on accuracy, especially with limited access to the posterior jaw or limited mouth opening. This factor may be of clinical importance, affecting the overall accuracy.[52,53]

It may be concluded that fully guided surgery is more accurate than partially guided surgery.[2,23,24] Even with increased accuracy and efficacy, guided implant surgery is a technically demanding procedure and is not complication free. Hence, the belief that "less training is needed" is far from true.[54] However, the limited scientific evidence available suggests that guided placement has equal or greater implant and prosthesis survival rate compared with conventional protocols with an equivalent clinical complication rate.[2,55,56]

Table 2
Advantages and disadvantages of flap and flapless approaches

	Flapless	Flap
Advantages	Reduces patient postoperative discomfort, surgical time, postoperative bleeding, and healing period[3,44–46]	Improves intraoperative assessment[47,48]
Disadvantages and prerequisites	Less visualization and adequate keratinized tissue are necessary	Increases patient discomfort[3,44,47]

SUMMARY

Current guided technology enables implant planning and placement in a prosthetically driven manner. The digital workflow generally consists of 6 steps: (1) patient assessment, (2) data collection, (3) data manipulation, (4) virtual implant planning, (5) guide and prosthesis manufacture, and (6) execution of surgery and potential delivery of an immediate provisional prosthesis. However, sometimes a combination of analog and digital steps may be applied to the workflow.

Guided implant surgery is assumed to be accurate, precise, and reliable compared with free-handed implant surgery. However, deviation between implant virtual planning and implant real position may occur because of the surgical learning curve and the accumulated errors that may occur throughout the multiple steps of the digital workflow.

The reliability of computer-guided surgery does not justify a blind execution. The learning curve is undeniable and a clinician with basic surgical skills, including conventional implant dentistry, will be in a better position to address any unforeseen complications.

ACKNOWLEDGMENTS

The author would like to acknowledge Dr Ryan Rubino, who provided photos and radiographs for **Fig. 10**.

REFERENCES

1. Tahmaseb A, Wu V, Wismeijer D, et al. The accuracy of static computer-aided implant surgery: a systematic review and meta-analysis. Clin Oral Implants Res 2018;29(Suppl 16):416–35.

2. Tahmaseb A, Wismeijer D, Coucke W, et al. Computer technology applications in surgical implant dentistry: a systematic review. Int J Oral Maxillofac Implants 2014;29(Suppl):25–42.

3. Jung RE, Schneider D, Ganeles J, et al. Computer technology applications in surgical implant dentistry: a systematic review. Int J Oral Maxillofac Implants 2009; 24(Suppl):92–109.

4. D'Haese J, Van De Velde T, Komiyama A, et al. Accuracy and complications using computer-designed stereolithographic surgical guides for oral rehabilitation by means of dental implants: a review of the literature. Clin Implant Dent Relat Res 2012;14:321–35.

5. Oh JH, An X, Jeong SM, et al. Digital workflow for computer-guided implant surgery in edentulous patients: a case report. J Oral Maxillofac Surg 2017;75: 2541–9.

6. Pettersson A, Komiyama A, Hultin M, et al. Accuracy of virtually planned and template guided implant surgery on edentate patients. Clin Implant Dent Relat Res 2012;14:527–37.

7. Tadinada A, Jalali E, Jadhav A, et al. Artifacts in cone beam computed tomography image volumes: an illustrative depiction. J Mass Dent Soc 2015;64:12–5.

8. Schulze RK, Berndt D, d'Hoedt B. On cone-beam computed tomography artifacts induced by titanium implants. Clin Oral Implants Res 2010;21:100–7.

9. Flugge T, Derksen W, Te Poel J, et al. Registration of cone beam computed tomography data and intraoral surface scans—a prerequisite for guided implant surgery with CAD/CAM drilling guides. Clin Oral Implants Res 2017;28:1113–8.

10. Pauwels R, Nackaerts O, Bellaiche N, et al. Variability of dental cone beam CT grey values for density estimations. Br J Radiol 2013;86:20120135.
11. Katsumata A, Hirukawa A, Okumura S, et al. Effects of image artifacts on gray-value density in limited-volume cone-beam computerized tomography. Oral Surg Oral Med Oral Pathol Oral Radiol Endod 2007;104:829–36.
12. Silva IM, Freitas DQ, Ambrosano GM, et al. Bone density: comparative evaluation of Hounsfield units in multislice and cone-beam computed tomography. Braz Oral Res 2012;26:550–6.
13. Nackaerts O, Maes F, Yan H, et al. Analysis of intensity variability in multislice and cone beam computed tomography. Clin Oral Implants Res 2011;22:873–9.
14. Reeves TE, Mah P, McDavid WD. Deriving hounsfield units using grey levels in cone beam CT: a clinical application. Dentomaxillofac Radiol 2012;41:500–8.
15. Nackaerts O, Depypere M, Zhang G, et al. Segmentation of trabecular jaw bone on cone beam CT datasets. Clin Implant Dent Relat Res 2015;17:1082–91.
16. Arisan V, Karabuda ZC, Ozdemir T. Accuracy of two stereolithographic guide systems for computer-aided implant placement: a computed tomography-based clinical comparative study. J Periodontol 2010;81:43–51.
17. El Kholy K, Janner SFM, Schimmel M, et al. The influence of guided sleeve height, drilling distance, and drilling key length on the accuracy of static computer-assisted implant surgery. Clin Implant Dent Relat Res 2019;21(1):101–7.
18. Van Assche N, Quirynen M. Tolerance within a surgical guide. Clin Oral Implants Res 2010;21:455–8.
19. Migliorati M, Amorfini L, Signori A, et al. Internal bone temperature change during guided surgery preparations for dental implants: an in vitro study. Int J Oral Maxillofac Implants 2013;28:1464–9.
20. Markovic A, Lazic Z, Misic T, et al. Effect of surgical drill guide and irrigans temperature on thermal bone changes during drilling implant sites - thermographic analysis on bovine ribs. Vojnosanit Pregl 2016;73:744–50.
21. Jeong SM, Yoo JH, Fang Y, et al. The effect of guided flapless implant procedure on heat generation from implant drilling. J Craniomaxillofac Surg 2014;42:725–9.
22. Komiyama A, Pettersson A, Hultin M, et al. Virtually planned and template-guided implant surgery: an experimental model matching approach. Clin Oral Implants Res 2011;22:308–13.
23. Zhou W, Liu Z, Song L, et al. Clinical factors affecting the accuracy of guided implant surgery-a systematic review and meta-analysis. J Evid Based Dent Pract 2018;18:28–40.
24. Bover-Ramos F, Vina-Almunia J, Cervera-Ballester J, et al. Accuracy of implant placement with computer-guided surgery: a systematic review and meta-analysis comparing cadaver, clinical, and in vitro studies. Int J Oral Maxillofac Implants 2018;33:101–15.
25. Raico Gallardo YN, da Silva-Olivio IRT, Mukai E, et al. Accuracy comparison of guided surgery for dental implants according to the tissue of support: a systematic review and meta-analysis. Clin Oral Implants Res 2017;28:602–12.
26. Seo C, Juodzbalys G. Accuracy of guided surgery via stereolithographic mucosa-supported surgical guide in implant surgery for edentulous patient: a systematic review. J Oral Maxillofac Res 2018;9:e1.
27. Cassetta M, Pompa G, Di Carlo S, et al. The influence of smoking and surgical technique on the accuracy of mucosa-supported stereolithographic surgical guide in complete edentulous upper jaws. Eur Rev Med Pharmacol Sci 2012;16:1546–53.

28. D'Haese J, De Bruyn H. Effect of smoking habits on accuracy of implant placement using mucosally supported stereolithographic surgical guides. Clin Implant Dent Relat Res 2013;15:402–11.

29. Vasak C, Watzak G, Gahleitner A, et al. Computed tomography-based evaluation of template (NobelGuide)-guided implant positions: a prospective radiological study. Clin Oral Implants Res 2011;22:1157–63.

30. Sun Y, Luebbers HT, Agbaje JO, et al. Accuracy of dental implant placement using CBCT-derived mucosa-supported stereolithographic template. Clin Implant Dent Relat Res 2015;17:862–70.

31. Van den Bergh O, Zaman J, Bresseleers J, et al. Anxiety, pCO_2 and cerebral blood flow. Int J Psychophysiol 2013;89:72–7.

32. Ersoy AE, Turkyilmaz I, Ozan O, et al. Reliability of implant placement with stereolithographic surgical guides generated from computed tomography: clinical data from 94 implants. J Periodontol 2008;79:1339–45.

33. Di Giacomo GA, da Silva JV, da Silva AM, et al. Accuracy and complications of computer-designed selective laser sintering surgical guides for flapless dental implant placement and immediate definitive prosthesis installation. J Periodontol 2012;83:410–9.

34. Behneke A, Burwinkel M, Behneke N. Factors influencing transfer accuracy of cone beam CT-derived template-based implant placement. Clin Oral Implants Res 2012;23:416–23.

35. Ozan O, Orhan K, Turkyilmaz I. Correlation between bone density and angular deviation of implants placed using CT-generated surgical guides. J Craniofac Surg 2011;22:1755–61.

36. Pettersson A, Kero T, Gillot L, et al. Accuracy of CAD/CAM-guided surgical template implant surgery on human cadavers: part I. J Prosthet Dent 2010;103:334–42.

37. Cassetta M, Giansanti M, Di Mambro A, et al. Accuracy of positioning of implants inserted using a mucosa-supported stereolithographic surgical guide in the edentulous maxilla and mandible. Int J Oral Maxillofac Implants 2014;29:1071–8.

38. Van Assche N, Vercruyssen M, Coucke W, et al. Accuracy of computer-aided implant placement. Clin Oral Implants Res 2012;23(Suppl 6):112–23.

39. Valente F, Schiroli G, Sbrenna A. Accuracy of computer-aided oral implant surgery: a clinical and radiographic study. Int J Oral Maxillofac Implants 2009;24:234–42.

40. Cassetta M, Stefanelli LV, Giansanti M, et al. Accuracy of implant placement with a stereolithographic surgical template. Int J Oral Maxillofac Implants 2012;27:655–63.

41. Cassetta M, Bellardini M. How much does experience in guided implant surgery play a role in accuracy? A randomized controlled pilot study. Int J Oral Maxillofac Surg 2017;46:922–30.

42. Rungcharassaeng K, Caruso JM, Kan JY, et al. Accuracy of computer-guided surgery: a comparison of operator experience. J Prosthet Dent 2015;114:407–13.

43. Cassetta M, Stefanelli LV, Giansanti M, et al. Depth deviation and occurrence of early surgical complications or unexpected events using a single stereolithographic surgi-guide. Int J Oral Maxillofac Surg 2011;40:1377–87.

44. Fortin T, Bosson JL, Isidori M, et al. Effect of flapless surgery on pain experienced in implant placement using an image-guided system. Int J Oral Maxillofac Implants 2006;21:298–304.

45. Azari A, Nikzad S. Flapless implant surgery: review of the literature and report of 2 cases with computer-guided surgical approach. J Oral Maxillofac Surg 2008;66: 1015–21.
46. Arisan V, Karabuda CZ, Ozdemir T. Implant surgery using bone- and mucosa-supported stereolithographic guides in totally edentulous jaws: surgical and post-operative outcomes of computer-aided vs. standard techniques. Clin Oral Implants Res 2010;21:980–8.
47. Rosenfeld AL, Mandelaris GA, Tardieu PB. Prosthetically directed implant placement using computer software to ensure precise placement and predictable prosthetic outcomes. Part 2: rapid-prototype medical modeling and stereolithographic drilling guides requiring bone exposure. Int J Periodontics Restorative Dent 2006;26:347–53.
48. Abboud M, Wahl G, Calvo-Guirado JL, et al. Application and success of two stereolithographic surgical guide systems for implant placement with immediate loading. Int J Oral Maxillofac Implants 2012;27:634–43.
49. D'Haese J, Van De Velde T, Elaut L, et al. A prospective study on the accuracy of mucosally supported stereolithographic surgical guides in fully edentulous maxillae. Clin Implant Dent Relat Res 2012;14:293–303.
50. Ozan O, Turkyilmaz I, Ersoy AE, et al. Clinical accuracy of 3 different types of computed tomography-derived stereolithographic surgical guides in implant placement. J Oral Maxillofac Surg 2009;67:394–401.
51. Lal K, White GS, Morea DN, et al. Use of stereolithographic templates for surgical and prosthodontic implant planning and placement. Part I. The concept. J Prosthodont 2006;15:51–8.
52. Laederach V, Mukaddam K, Payer M, et al. Deviations of different systems for guided implant surgery. Clin Oral Implants Res 2017;28:1147–51.
53. Koop R, Vercruyssen M, Vermeulen K, et al. Tolerance within the sleeve inserts of different surgical guides for guided implant surgery. Clin Oral Implants Res 2013; 24:630–4.
54. Sicilia A, Botticelli D, Working G. Computer-guided implant therapy and soft- and hard-tissue aspects. The third EAO consensus conference 2012. Clin Oral Implants Res 2012;23(Suppl 6):157–61.
55. Hultin M, Svensson KG, Trulsson M. Clinical advantages of computer-guided implant placement: a systematic review. Clin Oral Implants Res 2012;23(Suppl 6):124–35.
56. Joda T, Derksen W, Wittneben JG, et al. Static computer-aided implant surgery (s-CAIS) analysing patient-reported outcome measures (PROMs), economics and surgical complications: a systematic review. Clin Oral Implants Res 2018; 29(Suppl 16):359–73.

What is the Optimum for Alveolar Ridge Preservation?

Firas Al Yafi, DDS[a],*, Basem Alchawaf, DMD, DrMedDent[b],
Katja Nelson, DMD, DrMedDent[c]

KEYWORDS

- Alveolar ridge preservation • Ridge augmentation • Socket preservation
- Socket grafting • Extraction socket classification

KEY POINTS

- Bone resorption after tooth extraction is inevitable.
- Alveolar ridge preservation is effective in reducing ridge volume alteration.
- Many factors may affect the healing pattern and the treatment outcomes of the alveolar ridge preservation.
- A clinical classification of extraction sockets and treatment guidelines is proposed.

INTRODUCTION

The alveolar ridge is a tooth-dependent structure that develops in conjunction with tooth eruption and undergoes volume and morphologic alteration subsequent to tooth loss.[1] Early and recent studies have shown that unassisted natural healing of the alveolar process postextraction leads to substantial loss of the ridge volume.[2–4] Volume and morphologic alteration of alveolar ridge occur rapidly within the first 3 months to 6 months of tooth extraction and continue gradually at a slower rate thereafter. At 6 months, the ridge may lose up to 63% of its width and up to 22% of its original height.[4] In addition, an estimated mean bone loss of 3.87 mm horizontally and 1.25 mm to 1.67 mm vertically can be expected.[4–6] Alveolar bone resorption usually is more pronounced on the facial side, which leads to relocation of the ridge to an

Disclosure: The authors have nothing to disclose.
[a] Arab Board of Oral Surgery, Division of Periodontology, Department of Oral Health Practice, College of Dentistry, University of Kentucky, 800 Rose Street, 4th floor, Room D436, Dental Science Bldg, Lexington, KY 40536-0297, USA; [b] Department of Oral and Maxillofacial Surgery, College of Dentistry, King Saud University, PO Box 60169, Riyadh 11545, Saudi Arabia; [c] Department of Dental and Craniofacial Sciences, Clinic of Oral and Maxillofacial Surgery, Freiburg University Hospital, Hugstetter Street 55, Freiburg im. Breisgau D-79106, Germany
* Corresponding author.
E-mail address: firasyafi@uky.edu

Dent Clin N Am 63 (2019) 399–418
https://doi.org/10.1016/j.cden.2019.02.007
0011-8532/19/© 2019 Elsevier Inc. All rights reserved.

dental.theclinics.com

unfavorable position (the bone is located in a more lingual and apical position).[7] Changes of the alveolar ridge after tooth extraction could have an impact on prosthetically driven dental implant placement and may necessitate augmentation procedures (**Table 1**).

RATIONALE FOR ALVEOLAR RIDGE PRESERVATION

The alveolar ridge assisted healing concept was proposed to minimize postextraction alveolar ridge alterations. Additionally, preservation of the ridge volume and contour facilitates de novo bone formation within the socket.[8,9] In the literature, different terms have been used to describe the procedure: socket preservation, socket grafting, ridge preservation, and site preservation. The term, *alveolar ridge preservation* (*ARP*), was coined due to the rationale of minimizing dimensional changes of the alveolar ridge after tooth extraction.[10] ARP involves the use of bone graft material, a membrane, and biological products either alone or in combination with one another. If the objective is to increase the width or the height of the ridge beyond its boundaries, however, the term, *ridge augmentation*, should be used.[9]

A plethora of literature (**Table 2**) suggests that ARP procedures might decrease the physiologic bone loss, facilitating delayed implant placement.[8,10–16] ARP techniques may limit but not prevent ridge resorption.[17] The quality of the newly formed bone also is not predictably improved.[10] ARP is effective, however, in reducing ridge width loss and ridge height loss after tooth extraction by 1.25 mm to 1.86 mm and 1.36 mm to 1.62 mm, respectively, compared with unassisted ridge healing.[17,18] Moreover, ridges with damaged extraction socket walls benefit more from ARP than ridges with intact extraction socket.[17]

Table 1 Systematic reviews on alveolar ridge dimensional changes after tooth extraction in humans				
Study	Type of Review	Follow-up	Results	Conclusions
Tan et al,[4] 2012	Systematic review 20 studies	1–12 m	32% of horizontal dimensional change occurred at 3 mo. 3.79 mm or approximately 29%–63% of horizontal bone loss appeared at 6 mo. 1.24 mm or approximately 11%–22% of vertical bone loss appeared at 6 mo. Soft tissue gains 0.4–0.5 mm of thickness at 6 mo	Rapid reductions of alveolar ridge occur in the first 3–6 mo, followed by gradual dimensional reductions thereafter. Bone reduction is more pronounced at buccal side.
Van der Weijden et al,[5] 2009	Systematic review 12 studies	3–12 m	3.87-mm reduction in width of the alveolar ridges is expected. 1.67-mm midbuccal height resorption is apparent. 1.53 mm of vertical loss assessed on the radiographs.	Alveolar ridge undergoes significant dimensional changes during the postextraction healing period. Amount of ridge width reduction is greater than the height reduction.

Table 2
Summary of literature review on the efficacy of alveolar ridge preservation in maintaining the tissues of the alveolar ridge after tooth extraction and the pattern of bone healing

Study	Type of Review	Follow-up	Results	Conclusions
Bassir et al,[17] 2018	Meta-analysis 21 studies	2–9 mo	1.86 mm decrease of horizontal ridge resorption in comparison to natural healing 1.36-mm decrease of vertical ridge resorption	ARP is effective method in minimizing the dimensional changes after extraction. ARP outcomes are improved by the use of barrier membrane. Less favorable outcome with alloplasts APR is beneficial more in ridges with damaged extraction sockets compared with ridges with intact socket walls.
Troiano et al,[11] 2017	Meta-analysis 7 studies	3–9 mo	2.19-mm decrease of horizontal ridge resorption in comparison to natural healing 1.72-mm decrease of vertical ridge resorption	ARP using bone graft and restorable membrane can decrease the rate of alveolar ridge horizontal and vertical resorption after tooth extraction in comparison with spontaneous healing.
Corbella et al,[56] 2017	Quantitative synthesis 40 studies Meta-analysis 11 studies	3–9 mo	Bovine bone was related to a lower new bone formation compared with naturally healed sites. Porcine bone and magnesium-enriched hydroxyapatite were related to higher new bone formation. Allograft was not related to higher new bone formation than naturally healed sites.	No superiority of biomaterial over the others in terms of new bone formation; calcium sulfate and β-tricalcium phosphate show fastest resorption rate. Xenografts shows lower resorption rate and might be better in preserving bone size overtime than allograft.
Mardas et al,[8] 2015	Quantitative synthesis 40 studies Meta-analysis 27 studies	3–8 mo	There are no difference of survival, success, and marginal bone levels of implants placed in natural healed alveolar ridges or in ridges undergone ARP procedures.	ARP might lessen the need of bone augmentation during implant placement. No superiority of biomaterial or a treatment protocol to others

(continued on next page)

Table 2
(continued)

Study	Type of Review	Follow-up	Results	Conclusions
Le Risi et al,[13] 2015	Systematic review 38	3–7 mo	Xenografts and alloplasts presented the highest rate of residual particles after 7 mo of healing whereas allografts had the lowest amount. Allografts presented best amount of new bone formation at 3 mo. No differences between various ARP and natural healing in terms of percentage of bone and connective tissue	No histologic and histomorphometrical differences among different ARP protocols or in comparison to natural healing ARP is not effective in improving tissue quality. Unnecessary to wait more than 3–4 mo to insert implant in preserved sites from histologic stand point
Tomlin et al,[30] 2014	Review of the literature 14 studies	4–6 mo	No treatment: ridge width −2.51, ridge height −2.07, percentage of vital bone 42.2%. Bone graft only: ridge width −1.18, ridge height −1.31, percentage of vital bone 46.2%. Membrane only: ridge width −0.08, ridge height +0.14, percentage of vital bone N/A. Bone graft and membrane: ridge width +0.47, ridge height −0.15, percentage of vital bone 31.7%.	All ARP procedures are effective in reducing dimensional changes. Some bone graft interferes with healing inside the socket. No preference of some material over others
Avila-Ortiz et al,[12] 2014	Quantitative synthesis 8 studies Meta-analysis 6 studies	>3 mo	1.89-mm reduction of horizontal ridge resorption 2.07-mm and 1.18-mm reductions of midbuccal and midlingual vertical resorption, respectively 0.48-mm and 0.24-mm reductions of mesial and distal ridge resorption, respectively.	ARP using bone graft can be effective in reducing vertical and horizontal volume changes in comparison to natural healing. Flap elevation, usage of a membrane may enhance the outcomes. Xenograft or an allograft can be more effective than alloplastic materials.
Vittorini Orgeas et al,[14] 2013	Quantitative synthesis 13 studies Meta-analysis 6 studies	4–12 mo	Grafting materials and membranes together or alone may reduce resorption process.	ARP using bone graft can be effective in reducing vertical and horizontal volume changes in comparison to natural healing Use of barrier membranes alone might improve healing of extraction sockets. Flap elevation and soft tissue primary closure seem to have little effect on dimensional changes.

Horváth et al,[10] 2013	Systematic review 14 Studies	1.1–9 mo	(−1.0-mm and −3.5-mm ± 2.7-mm) horizontal ridge resorption in ARP group and (−2.5-mm and −4.6-mm ± 0.3-mm) in natural healing group (between +1.3-mm ± 2.0-mm and −0.7-mm ± 1.4-mm) vertical ridge changes in ARP group and (−0.8-mm ± 1.6-mm and −3.6-mm ± 1.5-mm) changes in natural healing group	Natural remodeling led to dimensional changes of extraction socket, more pronounced horizontally. ARP may limit but not prevent resorption rate with no superiority of specific method. ARP might lessen the need of bone augmentation procedure at implant placement Some grafts interfered with the healing. The presence of intact socket walls and primary flap closure is often associated with favorable results.
Vignoletti et al,[15] 2012	Systemic review 14 studies Meta-analysis 9 studies	>3 mo	1.83-mm decrease of horizontal ridge resorption in comparison to natural healing 1.47-mm decrease of vertical ridge resorption	ARP can be effective in reducing vertical and horizontal volume changes in comparison to natural healing. No superior surgical procedure or material or membrane A flap and primary closure may enhance the outcome.
Hammerle et al,[9] 2012	Osteology consensus report after discussion of 4 comprehensive systematic reviews	—	3.8-mm alveolar ridge width reduction occurred within 6 mo. 1.24-mm vertical reduction expected within 6 mo	ARP using biomaterial and/or membrane is recommended. Raising flap and primary closure is preferable. No superiority of specific biomaterial or membrane on the outcome, except collagen plug revealed negative results. No comparison is available between primary closure methods (soft tissue punch, connective tissue graft, barrier membrane, and soft tissue replacement matrix).
Weng,[18] 2011	Literature review 10 studies DGI conference consensus	3–12 mo	1.25-mm reduction of horizontal ridge resorption in comparison to natural healing 1.62-mm reduction of vertical ridge resorption	ARP seems effective in maintaining ridge dimensions. ARP might lessen the need of bone augmentation at implant placement by 5 times. No superiority of specific surgical procedure or material is evident. Primary closure of the socket might not be essential.

(continued on next page)

Table 2
(continued)

Study	Type of Review	Follow-up	Results	Conclusions
Darby et al,[31] 2009	Literature review 37 studies	1 mo up to 15 y	Grafting materials and membranes together or alone may reduce resorption process.	ARP can be effective in reducing vertical and horizontal volume changes in comparison to natural healing. No superiority of specific surgical procedure No evidence that ridge preservation procedures reduce the need for augmentation at implant placement Bone material may interfere with bone formation in the socket. Primary closure is not always necessary; however, the use of membranes requires soft tissue coverage.

Abbreviation: DGI, The German Association of Oral Implantology.

Immediate implant placement with or without socket shielding (keeping a root remnant at the facial wall of extraction socket) is suggested to serve the same purpose of protecting alveolar ridge structures.[19–21] Immediate implant placement by itself may not prevent the remodeling of the alveolar ridge after extraction.[22] Careful selection criteria for immediate implant cases should be followed to avoid unfavorable outcomes.[23] Although the socket shield technique has promising potential in maintaining the alveolar ridge dimension, the presence of infection, root fracture, or decay is a limitation of this technique. Furthermore, long-term prognosis of implant installation in proximity to tooth-root fragment has yet to be proved.[24]

PRETREATMENT ASSESSMENT AND SURGICAL CONSIDERATIONS

The rate of volumetric changes, healing pattern, and quality and quantity of newly formed bone may be affected by several factors; these should be considered when choosing the appropriate treatment approach.

Soft Tissue and Hard Tissue Configuration

Interproximal bone

After tooth extraction, dimensional changes usually affect the central part of the facial wall, whereas the proximal aspect is preserved by the healthy periodontal ligament of the neighboring teeth.[25]

Thickness of buccal bone wall

Buccal bone with a thickness less than 2 mm is prone to a higher resorption rate after tooth extraction because it is composed solely of bundle bone.[15,26,27] It seems, however, that ARP can limit the reduction in the ridge dimension regardless of the thickness of the buccal bone.[28] Two millimeters of buccal bone thickness should be a prerequisite for immediate implant placement. This thickness allows for predictable remodeling of the alveolar ridge[29] **(Fig. 1)**.

Socket walls

In intact socket walls, containment and vascularity of the bone graft material are improved.

Bone fenestration or dehiscence

A socket with no fenestration or dehiscence is reported to be associated with more favorable clinical outcomes.[10,30,31]

The gingival phenotype

Thick gingival tissue is associated with better healing, along with decreased bone resorption and gingival recession.[32,33] This could be attributed to increased vascularity and a greater presence of extracellular matrix and collagen.[34] Phenotype conversion is believed to increase the overall peri-implant health state and reduce bone loss[35] **(Fig. 2)**.

Surgical Technique

Atraumatic extraction

Performing an atraumatic extraction results in minimal trauma to soft tissue and hard tissue and may play an important role in ridge preservation.[36,37]

Primary closure versus open barrier technique

Different techniques have been used for ARP, including primary wound closure,[38,39] partial wound closure,[40] no primary closure,[41] and soft tissue graft to seal the socket.[42] ARP can be effective regardless of the closure technique.[14,18]

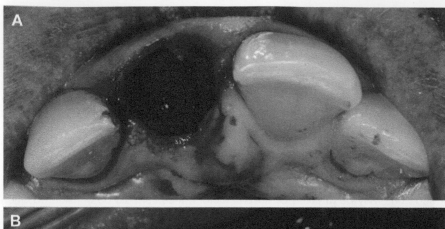
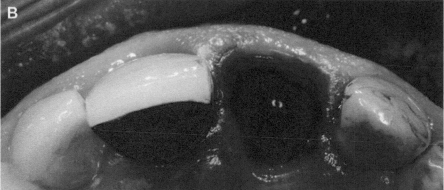

Fig. 1. (*A*) Thin buccal bone. (*B*) Thick buccal bone.

Flapless procedure

According to Fickl and colleagues,[43] reflection of the flap results in pronounced bone resorption compared with flapless procedures. Other researchers have disputed this finding and have demonstrated no significant difference between flapped and flapless extractions.[44] Vignoletti and colleagues[15] found a flap procedure in combination with ARP has a positive impact on the horizontal dimension of the ridge. These studies indicate a continued controversy in the literature with regard to flap design and its impact on the result of the ARP.

Location in the Mouth

The anterior maxilla frequently has a thin buccal bone phenotype (≤1 mm) causing pronounced facial bone remodeling.[45–47] Soft tissue and hard tissue grafting in conjunction with immediate implant placement or ARP to improve the esthetic outcome may be needed.[48]

Periodontal Status

If a tooth is extracted due to advanced periodontal disease, the postextraction healing process has been described as more complicated and less predictable compared to non-periodontally involved sites. Furthermore, slower bone regeneration is expected in infected sockets in comparison to disease-free sites.[40]

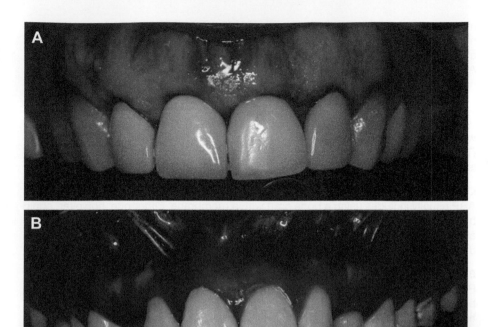

Fig. 2. (*A*) Thick gingival phenotype. (*B*) Thin gingival phenotype.

Biomaterial

Bone graft materials

Bone grafting materials are categorized into autogenous, allografts, xenografts, and alloplasts (**Table 3**). Each of these materials has shown its efficacy in reducing dimensional shrinkage after tooth extraction.[10,11] Current literature does not provide evidence for superiority of 1 material over another.[7–9,15,29,50] Nevertheless, some graft materials, such as xenografts and alloplasts, may resorb at a slower rate, with their remnant particles existing 7 months or more after the grafting procedure; thus, they

Table 3 Bone graft types		
Material	**Source**	**Examples**
Autogenous	The patient	• Intraoral: symphysis, ramus, and tuberosity • Extraoral: hip, rib, fibula, and tibia
Allografts	Same species, different individual	• Demineralized freeze-dried bone allograft • Freeze-dried bone allograft
Xenografts	Different species	• Bovine • Equine • Porcine
Alloplasts	Synthetic	• Hydroxyapatite • Calcium sulfate • Calcium phosphate • Bioglass

may be more suitable for long-term ARP.[10,13,50] On the other hand, allograft tends to resorb more rapidly with fewer residual particles and induces more newly formed bone after 3 months of healing.[13] These properties may be more favorable for short-term ARP. The long-term effect of residual grafting material on implant survival and success has not been reported.

Membranes types

Resorbable membranes and nonresorbable membranes with or without bone graft were effective on decreasing the alveolar ridge resorption after tooth extraction (**Table 4**).[10] ARP, however, has a more favorable outcome when a barrier membrane is used.[12,15,17]

Combination of bone graft and membrane

ARP usually includes using a bone graft with a membrane. Either one, however, could be used alone.[30] Nevertheless, Troiano and colleagues[11] stated that using a resorbable membrane with bone graft (the most common procedure used for ARP) can decrease both horizontal and vertical ridge shrinkage.

Biologics

Platelet concentrate products[51–53] and recombinant growth factors[50,54,55] have been used in ARP procedures. Their use may lead to accelerated bone regeneration and enhanced soft tissue healing, reducing the reentry time for implant placement.

CLASSIFICATION AND TREATMENT MODALITIES
Classification

An algorithm was developed by the authors to guide clinicians in an evidence-based approach for ARP. The algorithm classifies the single extraction socket according to the most critical factors that affect the predictability, esthetic outcomes, and functional results of the implant. Both hard tissue and soft tissue factors should be considered. Hard tissue examination should include the height of the interproximal bone, thickness and integrity of the buccal bone plate, and remaining extraction socket walls. The soft tissue contour and its relationship to underlying bone, gingival phenotype, and esthetics also should be considered (**Fig. 3**).

Using the classification decision tree (**Fig. 4**), a dentist is able to classify the extraction socket depending on the clinical examination, bone sounding, and periapical or bitewing radiographs. Based on the classification of the extraction socket, the appropriate treatment modality can be determined for each site.

Table 4 Membrane type	
Membrane Type	**Examples**
Resorbable	• Collagen (non–cross-linked and cross-linked) • Amnion chorion • Acellular dermal matrix grafts • Synthetic: organic aliphatic polymers and modifications
Nonresorbable	• Polytetrafluoroethylene • Titanium mesh

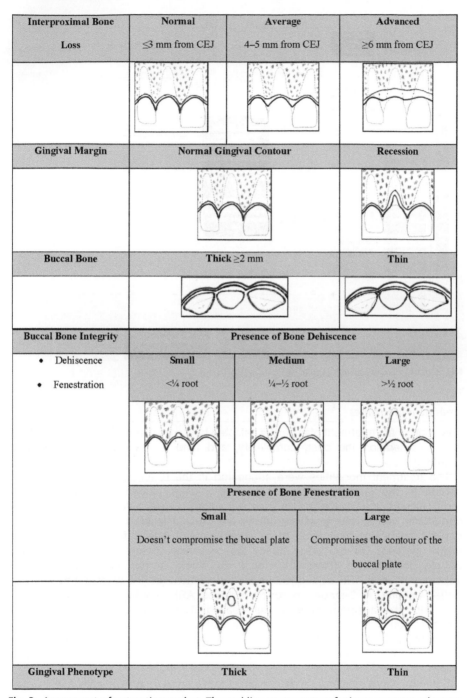

Interproximal Bone Loss	Normal ≤3 mm from CEJ	Average 4–5 mm from CEJ	Advanced ≥6 mm from CEJ
Gingival Margin	Normal Gingival Contour		Recession
Buccal Bone	Thick ≥2 mm		Thin
Buccal Bone Integrity • Dehiscence • Fenestration	Presence of Bone Dehiscence		
	Small <¼ root	Medium ¼–½ root	Large >½ root
	Presence of Bone Fenestration		
	Small Doesn't compromise the buccal plate		Large Compromises the contour of the buccal plate
Gingival Phenotype	Thick		Thin

Fig. 3. Assessment of extraction socket. The red line represents soft tissue contour, whereas the brown line represents the bone contour. CEJ, Cemento Enamel Junction.

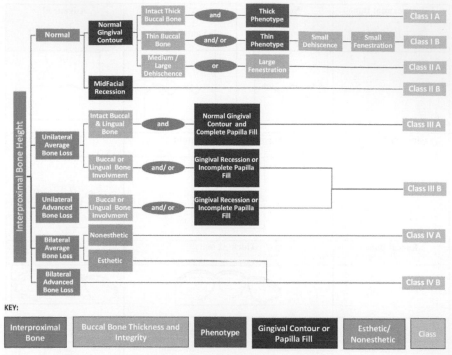

Fig. 4. Ridge preservation classification decision tree.

Treatment Modalities

The appropriate treatment plan can be selected based on these classifications, taking into consideration the cost, complexity, and time needed for each procedure (**Table 5**).

The treatment modalities were suggested in the order of the most favorable choice to the least favorable. Immediate implant placement at the time of tooth extraction is preferred in ideal situations (class I A). When suboptimal conditions with normal gingival contour are present (class I B or II A), however, implant installation may need to be supplemented with soft tissue and/or hard tissue grafting. On the other hand, the presence of any midfacial recession or big bony defect (class II A or II B) would compromise an immediate implant outcome; ARP or delayed implant placement (at 4–8 weeks) may become better options. A 3-stage approach includes ARP, implant site development, and implant placement after proper healing. This approach is recommended when esthetics are of concern in a site with a major tissue defect, especially locations lacking vertical bone height (class IV B). Moreover, recombinant growth factors and blood concentrate products are suggested in these challenging cases.

Esthetics play a major role in determining the preferred treatment approach. In a patient with a low smile line with minimal esthetic concerns, anterior implant placement may be considered as a nonesthetic site. In contrast, a posterior upper tooth, in a highly esthetically concerned patient with a wide smile, may be evaluated as an esthetic site (class IV A vs class IV B). A thorough patient assessment should be completed to determine the esthetic desires of a patient.

Table 5
Treatment decisions

	Treatment Option 1	Treatment Option 2	Treatment Option 3	Comments
Class I A	Immediate implant (**Fig. 5**)	Two-stage approach 1 ARP: bone graft + collagen plug or tissue punch (**Fig. 6**) 2 Implant placement after proper healing time	Two-stage approach 1 ARP: high-density polytetrafluoroethylene without bone graft 2 Implant placement after proper healing time (**Fig. 7**)	Flapless approach is recommended.
Class I B	Immediate implant Hard tissue and/or soft tissue graft is recommended	Two-stage approach 1 ARP: bone graft + membrane (resorbable/nonresorbable) 2 Implant placement after proper healing time	Delayed implant placement with simultaneous GBR if needed	The bony defect has to be completely included by the membrane. Flapless approach is recommended.
Class II A	Delayed implant placement with simultaneous GBR.	Two-stage approach 1 ARP: bone graft + membrane (resorbable/nonresorbable) 2 Implant placement with simultaneous GBR and soft tissue grafting as needed.	Immediate implant Hard tissue and/or soft tissue graft as needed	Immediate implant has less predictable esthetic outcomes. A flap might be needed to deal with the defect.
Class II B	Delayed implant placement with simultaneous GBR and soft tissue grafting	Two-stage approach 1 ARP: bone graft + membrane (resorbable/nonresorbable) 2 Implant placement with simultaneous GBR and soft tissue grafting as needed	Three-stage approach 1 ARP: bone graft + membrane (resorbable/nonresorbable) 2 Implant site development 3 Implant placement after the proper healing time	Immediate implant is not recommended. It is the clinician choice to do soft tissue grafting at the second phase or third phase of the 3-stage approach.
Class III A	Immediate implant Hard tissue and/or soft tissue graft as needed	Two-stage approach 1 ARP: bone graft + membrane (resorbable/nonresorbable) 2 Implant placement after the proper healing time		Enamel matrix derivative can be considered. The first treatment option is favorable in thick phenotype white; the second option is favorable in thin phenotype.

(continued on next page)

Table 5
(continued)

	Treatment Option 1	Treatment Option 2	Treatment Option 3	Comments
Class III B	Two-stage approach 1 ARP: bone graft + membrane (resorbable/nonresorbable) 2 implant placement with simultaneous GBR and soft tissue grafting as needed	Three-stage approach 1 ARP: bone graft + membrane (resorbable/nonresorbable) 2 Implant site development 3 Implant placement after the proper healing time.		Enamel matrix derivative is recommended. Immediate implant is not recommended. It is the clinician choice to do soft tissue grafting at the second phase or third phase of the 3-stage approach.
Class IV A	Two-stage approach 1 ARP: bone graft + membrane (resorbable/nonresorbable). 2 Implant placement with simultaneous GBR and soft tissue grafting as needed.	Delayed implant placement with simultaneous GBR and soft tissue graft as needed	Immediate implant hard tissue and/or soft tissue graft as needed	Immediate implant placement is not favorable and should be a case-by-case decision.
Class IV B	Three-stage approach 1 ARP: bone graft + membrane (resorbable/nonresorbable) 2 Implant site development 3 Implant placement after the proper healing time			Immediate implant is not recommended. It is the clinician choice to do soft tissue grafting at the second phase or third phase of the 3-stage approach. The use of bone enhancing products might be considered.

Abbreviation: GBR, Guided Bone Regeneration.

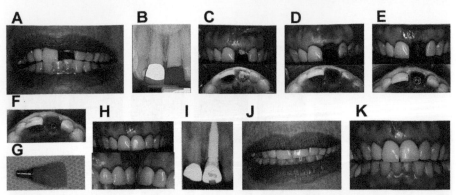

Fig. 5. (*A*) The patient smile shows the remaining root of tooth #9. (*B*) Preoperative periapical radiograph of tooth #9 showing intact interpoximal bone and (*C*) clinical frontal (*upper*) and occlusal (*lower*) views showing thick biotype. (*D*) Post-extraction frontal (*upper*) and occlusal (*lower*) views showing thick intact buccal bone. (*E*) The implant was installed (*lower*) and the metal screw retained provisional abutment was placed (*upper*). (*F*) The jumping space between the implant and the buccal bone was grafted with deproteinized bovine bone minerals. (*G*) The patient's failed crown was used to pick up the metal provisional abutment. (*H*) Frontal (*upper*) and lateral (*lower*) views of a screw retained implant provisional. (*I*) Postoperative radiograph of implant and the provisional crown. (*J*) The patient's smile. (*K*) Three-month follow-up showing the preservation of gingival architecture.

A flapless approach is recommended when possible to minimize the patient postoperative discomfort, unless a large defect exists and has to be visualized and contained with the membrane. The treatment options for each class are not limited to the suggested options. It is a clinician's choice to decide bone graft material and type of membrane to be used.

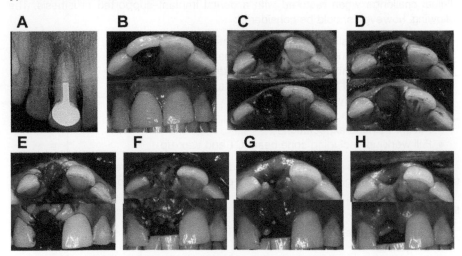

Fig. 6. (*A*) Preoperative radiograph of tooth #8 showing periapical lesion and intact interproximal bone. (*B*) Clinical frontal (*lower*) and occlusal (*upper*) views showing thin gingival phenotype. (*C*) Occlusal view before extraction (*lower*) and after extraction (*upper*) showing thin buccal bone. (*D*) The extraction socket was filled with a mixture of demineralized freeze-dried bone allograft and Deproteinized bovine bone (*upper*). Collagen plug was used to seal the orifice of the socket (*lower*). (*E*) An occlusal (*upper*) and frontal (*lower*) views of a PRF membrane which was used to cover the collagen plug and secured with a criss-cross suture. (*F*) Occlusal (*upper*) and frontal (*lower*) views, 2 days post operative. (*G*) Occlusal (*upper*) and frontal (*lower*) views, 8 days post operative. (*H*) Occlusal (*upper*) and frontal (*lower*) views, 30 days post operative.

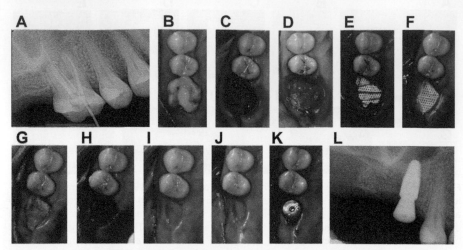

Fig. 7. (*A*) Preoperative periapical radiograph of tooth # 3 showing failed endodontic treatment. (*B*) Clinical occlusal photograph before extraction showing. (*C*) Occlusal view of the socket after atraumatic extraction. (*D*) The socket was filled with platelet-rich fibrin plugs. (*E*) Nonresorbable membrane covering the socket and secured with sutures. (*F*) Clinical occlusal view at 1-week follow-up showing uneventful soft tissue healing. (*G*) Four weeks follow up before membrane removal. (*H*) Four weeks follow up after membrane removal. (*I*) Twelve-week follow-up showing complete soft tissue healing. (*J*) Occlusal view at 14 week. (*K*) Occlusal view at 14 week post implant placement. (*L*) Postoperative radiograph with implant in place.

Multiple extraction sites are not considered in the proposed algorithm. They pose a clinical challenge when restored with a dental implant–supported prosthesis. The following, however, should be considered:

- Type of prosthesis, intraocclusal and interocclusal spaces
- The proximal bone adjacent to the remaining teeth
- The interproximal bone between the extracted teeth
- The integrity and thickness of the buccal and lingual plates
- The gingival biotype and architecture
- Patient smile line and lip support
- Patient esthetic expectations
- Full work-up, including cone beam CT and wax-up

In general, esthetic result of immediate adjacent implants is predictable only in ideal scenarios, and a staged approach for site development yields better outcomes.

SUMMARY

- ARP is an effective method to limit the dimensional changes after tooth extraction.
- No evidence has shown to support the superiority of a certain material or technique for ART. The chosen technique remains at the clinician discretion.
- Immediate implant placement should be done only in optimal conditions, especially in the esthetic zone.

REFERENCES

1. Schroeder HE. The periodontium. Berlin: Springer-Verlag; 1986.

2. Atwood DA, Coy WA. Clinical, cephalometric, and densitometric study of reduction of residual ridges. J Prosthet Dent 1971;26:280–95.
3. Schropp L, Wenzel A, Kostopoulos L, et al. Bone healing and soft tissue contour changes following single-tooth extraction: a clinical and radiographic 12-month prospective study. Int J Periodontics Restorative Dent 2003;23:313–23.
4. Tan WL, Wong TL, Wong MC, et al. A systematic review of post-extractional alveolar hard and soft tissue dimensional changes in humans. Clin Oral Implants Res 2012;23(Suppl 5):1–21.
5. Van der Weijden F, Dell'Acqua F, Slot DE. Alveolar bone dimensional changes of post-extraction sockets in humans: a systematic review. J Clin Periodontol 2009; 36:1048–58.
6. Lang NP, Pun L, Lau KY, et al. A systematic review on survival and success rates of implants placed immediately into fresh extraction sockets after at least 1 year. Clin Oral Implants Res 2012;23:39–66.
7. Misawa M, Lindhe J, Araujo MG. The alveolar process following single-tooth extraction: a study of maxillary incisor and premolar sites in man. Clin Oral Implants Res 2016;27:884–9.
8. Mardas N, Trullenque-Eriksson A, MacBeth N, et al. Does ridge preservation following tooth extraction improve implant treatment outcomes: a systematic review: Group 4: Therapeutic concepts & methods. Clin Oral Implants Res 2015; 26(Suppl 11):180–201.
9. Hammerle CH, Araujo MG, Simion M. Evidence-based knowledge on the biology and treatment of extraction sockets. Clin Oral Implants Res 2012;23(Suppl 5): 80–2.
10. Horváth A, Mardas N, Mezzomo LA, et al. Alveolar ridge preservation. A systematic review. Clin Oral Investig 2013;17:341–63.
11. Troiano G, Zhurakivska K, Lo Muzio L, et al. Combination of bone graft and resorbable membrane for alveolar ridge preservation: a systematic review, meta-analysis and trial sequential analysis. J Periodontol 2017;1–17 [Epub ahead of print].
12. Avila-Ortiz G, Elangovan S, Kramer KW, et al. Effect of alveolar ridge preservation after tooth extraction: a systematic review and meta-analysis. J Dent Res 2014; 93:950–8.
13. De Risi V, Clementini M, Vittorini G, et al. Alveolar ridge preservation techniques: a systematic review and meta-analysis of histological and histomorphometrical data. Clin Oral Implants Res 2015;26:50–68.
14. Vittorini Orgeas G, Clementini M, De Risi V, et al. Surgical techniques for alveolar socket preservation: a systematic review. Int J Oral Maxillofac Implants 2013;28: 1049–61.
15. Vignoletti F, Matesanz P, Rodrigo D, et al. Surgical protocols for ridge preservation after tooth extraction. A systematic review. Clin Oral Implants Res 2012; 23(Suppl 5):22–38.
16. Wang RE, Lang NP. Ridge preservation after tooth extraction. Clin Oral Implants Res 2012;23(Suppl 6):147–56.
17. Bassir SH, Alhareky M, Wangsrimongkol B, et al. Systematic review and meta-analysis of hard tissue outcomes of alveolar ridge preservation. Int J Oral Maxillofac Implants 2018;33:979–94.
18. Weng D, Stock V, Schliephake H. Are socket and ridge preservation techniques at the day of tooth extraction efficient in maintaining the tissues of the alveolar ridge? Systematic review, consensus statements and recommendations of the

1st DGI Consensus Conference in September 2010. Eur J Oral Implantol 2011;4: S59–66.

19. Paolantonio M, Dolci M, Scarano A, et al. Immediate implantation in fresh extraction sockets. A controlled clinical and histological study in man. J Periodontol 2001;72:1560–71.

20. Hurzeler MB, Zuhr O, Schupbach P, et al. The socket-shield technique: a proof-of-principle report. J Clin Periodontol 2010;37:855–62.

21. Gluckman H, Salama M, Du Toit J. Partial extraction therapies (PET) part 1: maintaining alveolar ridge contour at pontic and immediate implant sites. Int J Periodontics Restorative Dent 2016;36:681–7.

22. Araujo MG, Sukekava F, Wennstrom JL, et al. Ridge alterations following implant placement in fresh extraction sockets: an experimental study in the dog. J Clin Periodontol 2005;32:645–52.

23. Chen ST, Buser D. Esthetic outcomes following immediate and early implant placement in the anterior maxilla–a systematic review. Int J Oral Maxillofac Implants 2014;29(Suppl):186–215.

24. Langer L, Langer B, Salem D. Unintentional root fragment retention in proximity to dental implants: a series of six human case reports. Int J Periodontics Restorative Dent 2015;35:305–13.

25. Chappuis V, Araujo MG, Buser D. Clinical relevance of dimensional bone and soft tissue alterations post-extraction in esthetic sites. Periodontol 2000 2017;73: 73–83.

26. Spray JR, Black CG, Morris HF, et al. The influence of bone thickness on facial marginal bone response: stage 1 placement through stage 2 uncovering. Ann Periodontol 2000;5:119–28.

27. Araujo MG, Lindhe J. Dimensional ridge alterations following tooth extraction. An experimental study in the dog. J Clin Periodontol 2005;32:212–8.

28. Cardaropoli D, Tamagnone L, Roffredo A, et al. Relationship between the buccal bone plate thickness and the healing of postextraction sockets with/without ridge preservation. Int J Periodontics Restorative Dent 2014;34:211–7.

29. Qahash M, Susin C, Polimeni G, et al. Bone healing dynamics at buccal peri-implant sites. Clin Oral Implants Res 2008;19:166–72.

30. Tomlin EM, Nelson SJ, Rossmann JA. Ridge preservation for implant therapy: a review of the literature. Open Dent J 2014;8:66–76.

31. Darby I, Chen ST, Buser D. Ridge preservation techniques for implant therapy. Int J Oral Maxillofac Implants 2009;24(Suppl):260–71.

32. Vervaeke S, Dierens M, Besseler J, et al. The influence of initial soft tissue thickness on peri-implant bone remodeling. Clin Implant Dent Relat Res 2014;16: 238–47.

33. Giannobile WV, Jung RE. Evidence-based knowledge on the aesthetics and maintenance of peri-implant soft tissues: Osteology Foundation Consensus Report Part 1-Effects of soft tissue augmentation procedures on the maintenance of peri-implant soft tissue health. Clin Oral Implants Res 2018;29(Suppl 15):7–10.

34. Hwang D, Wang HL. Flap thickness as a predictor of root coverage: a systematic review. J Periodontol 2006;77:1625–34.

35. Thoma DS, Naenni N. Effects of soft tissue augmentation procedures on peri-implant health or disease: A systematic review and meta-analysis. Clin Oral Implants Res 2018;29(Suppl 15):32–49.

36. Oghli AA, Steveling H. Ridge preservation following tooth extraction: a comparison between atraumatic extraction and socket seal surgery. Quintessence Int 2010;41:605–9.

37. Bartee BK. Extraction site reconstruction for alveolar ridge preservation. Part 2: membrane-assisted surgical technique. J Oral Implantol 2001;27:194–7.
38. Froum S, Cho SC, Rosenberg E, et al. Histological comparison of healing extraction sockets implanted with bioactive glass or demineralized freeze-dried bone allograft: a pilot study. J Periodontol 2002;73:94–102.
39. Guarnieri R, Stefanelli L, De Angelis F, et al. Extraction socket preservation using porcine-derived collagen membrane alone or associated with porcine-derived bone. clinical results of randomized controlled study. J Oral Maxillofac Res 2017;8:1–9.
40. Iasella JM, Greenwell H, Miller RL, et al. Ridge preservation with freeze-dried bone allograft and a collagen membrane compared to extraction alone for implant site development: a clinical and histologic study in humans. J Periodontol 2003;74:990–9.
41. Kim DM, De Angelis N, Camelo M, et al. Ridge preservation with and without primary wound closure: a case series. Int J Periodontics Restorative Dent 2013;33: 71–8.
42. Tal H. Autogenous masticatory mucosal grafts in extraction socket seal procedures: a comparison between sockets grafted with demineralized freeze-dried bone and deproteinized bovine bone mineral. Clin Oral Implants Res 1999;10: 289–96.
43. Fickl S, Zuhr O, Wachtel H, et al. Tissue alterations after tooth extraction with and without surgical trauma: a volumetric study in the beagle dog. J Clin Periodontol 2008;35:356–63.
44. Araujo MG, Lindhe J. Ridge alterations following tooth extraction with and without flap elevation: an experimental study in the dog. Clin Oral Implants Res 2009;20: 545–9.
45. Ferrus J, Cecchinato D, Pjetursson EB, et al. Factors influencing ridge alterations following immediate implant placement into extraction sockets. Clin Oral Implants Res 2010;21:22–9.
46. Januario AL, Duarte WR, Barriviera M, et al. Dimension of the facial bone wall in the anterior maxilla: a cone-beam computed tomography study. Clin Oral Implants Res 2011;22:1168–71.
47. Huynh-Ba G, Pjetursson BE, Sanz M, et al. Analysis of the socket bone wall dimensions in the upper maxilla in relation to immediate implant placement. Clin Oral Implants Res 2010;21:37–42.
48. Kan JYK, Rungcharassaeng K, Deflorian M, et al. Immediate implant placement and provisionalization of maxillary anterior single implants. Periodontol 2000 2018;77:197–212.
49. Ahn JJ, Shin HI. Bone tissue formation in extraction sockets from sites with advanced periodontal disease: a histomorphometric study in humans. Int J Oral Maxillofac Implants 2008;23:1133–8.
50. Wallace SC, Snyder MB, Prasad H. Postextraction ridge preservation and augmentation with mineralized allograft with or without recombinant human platelet-derived growth factor BB (rhPDGF-BB): a consecutive case series. Int J Periodontics Restorative Dent 2013;33:599–609.
51. Anwandter A, Bohmann S, Nally M, et al. Dimensional changes of the post extraction alveolar ridge, preserved with Leukocyte- and platelet rich fibrin: a clinical pilot study. J Dent 2016;52:23–9.
52. Castro AB, Meschi N, Temmerman A, et al. Regenerative potential of leucocyte- and platelet-rich fibrin. Part B: sinus floor elevation, alveolar ridge preservation and implant therapy. A systematic review. J Clin Periodontol 2017;44:225–34.

53. Temmerman A, Vandessel J, Castro A, et al. The use of leucocyte and platelet-rich fibrin in socket management and ridge preservation: a split-mouth, randomized, controlled clinical trial. J Clin Periodontol 2016;43:990–9.

54. Howell TH, Fiorellini J, Jones A, et al. A feasibility study evaluating rhBMP-2/absorbable collagen sponge device for local alveolar ridge preservation or augmentation. Int J Periodontics Restorative Dent 1997;17:124–39.

55. Fiorellini JP, Howell TH, Cochran D, et al. Randomized study evaluating recombinant human bone morphogenetic protein-2 for extraction socket augmentation. J Periodontol 2005;76:605–13.

56. Corbella S, Taschieri S, Francetti L, et al. Histomorphometric results after postextraction socket healing with different biomaterials: a systematic review of the literature and meta-analysis. Int J Oral Maxillofac Implants 2017;32:1001–17.

Resorbable Versus Nonresorbable Membranes
When and Why?

Noel Ye Naung, BDS, Higher Grad Dip Clin Sc (OMFS), MSc (OMFS), FIAOMS[a],*,
Ehab Shehata, DDS, MD, MSc (GS), PhD[a,b], Joseph E. Van Sickels, DDS[a]

KEYWORDS

- Resorbable membrane • Nonresorbable membrane • Guided tissue regeneration
- Guided bone regeneration • Barrier membrane

KEY POINTS

- Guided tissue engineering has been proved successful for alveolar ridge augmentation, maxillary sinus implant site development, periodontal furcation defects, and treatment of intrabony pockets and socket preservation.
- Numerous factors play a role in the success of guided bone regeneration, such as the choice of resorbable or nonresorbable membranes and the timing of membrane removal.
- The type of membrane chosen depends on the requirements needed for space creation.
- Nonresorbable membranes are required at load-bearing regions, such as in vertical ridge augmentation.
- Resorbable membranes are recommended to be used in non–load-bearing regions, such as in maxillary sinus augmentation.

INTRODUCTION

It is difficult to study resorbable versus nonresorbable membranes because the use of these 2 types of membrane are intimately tied to the site of augmentation and the material used. Aghaloo and Moy,[1] in their 2007 meta-analysis of literature on hard-tissue augmentation techniques, noted that implant survival rate was the highest for guided bone regenerations (95.5%) versus the other techniques used.

The use of guided membranes in an attempt to improve the quality of bone grafting is not a new concept. In 1957, Murray and colleagues[2] demonstrated new bone

Disclosure Statement: The authors have nothing to disclose.
[a] Division of Oral and Maxillofacial Surgery, Chandler Medical Center, College of Dentistry, University of Kentucky, D508, 800 Rose Street, Lexington, KY 40536-0297, USA; [b] Maxillofacial and Plastic surgery department, College of Dentistry, Alexandria University, Champilion street, Al-Azarita, Egypt
* Corresponding author.
E-mail address: noel.naung@uky.edu

Dent Clin N Am 63 (2019) 419–431
https://doi.org/10.1016/j.cden.2019.02.008
0011-8532/19/© 2019 Elsevier Inc. All rights reserved.

growth in dog femur, ileum, and spinal column using a plastic fenestrated cage as a barrier to soft-tissue invasion. Recognizing potential benefits of guided bone regeneration (GBR) in dentistry, in 1960 Linghorne[3] presented the sequence of osteogenesis events, which he described as "pathologic and physiologic phases," after bridging a 15-mm ostectomy site in dog fibula. In 1969, Richter and Boyne[4] published a paper on new concepts in facial bone healing and grafting procedures, in which they presented the use of hematopoietic bone marrow placed in a vitallium meshwork lined with a Millipore filter to stabilize and discourage the ingrowth of fibrous tissue.

In the intervening period, the evolution of these bone-volume growth techniques has improved. According to Jimenez Garcia and colleagues,[5] the use of a membrane technique prevents the migration of fibroblasts and soft connective tissue cells into the intended regeneration site. In 1996, Hermann and Buser[6] discussed the critical surgical factors for adequate and predictable regeneration: use of an appropriate membrane, attaining primary soft-tissue healing, creation and maintenance of a membrane-protected space, close adaptation and stabilization of the membrane to the surrounding bone, and sufficient length of healing period. In 2006 Wang and Boyapati[7] published the PASS principles: primary wound closure without tension to enable proper healing by means of first intention and reduction of the risk of membrane exposure, angiogenesis to promote blood supply, space maintenance to create a bed for the undifferentiated mesenchymal cells, and clot stability to allow for the proper development of these cells.

CONCEPTS OF GUIDED TISSUE MEMBRANES AND IDEAL PROPERTIES

Current concepts to increase the outcome of successful bone regeneration are built on those already discussed and are broken down into ideal properties anticipated from the barrier membranes.[8–10]

Biocompatibility: the membrane should not trigger host immune response, sensitization, or chronic inflammatory reaction and not adversely affect healing.

Space creation and maintenance: the membrane should have adequate toughness to create and maintain space to allow the ingrowth of nearby osteoblasts to regenerate bone, and have adequate strength to withstand the pressures from nearby muscles of mastication and the tongue.

Occlusivity and selective permeability: the membrane should prevent unwanted cells such as epithelial cells, fibrous tissue, or granulation tissue from entering into the intended bone-healing space, while permitting nearby osteoprogenitors, osteoblasts, and cells responsible for neovascularization as well as facilitating diffusion of the growth factors, signaling molecules, nutrients, and bioactive substances.

Tissue integration: membrane should fully integrate with the host tissue to provide structural integrity and provide mucosal support and stability. It should also have a sufficient adaptability between the bone-membrane border by sealing off the cavity, preventing fibrous tissue infiltration and encapsulation of the membrane.

Clinical manageability: the membrane should be easy to handle and should maintain its shape and position for easy placement.

TYPES OF MEMBRANES: ADVANTAGES AND DISADVANTAGES

Various materials have been used to fabricate GBR membranes over the last decades. The types of membrane can vary widely from titanium mesh that is very rigid to membranes that are very flexible, and which may be bioresorbable or might require a second surgery to remove it at a later stage.[11]

Nonresorbable Membranes

Cellulose acetate (Millipore) was the first material used to keep gingival connective tissue away from the root surface and allow periodontal regeneration.[12] Commercially available nonresorbable guided tissue regeneration (GTR) membranes for periodontal regeneration and GBR membranes for alveolar bone regeneration are expanded polytetrafluoroethylene (e-PTFE) and high-density PTFE (d-PTFE), both of which are available with or without titanium reinforcement.[13-16]

Numerous studies have shown positive results with the use of e-PTFE membranes, widely known as Gore-tex (W.L. Gore & Associates, Flagstaff, AZ, USA).[17-20] However, premature exposure of e-PTFE membranes is relatively common and is reported to be around 30% to 40%. Membrane exposure may lead to infection and lack of new bone formation as a result of fibrous tissue ingrowth.[21] Primary closure is necessary over e-PTFE membranes, which can be challenging in larger defects.[22] Another disadvantage of nonresorbable membranes is the need for additional surgery to remove the membrane, increasing the risk of exposing newly regenerated bone to bacteria. Timing of membrane removal is also important because early removal can lead to resorption of regenerated bone, whereas late removal can increase the risks of bacterial contamination and infection.[23]

The e-PTFE membrane has been replaced with d-PTFE, marketed as Cytoplast barrier membranes (Osteogenic Biomedical, Lubbock, TX, USA). This membrane has high density and smaller pore size (0.2 μm), preventing bacterial infiltration and leading to lower risks of infection when exposed. In addition, primary closure over the membrane is not necessary.[22,24] In a randomized controlled trial, no difference was detected in the mean vertical bone defect fill after 6 months with either e-PTFE and d-PTFE membrane; however, d-PTFE membrane was easier to remove than e-PTFE.[25]

Titanium mesh (eg, Ti-Micromesh; ACE, Brockton, MA, USA) is also commercially available as nonresorbable GBR membrane. Various studies have demonstrated that titanium mesh membranes have sufficient strength and toughness to provide space maintenance and prevent contour collapse from mucosal compression because of its elasticity.[26] In addition, they are less susceptible to bacterial contamination secondary to its smooth surface.[27] However, stiffness of the material and sharp edges caused by trimming and contouring can cause mucosal irritation and are associated with higher risk of membrane exposure.[27-29] In addition, the removal of titanium mesh can be challenging. In a randomized clinical treatment trial of atrophic alveolar bone in the posterior mandible, similar vertical bone gain and implant stability was achieved by using either titanium mesh or d-PTFE membrane.[30]

Resorbable Membranes

Requirement for a second surgical procedure to remove a barrier membrane is the major disadvantage of nonresorbable membranes. Since the early 1990s, bioresorbable membranes have been successfully used clinically.[31-33] Resorbable membranes are available as natural and synthetic membranes. Natural membranes are manufactured using bovine or porcine collagen or chitosan.[34,35] Commercially available synthetic membranes are made up of organic aliphatic polymers such as polyglycolic acid or polylactic acid, and their modifications. These include poly-DL-lactic acid, polylactic-glycolic acid, polyglycolic acid-trimethylene carbonate, poly-LD-lactic-glycolic acid-trimethylene carbonate, and poly-DL-caprolactone.[23]

Collagen has the ability to attract and activate gingival fibroblast cells and stimulate fibroblast DNA synthesis.[31,34,36] Biocompatible type 1 and type 3 collagen membranes are commercially available with varying rates of resorption ranging from

0.5 month (CollaPlug; Zimmer Biomet, Warsaw, IN, USA) up to 10 months (Mem-Lok RCM; BioHorizons, Birmingham, AL, USA).[23] Chitosan is biodegradable and biocompatible, and possesses antimicrobial and osteoinductive properties.[35] Synthetic membranes have advantages of biocompatibility and complete hydrolysis as well as removal by proteolytic enzymes from the body.[23,37] These membranes are resorbed by the body with variable resorption time from 1.5 to 24 months depending on the type and properties of the materials.[23,37]

More recently, resorbable allograft membranes derived from natural biological materials such as human placental amnion chorion tissue (BioXclude; Snoasis Medical, Golden, CO, USA), human pericardium (Mem-Lok Pericardium; BioHorizons), human fascia lata (Fascia Lata Tissuenet; TissueNet, Orlando, FL, USA), and human fascia temporalis (Tutoplast Fascia Temporalis; Biodynamics International, Milwaukee, WI, USA) has become commercially available. As processed biological materials, they carry minimal risk of inflammatory or foreign body reactions. In a study comparing different types of membranes on New Zealand white rabbits, fascia lata, pericardium, and e-PTFE membranes showed significantly better bone regeneration than fascia temporalis.[38]

Because resorbable membranes do not require secondary surgery for their removal, there is a reduced risk of infection and less tissue damage. As such, there is decreased pain and discomfort, along with decreased costs associated with a second surgery.[26,39] However, the timing and degree of resorption of the membrane can be unpredictable.[40] Premature resorption can lead to gradual loss of strength, membrane collapse, and loss of the ability to maintain space. Loss of strength can decrease bone regeneration, allowing fibrous tissue ingrowth, and prolonged or incomplete resorption can be associated with membrane exposure, inflammation, and bacterial contamination. These disorders can jeopardize the healing of the newly formed bone. In general, as resorbable membranes are not as stiff as nonresorbable membranes they do not allow tenting of the tissues.

STUDIES COMPARING RESORBABLE AND NONRESORBABLE MEMBRANES

There are multiple comparative studies of resorbable versus nonresorbable membranes, each with its strengths and weaknesses. To facilitate the understanding of the topic, this section focuses firstly on a systematic review and meta-analysis and secondly on clinical trials that address GBR in different sites.

Systematic Review and Meta-Analysis

Lim and colleagues[41] retrospectively reviewed and performed a meta-analysis of 21 qualitative and 15 qualitative clinical trials to compare the wound-healing complications among resorbable and nonresorbable membranes, and found no statistically significant difference between the types of membrane used.

Clinical Trials

Class II furcation defects

A substantial number of comparative studies of resorbable and nonresorbable membranes exists regarding the treatment of class II furcation defects. Coffesse and colleagues[42] (1997), Scott and colleagues (1997)[43], Eickholz and colleagues[44] (1997), and Karapataki and colleagues[45] (1999) found no significant difference in probing depth reduction, clinical attachment gain, and vertical and horizontal bone fill between groups. Both resorbable membrane groups and nonresorbable membrane groups showed significant clinical and radiographic improvements. In a randomized multicenter study of 38 patients conducted in 1995, Hugoson and colleagues[46] found a statistically significant improvement in clinical attachment level in both horizontal and vertical direction in the resorbable membrane group. The nonresorbable membrane group showed improvement in clinical attachment in the vertical direction only. Gingival recession was significantly higher in the nonresorbable membrane group compared with resorbable membranes. In a long-term study in 2006, Eickholz and colleagues[47] found that treatment of class II furcation defects demonstrated stable horizontal attachment gain after 10 years with no statistically significant difference among the types of membrane used.

Class III furcation defects
Class III through-and-through furcation defects respond poorly to GTR techniques. No significant gain in pocket depth or vertical probing attachment levels were observed in both type of barrier membranes when used in class III furcations.[48]

Intrabony periodontal defects
Multiple clinical trials conducted to compare absorbable and nonresorbable barrier membranes in the treatment of intrabony periodontal defects failed to show statistically significant differences in probing depth reduction, clinical attachment level gain, and bone fill.[44,49–52] In a 10-year follow-up study on treatment of intrabony defects conducted in 2008, Pretzl and colleagues[53] found no statistically significant difference in the stability of vertical attachment gain between the 2 membranes groups after GTR therapy.

Ridge preservation procedures
In 2012, Arbab and colleagues[54] found no statistically significant differences in horizontal and vertical ridge dimension changes between the use of resorbable and nonresorbable membrane for ridge preservation. In addition, the viable bone gain in the extraction sockets was histologically found to be the same for both membrane groups. The investigators concluded that the choice of barrier membrane has no effect on the outcome of the ridge preservation both clinically and histologically.

Implant site development
In a 2014 double-blind randomized clinical trial, Merli and colleagues[55] compared the efficacy of resorbable and nonresorbable barriers for vertical ridge augmentation procedure with simultaneous implant placement, and found no significant differences in radiographic vertical bone gain at the 6-year follow-up visit.

Maxillary sinus augmentation
A study comparing the use of resorbable versus nonresorbable barrier membranes for maxillary sinus augmentation revealed uneventful healing and successful closure of the lateral sinus walls. At the microscopic level, higher amount of fibrous connective tissue ingrowth was observed in the bone samples obtained from the resorbable membrane group; however, the difference did not affect the clinical outcome.[56]

Peri-implant bony defects
Randomized controlled trials comparing the efficacy of resorbable and nonresorbable membrane in the treatment of bony defects around endosseous dental implants revealed no statistically significant difference in clinical parameters between the 2 membrane types. Both membranes were proved to be successful when used in combination with particulate bone grafts.[57,58]

CRITERIA FOR MEMBRANE SELECTION

In routine practice, the type of membrane used will vary with the choice of grafting material and the nature of the bony defect. When a cortical or corticocancellous block graft is used, the graft material will act as a tenting device; therefore, the use of resorbable membrane is recommended (**Fig. 1**), whereby a large anterior defect was reconstructed with a combination of cortical and cancellous grafts augmented with a bone morphogenetic protein (BMP) sponge and a resorbable membrane. Extensive undermining of mucosa of the lip was done before placement of the grafts. The cortical grafts and autogenous marrow were obtained from the patient's hip. The cortical grafts were held in place with titanium screws that act as their own tenting of the graft site. The space was created and maintained by the cortical blocks stabilized by the titanium screws. The membrane was occlusive and did not need to be rigid, as the grafting provided this aspect of GBR. With the necessary undermining to provide a tension-free closure, the anterior vestibule was eliminated. At a secondary stage after implants were placed, a maxillary vestibuloplasty was performed.

Likewise, with a sinus lifts the authors prefer a resorbable GBR because there is no pressure on the graft after it is placed. In **Fig. 2** the patient has a long-standing defect from the loss of the upper first molar and second bicuspid. The maxillary sinus is approached from a standard lateral window technique. Once the maxillary membrane has been lifted and inspected for perforations, the sinus is lifted and a resorbable membrane is placed, creating a space for the bone graft. In this case, demineralized bone was packed against the maxillary floor and the membrane. A second membrane was placed on the labial to provide an occlusive barrier laterally, and the flap was closed.

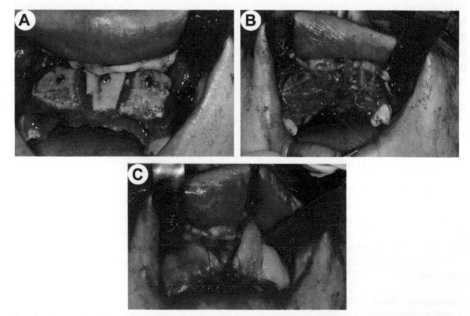

Fig. 1. Augmentation of maxillary anterior region in preparation for implant placement using resorbable membrane. (*A*) Cortical grafts stabilized with titanium screws. (*B*) Cancellous graft with autogenous marrow segment with autogenous marrow. (*C*) Resorbable membrane placed over collagen sponge membrane with BMP-2, both placed before closure of the wound.

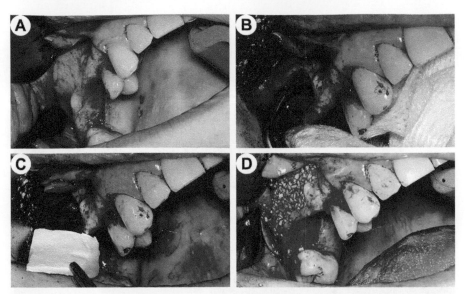

Fig. 2. Maxillary sinus augmentation using resorbable membrane. (*A*) Exposure of bone defect in the first M second bicuspid region. (*B*) Window developed, sinus lifted, and sinus membrane visible above elevator. (*C*) Resorbable membrane about to be placed against the sinus membrane. (*D*) Sinus packed, surgical site just before placement of a second resorbable membrane on the labial surface.

For ridge augmentation when there is adequate interocclusal space, a nonresorbable membrane is preferred. Types will vary from a titanium-reinforced mesh, to a plain titanium mesh, to a d-PTFE membrane that is tented. In **Fig. 3** there is a horizontal defect on the posterior mandibular ridge that was addressed with a nonresorbable membrane with tenting. Because of the defect and its location, it was necessary to have a more rigid membrane system to create space while providing an occlusive cover. The flap was elevated and undermined, anticipating the volume of bone needed to reconstruct the ridge. The postoperative panorex illustrates the tenting provided by a tenting screw and the tacking down of the edges of the membrane. Two implants were placed in the bone-grafting site and a third implant anterior to the site. The periapical film was obtained 1.5 years later and illustrates the excellent bone fill that occurred around the 2 posterior implants.

The authors consider it important to emphasize that when performing a ridge augmentation, preparation of the bed is critical. In the authors' experience, the flaps must be adequately mobilized before placement of the graft material. Failure to achieve a tension-free closure almost always results in exposure of the membrane and loss of the graft. In some cases, as in the first one, extensive undermining will result in loss of the vestibule, necessitating a secondary vestibuloplasty. In others, as in the last case, the loss of vestibule is minimal and will not require a secondary procedure.

Failure to achieve a tension-free closure, especially when a nonresorbable membrane is being used, will often result in early membrane exposure. The time when a membrane becomes exposed is important. If the membrane is exposed early—for example, in the first few weeks after the surgical intervention—antibiotics and chlorhexidine may help but the membrane will have to be removed. It is the authors' experience that when this occurs the results of the augmentation are likely to be very poor.

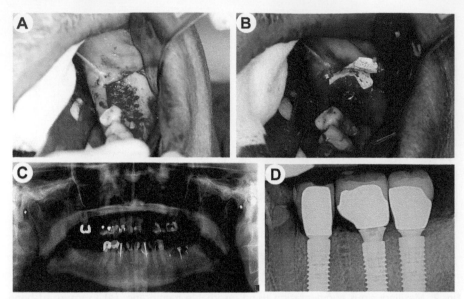

Fig. 3. Vertical ridge augmentation of the posterior mandibular alveolar ridge using nonresorbable membrane. (*A*) Horizontal defect mandible site developed. (*B*) Placement of demineralized bone and a nonresorbable membrane secured with tenting screw. (*C*) Postoperative panorex of grafted site. (*D*) Impacts placed and restored 1 year 6 months later.

When the exposure is late—for example, after a month or two—antibiotic use and chlorhexidine use will be required along with removal of the membrane. When exposures occur late in the course of treatment, there will usually be some success with the augmentation (**Table 1**).

Table 1 Criteria for the choice of membranes		
Treatment	**Resorbable Membrane**	**Nonresorbable Membrane**
Sinus graft	Underneath schneiderian membrane and over the lateral window osteotomy	Not recommended
GTR (periodontal defects)	If particulate bone is used	Not generally recommended, May be used if no particulate bone is used
Ridge preservation	✔	✔
Alveolar ridge augmentation		
Monocortical block	If autogenous bone graft is used	Large bone defects If allograft is used Vertical augmentation with bone blocks
GBR	Horizontal ridge augmentation • If xenograft or combination of allograft and xenograft is used	Horizontal ridge augmentation if only autograft or allograft is used Vertical ridge augmentation
Ridge split	✔	✗
Biologics (growth factors)	With particulate bone graft	Without particulate bone graft

SUMMARY

The use of guided membranes in an attempt to improve the quality of bone grafting is not a new concept. However, the evolution of these bone-volume growth techniques has improved and most likely will continue to improve with time.[5] In routine daily practice, both types of membranes will be used depending on the needs of the case. Whether a nonresorbable or a resorbable membrane is used, it should be biocompatible, allow selective permeability with good tissue integration, and have satisfactory handling properties. Surgical techniques to attain primary soft-tissue healing, the creation and maintenance of a membrane-protected space with close adaptation and stabilization of the membrane to the surrounding bone, and sufficient length of healing period are very important.[6]

Commercially available nonresorbable GTR membranes comprise e-PTFE and d-PTFE, both of which are available with or without titanium reinforcement.[13–16] In addition to titanium mesh membranes, these have sufficient strength and toughness to provide space maintenance and prevent contour collapse while preventing mucosal compression caused by its elasticity.[26] The authors' preference is to use such membranes when vertical augmentation is needed. The biggest disadvantages of nonresorbable membranes are early exposure, infection, and loss of graft material. Gortex (e-PTFE) has a 30% to 40% risk of exposure with subsequent infection and suppuration. d-PTFE, marketed as Cytoplast barrier membranes, has high density and smaller pore size (0.2 μm), eliminating bacterial infiltration, and poses a lower risk of infection when exposed. Currently the authors use d-PTFE when we nonresorbable membrane is required.

There are numerous resorbable membranes available as natural and synthetic membranes. Natural membranes are manufactured using bovine or porcine collagen or chitosan. Resorbable allograft membranes derived from natural biologics are currently available. Synthetic membranes are made of organic aliphatic polymers (polyglycolide or polylactide) and are commercially available.[26] The biggest advantage of resorbable membranes is that they do not require secondary surgery and usually have less tissue damage with less pain and discomfort. However, the timing and degree of membrane resorption are unpredictable. Premature resorption can lead to loss of membrane strength and space collapse. Resorbable membranes are preferred in the authors' practice when the graft material will function to maintain the space (eg, corticocancellous bone graft), when there is no pressure on the graft after its placement (eg, as in sinus lift procedures), or when occlusion is needed, as in socket preservation. It is clear that one type of membrane will not fit all clinical needs, and further work on this valuable clinical tool is warranted.

REFERENCES

1. Aghaloo TL, Moy PK. Which hard tissue augmentation techniques are the most successful in furnishing bony support for implant placement? Int J Oral Maxillofac Implants 2007;22(Suppl):49–70.
2. Murray G, Holden R, Roschlau W. Experimental and clinical study of new growth of bone in a cavity. Am J Surg 1957;93(3):385–7.
3. Linghorne WJ. The sequence of events in osteogenesis as studied in polyethylene tubes. Ann N Y Acad Sci 1960;85:445–60.
4. Richter HE, Boyne PJ. New concepts in facial bone healing and grafting procedures. J Oral Surg 1969;27(7):557–9.

5. Jimenez Garcia J, Berghezan S, Carames JMM, et al. Effect of cross-linked vs non-cross-linked collagen membranes on bone: a systematic review. J Periodontal Res 2017;52(6):955–64.
6. Hermann JS, Buser D. Guided bone regeneration for dental implants. Curr Opin Periodontol 1996;3:168–77.
7. Wang HL, Boyapati L. "PASS" principles for predictable bone regeneration. Implant Dent 2006;15(1):8–17.
8. Sam G, Pillai BRM. Evolution of barrier membranes in periodontal regeneration—"are the third generation membranes really here?". J Clin Diagn Res 2014;8(12): ZE14–7.
9. Scantlebury TV. 1982-1992: a decade of technology development for guided tissue regeneration. J Periodontol 1993;64(11 Suppl):1129–37.
10. Gottlow J. Guided tissue regeneration using bioresorbable and non-resorbable devices: initial healing and long-term results. J Periodontol 1993;64(11 Suppl): 1157–65.
11. Alagl AS, Madi M. Localized ridge augmentation in the anterior maxilla using titanium mesh, an alloplast, and a nano-bone graft: a case report. J Int Med Res 2018;46(5):2001–7.
12. Nyman S, Gottlow J, Karring T, et al. The regenerative potential of the periodontal ligament. An experimental study in the monkey. J Clin Periodontol 1982;9(3): 257–65.
13. Aaboe M, Pinholt EM, Hjorting-Hansen E. Healing of experimentally created defects: a review. Br J Oral Maxillofac Surg 1995;33(5):312–8.
14. Jovanovic SA, Nevins M. Bone formation utilizing titanium-reinforced barrier membranes. Int J Periodontics Restorative Dent 1995;15(1):56–69.
15. Bottino MC, Thomas V. Membranes for periodontal regeneration—a materials perspective. Front Oral Biol 2015;17:90–100.
16. Wolff LF. Guided tissue regeneration in periodontal therapy. Northwest Dent 2000; 79(6):23–8, 40.
17. Wadhawan A, Gowda TM, Mehta DS. Gore-tex((R)) versus resolut adapt((R)) GTR membranes with perioglas((R)) in periodontal regeneration. Contemp Clin Dent 2012;3(4):406–11.
18. Rocchietta I, Fontana F, Simion M. Clinical outcomes of vertical bone augmentation to enable dental implant placement: a systematic review. J Clin Periodontol 2008;35(8 Suppl):203–15.
19. Bernstein S, Cooke J, Fotek P, et al. Vertical bone augmentation: where are we now? Implant Dent 2006;15(3):219–28.
20. Merli M, Migani M, Bernardelli F, et al. Vertical bone augmentation with dental implant placement: efficacy and complications associated with 2 different techniques. A retrospective cohort study. Int J Oral Maxillofac Implants 2006;21(4): 600–6.
21. Vroom M, Gründemann L. Non-resorbable membranes. Tandartspraktijk 2014; 35(1):8–13.
22. Barber HD, Lignelli J, Smith BM, et al. Using a dense PTFE membrane without primary closure to achieve bone and tissue regeneration. J Oral Maxillofac Surg 2007;65(4):748–52.
23. Rodriguez I, Selders GS, Fetz A, et al. Barrier membranes for dental applications: a review and sweet advancement in membrane developments. Mouth and Teeth 2018;2(1):1–9.

24. Bartee BK, Carr JA. Evaluation of a high-density polytetrafluoroethylene (n-PTFE) membrane as a barrier material to facilitate guided bone regeneration in the rat mandible. J Oral Implantol 1995;21(2):88–95.
25. Ronda M, Rebaudi A, Torelli L, et al. Expanded vs. dense polytetrafluoroethylene membranes in vertical ridge augmentation around dental implants: a prospective randomized controlled clinical trial. Clin Oral Implants Res 2014;25(7):859–66.
26. Rakhmatia YD, Ayukawa Y, Furuhashi A, et al. Current barrier membranes: Titanium mesh and other membranes for guided bone regeneration in dental applications. J Prosthodont Res 2013;57(1):3–14.
27. Schopper C, Goriwoda W, Moser D, et al. Long-term results after guided bone regeneration with resorbable and microporous titanium membranes. Oral Maxillofac Surg Clin North Am 2001;13(3):449–58.
28. Watzinger F, Luksch J, Millesi W, et al. Guided bone regeneration with titanium membranes: a clinical study. Br J Oral Maxillofac Surg 2000;38(4):312–5.
29. Becker W, Becker BE, Mellonig J, et al. A prospective multi-center study evaluating periodontal regeneration for class II furcation invasions and intrabony defects after treatment with a bioabsorbable barrier membrane: 1-year results. J Periodontol 1996;67(7):641–9.
30. Cucchi A, Vignudelli E, Napolitano A, et al. Evaluation of complication rates and vertical bone gain after guided bone regeneration with non-resorbable membranes versus titanium meshes and resorbable membranes. A randomized clinical trial. Clin Implant Dent Relat Res 2017;19(5):821–32.
31. Lundgren D, Sennerby L, Falk H, et al. The use of a new bioresorbable barrier for guided bone regeneration in connection with implant installation. Case reports. Clin Oral Implants Res 1994;5(3):177–84.
32. Mayfield L, Nobreus N, Attstrom R, et al. Guided bone regeneration in dental implant treatment using a bioabsorbable membrane. Clin Oral Implants Res 1997;8(1):10–7.
33. Hurzeler MB, Strub JR. Guided bone regeneration around exposed implants: a new bioresorbable device and bioresorbable membrane pins. Pract Periodontics Aesthet Dent 1995;7(9):37–47.
34. Bunyaratavej P, Wang HL. Collagen membranes: a review. J Periodontol 2001; 72(2):215–29.
35. Xu C, Lei C, Meng L, et al. Chitosan as a barrier membrane material in periodontal tissue regeneration. J Biomed Mater Res B Appl Biomater 2012;100(5): 1435–43.
36. Sheikh Z, Hamdan N, Ikeda Y, et al. Natural graft tissues and synthetic biomaterials for periodontal and alveolar bone reconstructive applications: a review. Biomater Res 2017;21:9.
37. Vert M, Li SM, Spenlehauer G, et al. Bioresorbability and biocompatibility of aliphatic polyesters. J Mater Sci Mater Med 1992;3(6):432–46.
38. Thomaidis V, Kazakos K, Lyras DN, et al. Comparative study of 5 different membranes for guided bone regeneration of rabbit mandibular defects beyond critical size. Med Sci Monit 2008;14(4):Br67–73.
39. McGinnis M, Larsen P, Miloro M, et al. Comparison of resorbable and nonresorbable guided bone regeneration materials: a preliminary study. Int J Oral Maxillofac Implants 1998;13(1):30–5.
40. Gutta R, Baker RA, Bartolucci AA, et al. Barrier membranes used for ridge augmentation: is there an optimal pore size? J Oral Maxillofac Surg 2009;67(6): 1218–25.

41. Lim G, Lin GH, Monje A, et al. Wound healing complications following guided bone regeneration for ridge augmentation: a systematic review and meta-analysis. Int J Oral Maxillofac Implants 2018;33(1):41–50.

42. Caffesse RG, Mota LF, Quinones CR, et al. Clinical comparison of resorbable and non-resorbable barriers for guided periodontal tissue regeneration. J Clin Periodontol 1997;24(10):747–52.

43. Scott TA, Towle HJ, Assad DA. Comparison of bioabsorbable laminar bone membrane and non-resorbable ePTFE membrane in mandibular furcations. J Periodontol 1997;68(7):679–86.

44. Eickholz P, Kim TS, Holle R. Guided tissue regeneration with non-resorbable and biodegradable barriers: 6 months results. J Clin Periodontol 1997;24(2): 92–101.

45. Karapataki S, Falk H, Hugoso A, et al. Treatment of class II furcation defects using resorbable and non-resorbable GTR barriers. Swed Dent J 1999;23(5–6): 173–83.

46. Hugoson A, Ravald N, Fornell J, et al. Treatment of class II furcation involvements in humans with bioresorbable and nonresorbable guided tissue regeneration barriers. A randomized multi-center study. J Periodontol 1995;66(7):624–34.

47. Eickholz P, Pretzl B, Holle R, et al. Long-term results of guided tissue regeneration therapy with non-resorbable and bioabsorbable barriers. III. Class II furcations after 10 years. J Periodontol 2006;77(1):88–94.

48. Eickholz P, Kim TS, Holle R. Regenerative periodontal surgery with non-resorbable and biodegradable barriers: results after 24 months. J Clin Periodontol 1998;25(8):666–76.

49. Corinaldesi G, Lizio G, Badiali G, et al. Treatment of intrabony defects after impacted mandibular third molar removal with bioabsorbable and non-resorbable membranes. J Periodontol 2011;82(10):1404–13.

50. Karapataki S, Hugoson A, Falk H, et al. Healing following GTR treatment of intrabony defects distal to mandibular 2nd molars using resorbable and non-resorbable barriers. J Clin Periodontol 2000;27(5):333–40.

51. Smith MacDonald E, Nowzari H, Contreras A, et al. Clinical and microbiological evaluation of a bioabsorbable and a nonresorbable barrier membrane in the treatment of periodontal intraosseous lesions. J Periodontol 1998;69(4): 445–53.

52. Christgau M, Schmalz G, Wenzel A, et al. Periodontal regeneration of intrabony defects with resorbable and non-resorbable membranes: 30-month results. J Clin Periodontol 1997;24(1):17–27.

53. Pretzl B, Kim TS, Holle R, et al. Long-term results of guided tissue regeneration therapy with non-resorbable and bioabsorbable barriers. IV. A case series of infrabony defects after 10 years. J Periodontol 2008;79(8):1491–9.

54. Arbab H, Greenwell H, Hill M, et al. Ridge preservation comparing a nonresorbable PTFE membrane to a resorbable collagen membrane: a clinical and histologic study in humans. Implant Dent 2016;25(1):128–34.

55. Merli M, Moscatelli M, Mariotti G, et al. Bone level variation after vertical ridge augmentation: resorbable barriers versus titanium-reinforced barriers. A 6-year double-blind randomized clinical trial. Int J Oral Maxillofac Implants 2014;29(4): 905–13.

56. Avera SP, Stampley WA, McAllister BS. Histologic and clinical observations of resorbable and nonresorbable barrier membranes used in maxillary sinus graft containment. Int J Oral Maxillofac Implants 1997;12(1):88–94.

57. Carpio L, Loza J, Lynch S, et al. Guided bone regeneration around endosseous implants with anorganic bovine bone mineral. A randomized controlled trial comparing bioabsorbable versus non-resorbable barriers. J Periodontol 2000; 71(11):1743–9.
58. Zitzmann NU, Naef R, Scharer P. Resorbable versus nonresorbable membranes in combination with Bio-Oss for guided bone regeneration. Int J Oral Maxillofac Implants 1997;12(6):844–52.

Tissue Engineering
What is New?

Dolphus R. Dawson III, DMD, MS, MPH[a],*,
Ahmed El-Ghannam, PhD[b], Joseph E. Van Sickels, DDS[c],
Noel Ye Naung, BDS, Higher Grad Dip Clin Sc (OMFS), MSc (OMFS), FIAOMS[c]

KEYWORDS

- Tissue engineering • Soft tissue grafts • Dental implants • Bone grafts
- Regeneration • Biologics

KEY POINTS

- Soft tissue engineering includes the use of mesenchymal stem cells to develop tissue sheets for donor soft tissue graft and incorporate other cell types to create new vascular structures within the graft.
- Osteoconductive scaffolds mixed with osteoinductive growth factors, including osteogenic stem and osteoprogenitor cells, enhance maxillofacial bone reconstruction.
- Hard tissue engineering of bone grafts, such as those with a silica-calcium phosphate composite seeded with human adipose-derived stem cells, creates better grafts with enhanced resorption profiles.

SOFT TISSUE ENGINEERING

Oral soft tissue engineering has long been associated with the reconstruction of mucosal or gingival defects associated with chronic disease or trauma, as well as congenital defects. The premise of the tissue engineering follows a requisite triad of cells, scaffolds, and physiologically active substances, along with angiogenesis and proper environmental factors/stimuli to induce tissue regeneration.[1] This tenet holds true for both hard and soft tissues. Soft tissue augmentation has evolved beyond conventional autogenous-only grafts to a variety of donor grafts. The regeneration of soft tissue has just begun to tap its potential through advancements in stem cell

Disclosure statement: The authors have nothing to disclose.
[a] Division of Periodontology, Department of Oral Health Practice, College of Dentistry, University of Kentucky, 800 Rose Street, D-444 Dental Sciences Building, Lexington, KY 40536-0297, USA; [b] Department of Mechanical Engineering and Engineering Science, University of North Carolina at Charlotte, 9201 University City Boulevard, Charlotte, NC 28223-0001, USA; [c] Division of Oral and Maxillofacial Surgery, College of Dentistry, University of Kentucky, 800 Rose Street, Lexington, KY 40536-0297, USA
* Corresponding author.
E-mail address: dolph.dawson@uky.edu

Dent Clin N Am 63 (2019) 433–445
https://doi.org/10.1016/j.cden.2019.02.009
0011-8532/19/© 2019 Elsevier Inc. All rights reserved.

dental.theclinics.com

technologies as well as cell signaling and cell trafficking. The focus here is to provide an overview of some key areas of these advancements.

Soft Tissue Augmentation

Soft tissue augmentation around implants has, for many years, focused on autogenous conventional epithelialized, free gingival grafts, or connective tissue grafts to gain keratinized tissue or address mucosal recession.[2] Studies indicate that shallow recession defects (≤ 2 mm) have shown success; there is no support for larger defects.[3] The adaptation of various tunneling techniques have led to minimal surgical access that produce both successful root coverage and esthetics.[4] These minimally invasive procedures, such as the vestibular incision supraperiosteal tunnel access or modified vestibular incision supraperiosteal tunnel access technique, have been used to address defects around dental implants.[5] Further studies are needed to better address outcomes in the esthetic zone.[6]

Autogenous soft tissue grafts rely on donor sites, usually the hard palate, which can have significant sequelae, such as postoperative pain or bleeding after the procedure. A number of commercially available soft tissue grafts allow the elimination of harvesting the graft from the donor as well as the grafting of multiple sites in 1 visit. Allogenic human acellular dermal matrix is commonly used for soft tissue augmentation and has similar results to autogenous grafts.[7] A common feature of several of these allogenic grafts is the preservation of the basement membrane. Xenografts, or those derived from other species, such as porcine or bovine species, have also been used. One such porcine collagen matrix studied in comparison to a free gingival graft showed mature collagen in the tissue samples from the porcine graft, whereas a more fragmented collagen tissue was seen in the free gingival graft samples.[8]

Although enhancements of harvested donor tissues allow for a greater extent of grafting and less patient morbidity, regeneration relies on the manipulation of cells and tissues to maximize gain of lost tissues.

Soft Tissue Regeneration

Soft tissue regeneration blends the processes of wound healing with the enhancement of cell types and functions present during the phase of regeneration. A number of key cell processes, including proliferation, viability, migration, gene expression, and differentiation have been studied in in vitro monolayer models and 3-dimensional (3D) models provide insight into higher order activity, such as cell contractility in a fibroblast model.[9] A 3D model was used to generate autologous cell sheets in a rat model.[10] Oral mucosal cells, specifically fibroblasts, as well as fibrin were used to create scaffolds for mucosal keratinocytes. In this rat model, reepithelization via cell sheets with fibroblasts was much faster than those without fibroblasts. The authors concluded that not only was the overall process relatively fast, but also that the outcome included no scarring. The 3D tissue models have also provided a platform to study various oral infection models, such as oral candidiasis, allowing for a better understanding of cytokine release and gene expression of the tissues as well as the process of invasion of the epithelium by the candidiasis.[11]

Tissue models rely on selected cells for specific applications. Mesenchymal stem cells (MSCs) give rise to various specialized cells. Recent efforts have focused on progenitor cells of the periodontal ligament (PDL) because these cells can form cementoblasts, osteoblasts, or fibroblasts.[12–15] Differentiated induced pluripotent stem cells that turn into MSCs are generally safer than undifferentiated pluripotent stem cells, but there are limitations on obtaining adequate quantities of cells.[16,17] Further research is needed to develop more sources of stem cells. Once an adequate source and quantity of therapeutic stem cells can be generated, the next challenge is getting the cells where they are needed. Local delivery may suffice if the defects are large and are accessed surgically; however, early defects may require attracting cells to the site. Enhancing attraction of the patient's own cells may be done through endogenous cell homing via chemokines or scaffolds that influence the recruitment of specific cells.[18] In a rat model, systemically transplanted MSCs were harvested from donor rats and implants were placed after tooth extractions.[19] The authors noted improved attachment and proliferation of oral mucous epithelial cells. The PDL is known for its regenerative capacity to enhance the replacement of lost cementum and bone on natural teeth. A novel concept of developing a PDL on dental implants has been investigated. In a rat model, dental progenitor cells were used to seed and develop a PDL on titanium implants.[20] Advancements in obtaining and maintaining a PDL on implants would be significant for regeneration around implant surfaces.

All augmentation procedures, both soft and hard tissue, rely on the establishment of vascular and nutrient supply after augmentation. The collection, harvesting, and delivery of specific cells would be of little use without an environment that allows proliferation and maturation. Assessment of various scaffolds via micro-computed tomography evaluation of perfusion can be done using a chorioallantoic membrane that allows for 3D imaging of the tissue engineered construct while reducing extensive animal use in research.[21] Vascularized connective tissue grafts in humans, when compared with conventional subepithelial connective tissue grafts, showed less shrinkage and maintained their initial volume better.[22] In another study, human adipose-derived cells and human umbilical vein endothelial cells were used to create vessel structures for vascularization of the engineered soft tissue flap.[23]

BONE ENGINEERING

Repair of bone defects, both large and small, in the maxillofacial skeleton have proved to be a treatment challenge for many years. Although autogenous bone grafts have been considered the mainstay and gold standard of treatment, allografts, xenografts, and alloplastic substitutes have been used with success for resolving bony defects in the maxilla and the mandible.[24–28] The traditional autogenous bone graft often required a donor site that added another source of morbidity to the patient. Searches for alternative methods that eliminate a donor site have been many and led to the understanding of osteoconductive and osteoinductive materials. Autogenous bone grafts stimulate bone regeneration through its osteogenic, osteoinductive, and osteoconductive properties, and avoid an immune reaction. In addition, autogenous grafts contain live stem or osteoprogenitor cells that can migrate, proliferate, and potentiate bone healing.[29] An osteoinductive material can recruit immature cells and stimulate them to develop into osteoblasts.[26,27,30] Although well beyond the scope of this article, several growth factors are involved in bone healing. They include vascular endothelial growth factor, fibroblastic growth factors, insulin-like growth factors, platelet-derived growth factor, and bone morphogenic proteins (BMP), to name a few.[31] Their concentration, interaction with other growth factors, and the timing of their application is critical in normal bone regeneration.[25]

Osteoconductive materials allow bone to grow on a surface and act as a scaffold. A scaffold should not only provide structural support, but also should be biodegradable at a rate comparable with that of newly formed bone and should have a porous structure similar to bone to promote capillary infiltration and cell proliferation.[28] Tricalcium phosphate is an example of an osteoconductive material that will resorb with time.[32]

Bone Morphogenic Proteins

BMPs are widely recognized for their important role in the postnatal bone formation. They are members of transforming growth factor-β group.[33,34] Out of nearly 20 different BMPs that have been identified, BMP-2 and BMP-7 are the most extensively studied and are considered to possess the most significant osteoinductive properties.[34–36]

Recombinant human BMP-2 (rhBMP-2) with an absorbable collagen sponge carrier is commercially available in the United States as INFUSE bone graft (Medtronic, Minneapolis, MN) and is approved by the US Food and Drug Administration. Current indications include sinus augmentations, alveolar ridge augmentation, and socket preservation procedures.[37] A series of clinical trials have demonstrated the effectiveness of rhBMP-2/absorbable collagen sponge for maxillary sinus augmentation and alveolar ridge augmentation procedures.[38–40] Separately, complete healing of alveolar grafting of premaxillary clefts was demonstrated in 10 patients treated with BMP-2/collagen sponges when compared with 2 control patients treated with conventional autogenous cancellous bone grafts.[41]

Even though good evidence exists regarding the effectiveness of rhBMP-2, its safety has been questioned based on a metaanalysis of individual participant data by Simmonds and colleagues[42] (2013). Their research was conducted in response to the finding from a review of clinical trials conducted by of Carragee and colleagues[43] (2011), where the risk of adverse events seemed to be significantly higher than original estimates when study bias was taken into consideration.

Conway and associates[44] (2014) compared the treatment of long bone union in 63 patients treated with BMP-2 versus 112 patients treated with BMP-7. They found that treatment with BMP-2 showed a better healing (15 weeks vs 23 weeks average time to weight bearing) and faster recovery (19 weeks vs 30 weeks average healing time) than treatment with BMP-7.[44] In contrast, another comparison study discovered that rhBMP-7, especially in higher doses, showed less inflammation and soft tissue edema than rhBMP-2.[45]

To deliver rhBMP-7 into the bony defect, bovine collagen is reconstituted with saline to form a paste or carboxymethylcellulose is added into the rhBMP-7/bovine collagen/saline paste to form a putty as a carrier. These are available as OP-1 Putty (Skryker Biotech, Hopkinton, MA) under limited approval from the US Food and Drug Administration. However, its use was discontinued in the United States in 2014 because the product failed to clearly demonstrate its efficacy in comparison with autogenous bone grafting.[46] Nevertheless, the use of rhBMP-7 has continued in other countries with promising results. Ayoub and colleagues[47] (2016) described a successful regeneration of alveolar cleft with the use of rhBMP-7.

One of the challenges with collagen-based carrier systems is a lack of strength to withstand forces exerted by the muscles of mastication. With increased pressure, the slow controlled and sustained release of BMPs can be compromised. With pressure, there is also an increased risk of the release of high doses of rhBMPs.[33] Thus, BMPs and a collagen sponge have been studied in conjunction with porous solid osteoconductive scaffolds such as hydroxyapatite, tricalcium phosphate, and chitosan to achieve the required mechanical support.[33]

Herford and colleagues[30] (2012) combined recombinant BMP with a compression-resistant osteoconductive matrix in an animal model mandibular continuity defect. They showed a significantly higher bone density and space maintenance than just recombinant BMP2 and an absorbable collagen sponge.[30] Their compression resistant matrix was composed of 15% hydroxyapatite and 85% β-tricalcium phosphate.

A number of studies that advocated for the use of osteoconductive scaffolds in combination with osteoinductive materials showed successful bone healing or regeneration that is comparable with those with autogenous bone grafts. However, in patients with limited native viable osteoprogenitor cells (such as osteoporotic bone or radiation-induced hypocellular bone), the addition of bone marrow aspirate may be beneficial. Melville and colleagues[26] (2017) used recombinant BMP2 with an allogeneic avascular bone graft combined with a bone marrow aspirate with a poly-D, L-lactic acid mesh to reconstruct the maxillary alveolus in a patient following a traumatic maxillary defect. Six months later, they were able to successfully place 3 dental implants.

Clinical Examples

Previously, our group published a report on the use of reconstruction plates with the use of rhBMP2 and tricalcium phosphate for patients with fractures and continuity defects of the mandible.[48] A successful outcome was achieved for 2 patients with no significant medical comorbidities, thus avoiding a secondary donor site. In 1 case, the defect was 4 cm.[48] We present an additional case using a similar technique.

Six months after maxillary and mandibular osteotomies, a 40-year-old patient presented with an infection and shifting of the occlusion. After the resolution of the infection and loss of bone, a diagnosis of a nonunion on the left side of the mandible was made (**Fig. 1**). A cone beam computerized tomogram was obtained that allowed for the fabrication of a 3D model with the patient in the proper occlusion. Intraoperatively, a 2-mm reconstruction plate was contoured to stabilize the segments (**Fig. 2**). This patient is still under active treatment.

Bone Grafts: The Next Generation

Annually, more than 4 million bone grafting surgeries are performed worldwide, at an estimated cost of US$10 billion.[49–52] In 2016, the global market for craniomaxillofacial implants was US$1.79 billion and is expected to reach US$2.49 billion by 2021.[53] Despite the huge advances of the state-of-the-art bone graft technology, the reconstruction of large craniofacial and maxillofacial bone defects remains a major challenge. The use of autografts is currently the gold standard technique despite the associated mortality and morbidity problems.[54] Cadaver bone grafts from bone banks is second in popularity after autografts; however, it carries risks of decreases in

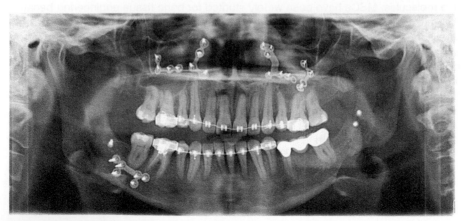

Fig. 1. Nonunion of the left mandible with significant loss of bone.

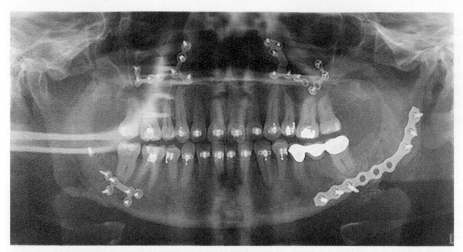

Fig. 2. Reconstruction plate and restoration of bone volume using rhBMP2, tricalcium phosphate, and demineralized bone.

mineral density owing to osteoclastic resorption and immune reaction because of genetic differences.[55–57] Synthetic grafts made of metals or polymers are not bioactive because they do not bond to bone or support bone cell function. The formation of discontinuous fibrous tissue at the interfaces with polymeric and metal implants has been reported in preclinical and clinical studies.[58–63] Several studies have shown that excessive fibrous capsule formation at the bone–implant interface can prevent tissue integration, and lead to bone resorption and fracture and implant failure.[64–67] Calcium phosphate ceramics such as hydroxyapatite and tricalcium phosphate are bioactive because they are able to enhance bone cell function and tissue formation. Nevertheless, a main concern in the application of hydroxyapatite bone grafts is the poor resorption. Several studies have reported fibrous encapsulation around hydroxyapatite ceramic particles inside alveolar bone.[68–70] These limitations create a significant need for improvements in bone graft technology.

Tissue engineering approaches for bone reconstruction use porous implant materials, like calcium phosphate ceramics, as a carrier for bone cells and/or osteoinductive molecules. MSCs have been widely studied for bone tissue engineering because they are able to differentiate to bone-forming cells (osteoblasts) and participate in fracture healing. Animal models have indicated that harvesting cells from bone marrow and delivering high numbers of cells into a graft site is inadequate to ensure appropriate healing and bon regenration.[71] Ideally, a bioactive ceramic carrier releases ions that signal the stem cells and induce their osteogenic differentiation. Culturing bone marrow MSCs onto osteoconductive or osteoinductive carrier matrix until they attach, spread, differentiate, and/or generate a specific amount of extracellular matrix in vitro before implantation has resulted in a significant improvement in outcomes.[72,73] The repair of a critical-sized femoral segmental defect using MSCs was accomplished without adverse immune responses and without the use of immunosuppressive therapy.[74] Other studies have shown the feasibility of treating children with osteogenesis imperfecta using isolated allogeneic bone marrow-derived mesenchymal cells without significant toxicity.[75–78]

The successful use of stem cells in bone reconstruction depends on the use of a suitable carrier. In a comparative study, the bone healing effect of MSCs seeded on

2 matrices, bovine bone hydroxyapatite and α-tricalcium phosphate, was compared with that of an autologous bone transfer.[79] Histomorphometric analyses showed that the bone volume in defects treated with tricalcium phosphate seeded with mesenchymal cells was comparable with that of defects treated with autogenous bone. However, although defects treated with autogenous bone showed uniform platforms of bone formation, bone formation in defects treated with tricalcium phosphate was associated with the ceramic particles. Defects treated with bovine bone hydroxyapatite (Bio-Oss) seeded with or without mesenchymal cells scored the lowest value of bone formation and highest value of fibrosis around the ceramic particles.

Human adipose-derived stem cells showed the ability to expand in vitro and to differentiate into osteogenic, chondrogenic, adipogenic, and myogenic mesenchymal cell lineage, in addition to others.[77] Adipose-derived stem cells are more favorable for bone regeneration than other multipotent stem cells such as bone marrow MSCs owing to the relative ease of collection, abundance, high proliferation, and fast robust mineralization.[80] The ability of silica-calcium phosphate composite (SCPC) scaffold seeded with human adipose-derived stem cells to regenerate bone in a critical size canine calvarial defect was evaluated (Ahmed El-Ghannam, Unpublished data, 2019). Bone tissue regeneration and graft material resorption was evaluated ay 3 and 6 months postoperative using computed tomography scanning and histology. Calvarial defects grafted with SCPC alone or SCPC-cell construct were grossly repaired, whereas a control ungrafted defect did not repair. Microscopically, the newly formed bone in the grafted defects was compact and integrated with the surrounding host tissues. Histomorphometric analysis demonstrated higher bone surface area and near complete graft material resorption in defects grafted with SCPC-cell hybrid compared with SCPC alone. Resorption of the graft material takes place by 2 mechanisms, solution mediated or cell mediated. These 2 mechanisms are intertwined; the dissolution of ions from bioactive ceramic into tissue fluids stimulates bone cell function and tissue formation. The enhanced resorbability of SCPC preseeded with differentiated osteoblasts points to the significant role played by these cells in the resorption of the graft material.

Vascularization of the newly formed bone is essential for tissue viability and functionality. The composition and porosity of the bone graft can facilitate vascularization and perfect the quality of the bone. Silicon ion release from the bioactive ceramic facilitates endothelization. Histologic analysis done on critical size saddle-type bone defects grafted with SCPC were noticeably vascularized.[81] In addition, in vivo and in vitro studies showed that silica plays an important role in bone cell differentiation and mineralized tissue formation.[82–86] A systematic increase of silica in calcium phosphate ceramic showed a significant increase in alkaline phosphatase activity and collagenous protein synthesis.[87] Other studies have showed that silica plays important role in the synthesis and stabilization of collagen I.[88] Calcium ions facilitate osteogenic gene expression and many cell functions, including mineralization of the collagenous bone matrix. Mineralization of the collagenous matrix is further enhanced by the alkaline pH created when the bioactive ceramic releases sodium ions into the surrounding tissue fluids.[89]

The efficacy of MSCs matrix graft in promoting healing is attributed to multiple mechanisms including osteoconduction, osteoinduction, and osteogenesis. The 3D porous scaffold provides guided bone growth in 3 dimensions, similar to natural bone. In addition, protein adsorption and surface characteristics enhance cell adhesion and osteoblastic differentiation. The high number of differentiated cells preseeded on the porous matrix provides more bone-forming cells necessary to expedite abundant bone formation. Nevertheless, barriers to the application of this bone engineering technology in bone grafting is related to the absence of a therapeutic strategy for the sterilization, packaging, and preservation of an MSC matrix hybrid to make it readily available for grafting applications. Culture and expansion of cells in vitro before seeding on the matrix is a lengthy process with complicated logistics; therefore, it presents operational hurdles at the clinical stage.[90,91] Moreover, the concentration of osteogenic cells from fresh bone marrow by selective adhesion is recommended to eliminate the remnant of the animal protein added to the tissue culture medium during cell expansion.[91,92] Cryopreservation has been used for the long-term storage of MSCs, enabling cells to be expanded in culture when needed, with full retention of functionality after thawing.[92,93] These studies clearly indicate that seeding porous biomaterial matrix with cryopreserved MSCs and using the MSC matrix construct as a bone graft is a promising approach that can enable enhanced bone reconstruction. Therefore, cryopreservation and storage of cell material constructs can maintain the osteogenic activities of stem cells and provide a strategy for unlimited supply of off-the-shelf tissue engineered bone graft for immediate use in craniofacial and maxillofacial surgeries.

SUMMARY AND FUTURE DIRECTIONS

Current soft and hard tissue engineering advancements, as discussed in this article, involve enhancements of the graft, that is, increased vascularization, the addition of stem cells for cellular proliferation, bone graft composite ratios, or improvements to the donor site (via scaffolds).Future directions include inducing human MSCs to proliferate into either soft or hard tissues via selective microRNA expression from mechanotransduction.[94] Nanotechnology presents exciting potential through developments in electrospun poly-L-lactic nanofiber meshes for stem cell culturing as well as nanofiber yarns that provide strong 3D scaffolds for interwoven cell lines.[95,96]

REFERENCES

1. Kim RY, Bae SS, Feinberg SE. Soft tissue engineering. Oral Maxillofacial Surg Clin N Am 2017;29(1):89–104.
2. Deeb GR, Deeb JG. Soft tissue grafting around teeth and implants. Oral Maxillofacial Surg Clin N Am 2015;27(3):425–48.
3. Sculean A, Chappuis V, Cosgarea R. Coverage of mucosal recessions at dental implants. Periodontol 2000 2017;73(1):134–40.
4. Reddy SSP. Pinhole surgical technique for treatment of marginal tissue recession: a case series. J Indian Soc Periodontol 2017;21(6):507–11.
5. Lee CT, Hamalian T, Schulze-Spate U. Minimally invasive treatment of soft tissue deficiency around an implant-supported restoration in the esthetic zone: modified VISTA technique case report. J Oral Implantol 2015;41(1):71–6.
6. Levine RA, Huynh-Ba G, Cochran DL. Soft tissue augmentation procedures for mucogingival defects in esthetic sites. Int J Oral Maxillofac Implants 2014; 29(Suppl):155–85.
7. Wolff J, Farre-Guasch E, Sandor GK, et al. Soft tissue augmentation techniques and materials used in the oral cavity: an overview. Implant Dent 2016;25(3): 427–34.
8. Menceva Z, Dimitrovski O, Popovska M, et al. Free gingival graft versus mucograft: histological evaluation. Open Access Maced J Med Sci 2018;6(4):675–9.
9. Weinreb M, Nemcovsky CE. In vitro models for evaluation of periodontal wound healing/regeneration. Periodontol 2000 2015;68(1):41–54.
10. Roh JL, Loo J, Jang H, et al. Use of oral mucosal cell sheets for accelerated oral surgical wound healing. Head Neck 2018;40(2):394–401.

11. Moharamzadeh K, Colley H, Murdoch C, et al. Tissue-engineered oral mucosa. J Dent Res 2012;91(7):642–50.
12. Han J, Menicanin D, Gronthos S, et al. Stem cells, tissue engineering and periodontal regeneration. Aust Dent J 2014;59(Suppl 1):117–30.
13. Fu Y, Deng S, Wang J, et al. Potential replication of induced pluripotent stem cells for craniofacial reconstruction. Curr Stem Cell Res Ther 2014;9(3):205–14.
14. Chamila Prageeth Pandula PK, Samaranayake LP, Jin LJ, et al. Periodontal ligament stem cells: an update and perspectives. J Investig Clin Dent 2014;5(2): 81–90.
15. Bojic S, Volarevic V, Ljujic B, et al. Dental stem cells–characteristics and potential. Histol Histopathol 2014;29(6):699–706.
16. Hynes K, Menichanin D, Bright R, et al. Induced pluripotent stem cells: a new frontier for stem cells in dentistry. J Dent Res 2015;94(11):1508–15.
17. Mitsiadis TA, Orsini G, Jimenez-Rojo L. Stem cell-based approaches in dentistry. Eur Cell Mater 2015;30:248–57.
18. Yin Y, Li X, He XT, et al. Leveraging stem cell homing for therapeutic regeneration. J Dent Res 2017;96(6):601–9.
19. Kondo R, Atsuta I, Ayukawa Y, et al. Therapeutic interaction of systemically-administered mesenchymal stem cells with peri-implant mucosa. PLoS One 2014;9(3):e90681.
20. Lin Y, Gallucci GO, Buser D, et al. Bioengineered periodontal tissue formed on titanium dental implants. J Dent Res 2011;90(2):251–6.
21. Woloszyk A, Liccardo D, Mitsiadis TA. Three-dimensional imaging of the developing vasculature within stem cell-seeded scaffolds cultured in ovo. Front Physiol 2016;7:146.
22. Akcali A, Schneider D, Unlu F, et al. Soft tissue augmentation of ridge defects in the maxillary anterior area using two different methods: a randomized controlled clinical trial. Clin Oral Implants Res 2015;26(6):688–95.
23. Zhang Q, Johnson JA, Dunne LW, et al. Decellularized skin/adipose tissue flap matrix for engineering vascularized composite soft tissue flaps. Acta Biomater 2016;35:166–84.
24. Sculean A, Nikolidakis D, Nikou G, et al. Biomaterials for promoting periodontal regeneration in human intrabony defects: a systematic review. Periodontol 2000 2015;68(1):182–216.
25. Herford AS, Miller M, Signorino F. Maxillofacial defects and the use of growth factors. Oral Maxillofacial Surg Clin N Am 2017;29(1):75–88.
26. Melville JC, Tursun R, Green JM 3rd, et al. Reconstruction of a post-traumatic maxillary ridge using a radial forearm free flap and immediate tissue engineering (bone morphogenetic protein, bone marrow aspirate concentrate, and cortical-cancellous bone): case report. J Oral Maxillofac Surg 2017;75(2):438.e1-6.
27. Jan A, Sandor GK, Brkovic BB, et al. Effect of hyperbaric oxygen on demineralized bone matrix and biphasic calcium phosphate bone substitutes. Oral Surg Oral Med Oral Pathol Oral Radiol Endod 2010;109(1):59–66.
28. Shao H, Sun M, Zhang F, et al. Custom repair of mandibular bone defects with 3D printed bioceramic scaffolds. J Dent Res 2018;97(1):68–76.
29. Pandit N, Pandit I. Autogenous bone grafts in periodontal practice: a literature review. J Int Clin Dent Res Organ 2016;8(1):27–33.
30. Herford AS, Lu M, Buxton AN, et al. Recombinant human bone morphogenetic protein 2 combined with an osteoconductive bulking agent for mandibular continuity defects in nonhuman primates. J Oral Maxillofac Surg 2012;70(3):703–16.

31. Devescovi V, Leonardi E, Ciapetti G, et al. Growth factors in bone repair. Chir Organi Mov 2008;92(3):161–8.

32. Tripathi G, Sugiura Y, Kareiva A, et al. Feasibility evaluation of low-crystallinity β-tricalcium phosphate blocks as a bone substitute fabricated by a dissolution–precipitation reaction from α-tricalcium phosphate blocks. J Biomater Appl 2018;33(2):259–70.

33. El Bialy I, Jiskoot W, Reza Nejadnik M. Formulation, delivery and stability of bone morphogenetic proteins for effective bone regeneration. Pharm Res 2017;34(6): 1152–70.

34. Chen D, Zhao M, Mundy GR. Bone morphogenetic proteins. Growth Factors 2004;22(4):233–41.

35. Lissenberg-Thunnissen SN, de Gorter DJ, Sier CF, et al. Use and efficacy of bone morphogenetic proteins in fracture healing. Int Orthop 2011;35(9):1271–80.

36. Herford AS. The use of recombinant human bone morphogenetic protein-2 (rhBMP-2) in maxillofacial trauma. Chin J Traumatol 2017;20(1):1–3.

37. McKay WF, Peckham SM, Badura JM. A comprehensive clinical review of recombinant human bone morphogenetic protein-2 (INFUSE Bone Graft). Int Orthop 2007;31(6):729–34.

38. Fiorellini JP, Howell TH, Cochran D, et al. Randomized study evaluating recombinant human bone morphogenetic protein-2 for extraction socket augmentation. J Periodontol 2005;76(4):605–13.

39. Boyne PJ, Marx RE, Nevins M, et al. A feasibility study evaluating rhBMP-2/absorbable collagen sponge for maxillary sinus floor augmentation. Int J Periodontics Restorative Dent 1997;17(1):11–25.

40. Boyne PJ, Lilly LC, Marx RE, et al. De novo bone induction by recombinant human bone morphogenetic protein-2 (rhBMP-2) in maxillary sinus floor augmentation. J Oral Maxillofac Surg 2005;63(12):1693–707.

41. Herford AS, Boyne PJ, Rawson R, et al. Bone morphogenetic protein-induced repair of the premaxillary cleft. J Oral Maxillofac Surg 2007;65(11):2136–41.

42. Simmonds MC, Brown JV, Heirs MK, et al. Safety and effectiveness of recombinant human bone morphogenetic protein-2 for spinal fusion: a meta-analysis of individual-participant data. Ann Intern Med 2013;158(12):877–89.

43. Carragee EJ, Hurwitz EL, Weiner BK. A critical review of recombinant human bone morphogenetic protein-2 trials in spinal surgery: emerging safety concerns and lessons learned. Spine J 2011;11(6):471–91.

44. Conway JD, Shabtai L, Bauernschub A, et al. BMP-7 versus BMP-2 for the treatment of long bone nonunion. Orthopedics 2014;37(12):e1049–57.

45. Lee KB, Taghavi CE, Murray SS, et al. BMP induced inflammation: a comparison of rhBMP-7 and rhBMP-2. J Orthop Res 2012;30(12):1985–94.

46. Vaccaro AR, Whang PG, Patel T, et al. The safety and efficacy of OP-1 (rhBMP-7) as a replacement for iliac crest autograft for posterolateral lumbar arthrodesis: minimum 4-year follow-up of a pilot study. Spine J 2008;8(3):457–65.

47. Ayoub A, Roshan CP, Gillgrass T, et al. The clinical application of rhBMP-7 for the reconstruction of alveolar cleft. J Plast Reconstr Aesthet Surg 2016;69(1):101–7.

48. Castro-Nunez J, Cunningham LL, Van Sickels JE. Atrophic mandible fractures: are bone grafts necessary? An update. J Oral Maxillofac Surg 2017;75(11): 2391–8.

49. Wang W, Yeung KWK. Bone grafts and biomaterials substitutes for bone defect repair: a review. Bioact Mater 2017;2(4):224–47.

50. Campana V, Milano G, Pagano E, et al. Bone substitutes in orthopaedic surgery: from basic science to clinical practice. J Mater Sci Mater Med 2014;25(10): 2445–61.

51. Dickson G, Buchanan F, Marsh D, et al. Orthopaedic tissue engineering and bone regeneration. Technol Health Care 2007;15(1):57–67.

52. Hollinger JO, Winn S, Bonadio J. Options for tissue engineering to address challenges of the ageing skeleton. Tissue Eng 2000;6(4):341–50.

53. Craniomaxillofacial Implants Market by Type (Mid Face, Plates, Screws, Mandibular Orthognathic Implants, Neuro, Mesh, Bone Graft, Dural Repair), by Material of construction (titanium, polymer), by application site & property - global Forecasts to 2021.

54. Ludwig SC, Kowalski JM, Boden SD. Osteoinductive bone graft substitutes. Eur Spine J 2000;9(Suppl 1):S119–25.

55. De Long WG Jr, Einhorn TA, Koval K, et al. Bone grafts and bone graft substitutes in orthopaedic trauma surgery. A critical analysis. J Bone Joint Surg Am 2007; 89(3):649–58.

56. Jahangir AA, Nunley RM, Mehta S, et al. Bone-graft substitutes in orthopaedic surgery. AAOS Now 2008.

57. Stevenson S, Horowitz M. The response to bone allografts. J Bone Joint Surg Am 1992;74(6):939–50.

58. Pelletier MH, Cordaro N, Punjabi VM, et al. PEEK versus Ti interbody fusion devices: resultant fusion, bone apposition, initial and 26-week biomechanics. Clin Spine Surg 2016;29(4):E208–14.

59. Phan K, Hogan JA, Assem Y, et al. PEEK-Halo effect in interbody fusion. J Clin Neurosci 2016;24:138–40.

60. Rao PJ, Pelletier MH, Walsh WR, et al. Spine interbody implants: material selection and modification, functionalization and bioactivation of surfaces to improve osseointegration. Orthop Surg 2014;6(2):81–9.

61. Walsh WR, Bertollo N, Christou C, et al. Plasma-sprayed titanium coating to polyetheretherketone improves the bone-implant interface. Spine J 2015;15(5): 1041–9.

62. Walsh WR, Pelletier MH, Bertollo N, et al. Does PEEK/HA enhance bone formation compared with PEEK in a sheep cervical fusion model? Clin Orthop Relat Res 2016;474(11):2364–72.

63. Wu SH, Li Y, Zhang YQ, et al. Porous titanium-6 aluminum-4 vanadium cage has better osseointegration and less micromotion than a poly-ether-ether-ketone cage in sheep vertebral fusion. Artif Organs 2013;37(12):E191–201.

64. Decking R, Reuter P, Huttner M, et al. Surface composition analysis of failed cementless CoCr- and Ti-base-alloy total hip implants. J Biomed Mater Res B Appl Biomater 2003;64(2):99–106.

65. Meneghini RM, Daluga A, Soliman M. Mechanical stability of cementless tibial components in normal and osteoporotic bone. J Knee Surg 2011;24(3):191–6.

66. Pap T, Claus A, Ohtsu S, et al. Osteoclast-independent bone resorption by fibroblast-like cells. Arthritis Res Ther 2003;5(3):R163–73.

67. Yang J, Ni B, Liu J, et al. Application of liposome-encapsulated hydroxycamptothecin in the prevention of epidural scar formation in New Zealand white rabbits. Spine J 2011;11(3):218–23.

68. Lindhe J, Cecchinato D, Donati M, et al. Ridge preservation with the use of deproteinized bovine bone mineral. Clin Oral Implants Res 2014;25(7):786–90.

69. Stavropoulos A, Kostopoulos L, Mardas N, et al. Deproteinized bovine bone used as an adjunct to guided bone augmentation: an experimental study in the rat. Clin Implant Dent Relat Res 2001;3(3):156–65.

70. Piattelli M, Favero GA, Scarano A, et al. Bone reactions to anorganic bovine bone (Bio-Oss) used in sinus augmentation procedures: a histologic long-term report of 20 cases in humans. Int J Oral Maxillofac Implants 1999;14(6):835–40.

71. Bianco P, Robey PG. Stem cells in tissue engineering. Nature 2001;414(6859): 118–21.

72. Lennon DP, Haynesworth SE, et al. Human and animal mesenchymal progenitor cells from bone marrow: Identification of serum for optimal selection and proliferation. In Vitro Cellular & Developmental Biology - Animal 1996;32(10):602–11.

73. Ohgushi H, Goldberg VM, Caplan AI. Repair of bone defects with marrow cells and porous ceramic. Experiments in rats. Acta Orthop Scand 1989;60(3):334–9.

74. Arinzeh TL, Peter SJ, Archambault MP, et al. Allogeneic mesenchymal stem cells regenerate bone in a critical-sized canine segmental defect. J Bone Joint Surg Am 2003;85-a(10):1927–35.

75. Connolly JF. Injectable bone marrow preparations to stimulate osteogenic repair. Clin Orthop Relat Res 1995;(313):8–18.

76. Horwitz EM, Gordon PL, Koo WK, et al. Isolated allogeneic bone marrow-derived mesenchymal cells engraft and stimulate growth in children with osteogenesis imperfecta: implications for cell therapy of bone. Proc Natl Acad Sci U S A 2002;99(13):8932–7.

77. Levi B, James AW, Wan DC, et al. Regulation of human adipose-derived stromal cell osteogenic differentiation by insulin-like growth factor-1 and platelet-derived growth factor-alpha. Plast Reconstr Surg 2010;126(1):41–52.

78. Zuk PA, Zhu M, Mizuno H, et al. Multilineage cells from human adipose tissue: implications for cell-based therapies. Tissue Eng 2001;7(2):211–28.

79. Raposo-Amaral CE, Bueno DF, Almeida AB, et al. Is bone transplantation the gold standard for repair of alveolar bone defects? J Tissue Eng 2014;5. 2041731413519352.

80. Xu Y, Malladi P, Wagner DR, et al. Adipose-derived mesenchymal cells as a potential cell source for skeletal regeneration. Curr Opin Mol Ther 2005;7(4):300–5.

81. Fahmy RA, Mahmoud N, Soliman S, et al. Acceleration of alveolar ridge augmentation using a low dose of recombinant human bone morphogenetic protein-2 loaded on a resorbable bioactive ceramic. J Oral Maxillofac Surg 2015;73(12): 2257–72.

82. El-Ghannam A. Bone reconstruction: from bioceramics to tissue engineering. Expert Rev Med Devices 2005;2(1):87–101.

83. Gupta G, Zbib A, El-Ghannam A, et al. Characterization of a novel bioactive composite using advanced X-ray computed tomography. Compos Struct 2005;71(3): 423–8.

84. El-Ghannam A, Ning CQ. Effect of bioactive ceramic dissolution on the mechanism of bone mineralization and guided tissue growth in vitro. J Biomed Mater Res A 2006;76(2):386–97.

85. Gupta G, Kirakodu S, El-Ghannam A. Dissolution kinetics of a Si-rich nanocomposite and its effect on osteoblast gene expression. J Biomed Mater Res A 2007;80(2):486–96.

86. Gupta G, El-Ghannam A, Kirakodu S, et al. Enhancement of osteoblast gene expression by mechanically compatible porous Si-rich nanocomposite. J Biomed Mater Res B Appl Biomater 2007;81(2):387–96.

87. Ning CQ, Mehta J, El-Ghannam A. Effects of silica on the bioactivity of calcium phosphate composites in vitro. J Mater Sci Mater Med 2005;16(4):355–60.
88. Reffitt DM, Ogston N, Jugdaohsingh R, et al. Orthosilicic acid stimulates collagen type 1 synthesis and osteoblastic differentiation in human osteoblast-like cells in vitro. Bone 2003;32(2):127–35.
89. Galow AM, Rebl A, Koczan D, et al. Increased osteoblast viability at alkaline pH in vitro provides a new perspective on bone regeneration. Biochem Biophys Rep 2017;10:17–25.
90. Kruyt MC, de Bruijn JD, Yuan H, et al. Optimization of bone tissue engineering in goats: a peroperative seeding method using cryopreserved cells and localized bone formation in calcium phosphate scaffolds. Transplantation 2004;77(3): 359–65.
91. Muschler GF, Midura RJ. Connective tissue progenitors: practical concepts for clinical applications. Clin Orthop Relat Res 2002;(395):66–80.
92. Bruder SP, Jaiswal N, Haynesworth SE. Growth kinetics, self-renewal, and the osteogenic potential of purified human mesenchymal stem cells during extensive subcultivation and following cryopreservation. J Cell Biochem 1997;64(2): 278–94.
93. Wezeman FH, Guzzino KM. Retention of bone cell viability in mouse calvarial explants after cryopreservation. Cryobiology 1986;23(1):81–7.
94. Frith JE, Kusuma GD, Carthew J, et al. Mechanically-sensitive miRNAs bias human mesenchymal stem cell fate via mTOR signalling. Nat Commun 2018;9(1): 257.
95. Gualandi C, Bloise N, Mauro N, et al. Poly-l-Lactic acid nanofiber-polyamidoamine hydrogel composites: preparation, properties, and preliminary evaluation as scaffolds for human pluripotent stem cell culturing. Macromol Biosci 2016;16(10):1533–44.
96. Wu S, Duan B, Liu P, et al. Fabrication of aligned nanofiber polymer yarn networks for anisotropic soft tissue scaffolds. ACS Appl Mater Interfaces 2016;8(26): 16950–60.

What is the Best Micro and Macro Dental Implant Topography?

Khalid Almas, BDS, MSc, FRACDS, MSc, FDSRCS, DDPHRCS, FICD[a],*,
Steph Smith, BChD, BChD (Hons), MDent, MChD[a],
Ahmad Kutkut, DDS, MS, FICOI, DICOI[b]

KEYWORDS

- Implant topography • Micro topography • Macro topography • Osseointegration
- Implant surface characteristics • Implant surface roughness
- Nanorough implant surfaces • Implants biocompatibility

KEY POINTS

- Micro and macro properties of an implant surface determine the magnitude of the biologic response. Therefore, they influence the rate and quality of early osseointegration.
- Modifications to implant surfaces have enhanced long-term implant success. Because of the risk of peri-implantitis, the identification of an optimal implant surface topography is needed.
- Selection of an implant system and topography is based on the clinical circumstances, as well as the clinician's skills and familiarity with the manufacturer's protocols.

INTRODUCTION

The biological fixation between an implant surface and bone is defined as osseointegration (OI).[1] During OI, direct bone-to-implant contact (BIC) is established without an intervening connective tissue layer. Over the last few decades, the influence of implant surface characteristics on the biological response has been extensively investigated. The physicochemical properties of the implant surface influence the reaction of surrounding tissue. This occurs between 4 and 14 days after implant insertion.[2] The reactions include upregulation of gene expression and induction of angiogenesis, osteogenesis, and neurogenesis,[3] through cellular responses such as cell adhesion, proliferation, differentiation, and migration.[4] Enhancement of implant surfaces to improve early OI has led researchers to investigate OI in relation

Disclosure: The authors have nothing to disclose.
[a] Division of Periodontology, Department of Preventive Dental Sciences, College of Dentistry, Imam Abdulrahman Bin Faisal University, P O Box. 1982, Dammam 31441, Saudi Arabia;
[b] Division of Prosthodontics, University of Kentucky, College of Dentistry, D646, 800 Rose Street, Lexington, KY 40536, USA
* Corresponding author.
E-mail addresses: kalmas@iau.edu.sa; khalidalmas9@gmail.com

Dent Clin N Am 63 (2019) 447–460
https://doi.org/10.1016/j.cden.2019.02.010
0011-8532/19/© 2019 Elsevier Inc. All rights reserved.

dental.theclinics.com

to bone mineral precipitation, protein deposition, and cell stimulation.[5,6] The exact implant micro and macro surface characteristics necessary for optimum OI remain to be identified.

The topographic parameters that have been identified to determine the success of OI include (1) the chemical composition, (2) the hydrophobicity/hydrophilicity of the surface, and (3) the roughness of the implant surface.[7,8] This article focuses on the effect of implant surface designs and characteristics on cellular responses that relate directly to early OI. This is the basis for current treatment protocols, including immediate or early loading.[9,10]

CHEMICAL COMPOSITION
Biocompatibility

A biomaterial is determined to be biocompatible when the material or its degradation products do not induce inflammatory reactions.[11] A biocompatible material also allows for the regulation of adsorption and configuration of proteins within the extracellular matrix (ECM). The molecular composition and 3-dimensional structure of the ECM forms a tissue scaffold for cell migration and anchorage.[4] Extracellular matrix proteins, such as collagen, fibronectin, and vitronectin, bind to integrins on osteoblasts, stimulating intracellular signaling pathways within the cytoplasm, cytoskeleton, and nucleus.[4,12] These signaling pathways result in the upregulation of transcription factors that are responsible for the expression of bone matrix formation genes.[13]

Commercially Pure Titanium and Titanium Alloy Implants

The primary factor contributing to the biocompatibility of commercially pure titanium (cpTi) is the spontaneous build-up of a stable and inert oxide layer.[2] This oxide coating is highly adherent and is spontaneously capable of repairing itself if damaged by the surrounding environment.[13] However, physicochemical differences exist when a titanium alloy is created. **Table 1**.

Titanium (Ti) grade 1 has the lowest strength, but it has the highest formability and corrosion resistance. Titanium grade 4 has very high strength, with moderate formability.[2,13] On the other hand, Ti grade 5 (also known as Ti-6Al-4V alloy) is the strongest among other Ti alloys. It has superior corrosion resistance, high fatigue strength, improved fracture resistance,[14] and low elastic modulus, which reduces stress shielding.[13] The Ti-6Al-4V alloy is preferred in the posterior jaw, where occlusal forces are high.[13] However, cpTi implants have demonstrated higher removal torque values and higher bone contacts than Ti-6Al-4V implants.[15]

Studies have shown that osteoclasts corrode Ti surfaces. In addition, extracellular fluids contain metal-binding proteins. The combination of corrosion and metal-binding proteins causes the release of titanium debris into the surrounding soft tissues, thereby inducing inflammatory reactions.[16] Ti alloys release vanadium and aluminum (detectable locally and systemically in tissues), causing possible toxic effects.[17] Vanadium-free and aluminum-free Ti alloys have been introduced, and nontoxic elements such as zirconium, niobium, tantalum, palladium, and indium have been incorporated to enhance biocompatibility.[18] Binary titanium zirconium (TiZr) alloy has been shown to retain biocompatibility by maintaining the same alpha structure as cpTi. In addition, it is not affected by sandblasting, large grit, acid-etched (SLA), and SLActive treatments. TiZr is particularly indicated for use in small-diameter implant applications because of improved strength.[18] However, further ongoing comparative studies on the different surface characteristics need

Table 1
Physicochemical features of cpTi and Ti alloys

Grade	Composition	Physical Properties
1	Commercially pure titanium Oxygen 0.18% max Nitrogen 0.03% max Carbon 0.08% max Iron 0.2% max Hydrogen 0.015% max Titanium 99%	• Softest • Most ductile • Greatest formability • Excellent corrosion resistance • High impact toughness
4	Commercially pure titanium Oxygen 0.4% max Nitrogen 0.05% max Carbon 0.08% max Iron 0.5% max Hydrogen 0.015% max Titanium 99%	• Excellent corrosion resistance • Good formability and weldability
5	Ti 6Al-4V titanium alloys Oxygen 0.2% max Nitrogen 0.05% max Carbon 0.08% max Iron 0.4% max Hydrogen 0.015% max Aluminum 5.5%–6.75% Vanadium 3.5%–4.5% Titanium 90%	• Heat treated to increase its strength • Useful formability • High corrosion resistance

to be conducted to assess these new Ti alloys for their potential use in clinical application.[17,18]

Zirconium implants

Zirconium is highly reactive with water and oxygen. During this reaction, a crystalline dioxide, zirconia (ZrO_2), is formed.[1] The alloying of ZrO_2 with yttrium (Y_2O_3) produces a stable tetragonal structure at room temperature known as yttrium tetragonal zirconia polycrystal (Y-TZP).[19] Y-TZP has increased fracture strength and toughness,[20] increased corrosion and wear resistance, high flexural strength, and low thermal conductivity.[21] Y-TZP can also be toughened by adding alumina.[3] ZrO_2 has been shown to be as osteoconductive and biocompatible as Ti,[22] provoking less tissue reaction and minimum ion leakage when compared with Ti.[23]

Bone healing around ZrO_2 implants is similar to that around Ti implants. Intramembranous osteogenesis occurs and leads to the generation of woven bone. This process is initially accompanied by the formation of parallel-fibered and lamellar bone. Thus, trabecular bone is created earlier than compact bone.[23]

ZrO_2 has been suggested to be clinically suitable because of its tooth-like color, which has the advantage of avoiding the complication of a bluish discoloration of the overlying gingiva. This can be seen and ascribed to crestal bone loss and gingival recession associated with metal implants.[24] However, the clinical use of ZrO_2 dental implants is limited because surface modifications are difficult, and smooth ZrO_2 implant surfaces do not promote OI.[25] Clinical trials with long-term follow-ups are warranted to evaluate the clinical performance and predictability of ZrO_2 implants before recommending them for routine clinical use.[20,24]

HYDROPHOBICITY/HYDROPHILICITY (SURFACE WETTABILITY)

The property of hydrophobicity and/or hydrophilicity (surface wettability) of an implant surface is important to OI.[26] This is expressed by the water contact angle (CA) that ranges from 0° on very hydrophilic surfaces to greater than 90° on hydrophobic surfaces.[27] Wettability is directly influenced by surface free energy (SFE), which is defined as the interaction between the forces of adhesion and the forces of cohesion, that is, the spreading of a liquid over the implant surface.[28] Surface free energy is measured indirectly (quantified) by the liquid-solid CA.[29] It is affected by the surface chemical composition, surface charge, and microstructural topography.[30]

When surfaces are roughened by means of anodization, etching, blasting, or a combination of blasting and etching, CAs are changed, thus affecting the surface wetability.[29,31] Increased CAs are usually associated with increased roughness on nontreated surfaces. However, modified surfaces that incorporate differences in roughness can show different CAs.[30] A high SFE promotes increased wettability, thereby enhancing the interaction between the implant surface and the biologic environment.[32] Extremely high SFE can promote cell adhesion, but decreases cell motility and impairs subsequent cell functions.[29] Although hydrophilic surfaces maintain the function of proteins and possess a higher affinity for these proteins than hydrophobic surfaces, hydrophobic surfaces can cause partial denaturation of proteins by exerting conformational changes.[26] As a result, a disturbance of their tertiary structure occurs causing cell-binding sites to be less accessible, consequentially diminishing cell adhesion.[29] Furthermore, hydrophobic surfaces foster hydrocarbon contamination, which can lead to the entrapment of air bubbles thereby interfering with protein adsorption and cell receptor adhesion/activation.[29]

Surface Wettability and Initial Blood Protein/Cellular Interactions

Hydrophilicity influences the selective adhesion of blood proteins and their composition, bonding strength, conformation, and orientation.[29] This leads to the adhesion and activation of thrombocytes and subsequent formation of a blood clot.[33] Activated platelets interact with the implant surface as well as with the fibrin scaffold and then degranulate into the extracellular environment.[34] Degranulation causes the release of growth factors responsible for wound healing[35] as well as the release of differentiation factors responsible for the recruitment, differentiation and proliferation of undifferentiated mesenchymal stem cells (MSCs). This then enhances the differentiation of osteogenic cells and angiogenesis, which promote bone regeneration.[35]

Extracellular matrix proteins, such as fibronectin and albumin, bound to the conditioning layer of dental implants, show a marked reduction in their cell-adhesive function when adsorbed to hydrophobic surfaces.[36] However, the cell-adhesive functionality of fibronectin is enhanced on hydrophilic surfaces, thereby improving a cellular response.[37] The adsorption of type I collagen and vitronectin on hydrophilic surfaces is essential for osteoblast differentiation.[38]

The interaction between blood and biomaterial also initiates the migration of polymorphonuclear leukocytes (PMNs) and macrophages to the wound site, which induces wound healing.[39] Receptor expression and adhesion of PMNs are influenced by surface wettability. CD16 receptors on PMNs bind to hydrophilic surfaces, whereas CD162 receptors bind to hydrophobic surfaces.[40] Macrophages involved in inflammation and maintenance of tissue homeostasis are activated by Interferon gamma secreted from other inflammatory cells and lipopolysaccharide. A balance between pro-inflammatory macrophages (M1) and anti-inflammatory macrophages (regenerative) (M2) is also required for proper healing and biomaterial integration of the implant.[39]

Smooth Ti induces M1 activation, as indicated by increased levels of interleukin-1b (IL-1b), IL-6, and tumor necrosis factor alpha. Hydrophilic rough titanium surfaces induce M2 activation, as depicted by increased levels of IL-4 and IL-10.[39] M2 cells express fibroblast growth factors, transforming growth factors, epithelial growth factor, as well as bone morphogenetic proteins (BMPs), which induce angiogenesis.[39] A decrease in gene expression of M1 markers on hydrophilic rough Ti surfaces has been shown compared with rough hydrophobic surfaces.[41] In addition, increased wettability of microrough surfaces has shown to stimulate more anti-inflammatory cytokine released by macrophages than those on hydrophilic smooth surfaces.[39] The synergistic effect of increased surface roughness and hydrophilicity may induce a microenvironment that reduces healing time and accelerates OI.[39]

Dendritic cells remain in a more immature state when interacting with hydrophilic surfaces. As a result, there is a reduction in the innate immune response causing a noninflammatory environment, which promotes clinical peri-implant bone formation.[42] Multinucleated giant cells derived from either osteoclasts or macrophages have been quantified on different surfaces[43] and seem to be an integral part of the normal OI process.[3] However, whether these cells are responsible for any true foreign body reaction around dental implants is still not clear, and their presence may not predict any future implant loss.[3]

Surface Wettability and Cell Interactions with Preconditioned Surfaces

Adsorbed serum proteins possess cell-binding domains and function as biological signals that activate receptors (integrins) located on the outer membrane of cells.[26,44] Integrins, which recognize a particular amino acid sequence within a protein, may also vary based on cell type and differentiation stage.[45] After initial cellular adhesion, the short- and long-term processes of cellular proliferation and differentiation are determined.[29,44]

Mesenchymal stem cells initially invade the blood clot and colonize the implantation site.[46] The osteoblastic differentiation of MSCs is promoted when hydrophilic surfaces increase the expression of osteocalcin, osteoprotegerin, and integrins.[29] Surface nanomodification induced by differences in surface wettability may be partly responsible for different contributions from osteoblast lineage cells at different stages of osteoblast commitment.[47]

Increased osteogenic differentiation and maturation, as depicted by a significant upregulation of genes associated with the transforming growth factor β/BMP signaling cascade,[48] is associated with increased hydrophilicity, thereby contributing to accelerated OI.[36] Furthermore, implants with moderately rough surfaces with a high level of energy/wettability show greater trabecular density of newly formed woven bone, leading to an increase in the BIC ratio, as well as in the bonding strength of such contact.[35]

Superhydrophilic surfaces, such as smoother acid-etched surfaces, compared with rougher blasted ones, may positively influence the epithelial seal around implants, as well as enhance keratinocyte proliferation, cell spreading, and motility.[49] This results in faster surface coverage, leading to a faster restoration of a tight epithelial seal.[29] Surface nanomodification, enhancing keratinocyte adhesion and spreading and filopodium extension, has been shown on e-beam-evaporated (nanorough) surfaces with intermediate surface energy compared with anodized (nanotubular) surfaces.[50] Fibroblast morphology and activity may be enhanced on Ti surfaces coated with titanium nickel by physical vapor deposition compared with surfaces that were thermally oxidized or laser irradiated.[51]

Surface Wettability and Bacterial Adhesion

There are contradictory data regarding the influence of surface roughness (Ra), SFE, and chemical alterations of Ti implants on biofilm formation.[52] Ra values greater than 0.2 μm have been shown to lead to an increased rate of biofilm formation, whereas Ra values less than 0.2 μm may have no effect on supragingival and subgingival plaque formation, including no further quantitative or qualitative effects on the microflora.[28] Hydrophilicity and Ra have been shown to drive initial biofilm adhesion and formation, whereas superhydrophilic, chemically modified acid-etched surfaces have shown significantly less initial biofilm formation.[53] Moreover, hydrophobic SLA and machined surfaces increase hydrophobicity, which may be the main force for bacterial adhesion.[53] This is attributed to interactions between hydrophobic implant surface properties and bacterial hydrophobic cell membrane components, as well as adhesins located on fimbria or pili.[54]

Despite surfaces having high hydrophilicity, surface topography has the predominant effect on bacterial attachment, whereas surface charge and wetting have less influence.[55] Microtopography may have a highly erratic influence on supragingival plaque biofilm formation.[56] The attachment of certain bacteria has been shown to be higher on surfaces with nanophase topographies compared with conventional topographies. However, other studies have found nanophase materials to have a bacteria-repelling effect.[57]

Although specific oral bacteria may have high adhesion affinity for titanium surfaces,[58] the clinical situation is far more complex. The in vivo formation of conditioning films by serum proteins may alter the surface properties of biomaterials as soon as they encounter biofluids.[59] Serum proteins may exert a greater effect on the surface adhesion and biofilm formation of oral bacteria in vivo than that observed in vitro.[60] Bacteria use specific adhesion mechanisms to attach to specific serum proteins, such as fibrinogen, fibronectin, collagen, vitronectin, and laminin.[60] Any conformational changes of these proteins during implant surface conditioning may also influence bacterial adhesion.[59] Therefore, indirect biomaterial surface properties, such as chemical composition and nanoscale features, will influence the molecular conformation in the conditioning film during surface protein adsorption, with the latter having a greater influence on bacterial adhesion.[60] However, bacterial attachment remains dependent on multiple factors. Different preferences for attachment to implant surfaces may be attributed to the specific bacteria present, as well as the physicochemical properties of implant surfaces.[52,61]

Surface Wettability and Rate of Osseointegration

Hydrophilicity has a greater role in promoting early bone formation by enhancing osteoblastic differentiation in the early stages of OI compared with hydrophobic surfaces.[62] A synergistic effect has been described between surface microroughness, superhydrophilicity, and bioactive implant surfaces. This leads to enhanced OI, thereby facilitating early loading capacity.[63] Anodized surfaces displaying well-defined nanostructures, which have the lowest surface roughness and highest hydrophilicity, have been shown to promote the highest removal torque. This suggests that hydrophilicity elicits a stronger response compared with surface roughness.[14]

ROUGHNESS OF IMPLANT SURFACES

A positive correlation has been described between surface roughness and bone response compared with the mechanical quality of the BIC interface.[7,8,64] Surface-roughening procedures cause a modification of the surface chemistry.[8] Therefore, it is still unclear whether a predictable implant-to-bone response is mainly because of surface roughness or the related changes in surface chemistry.[8] Surface engineering methods (ie, mechanical, chemical, and physical) have been developed to create various surface compositions to potentially control the biological activity of the implant surface.[8] In vitro studies showed that surface roughness affects the spreading, proliferation, and differentiation of osteoblastic lineage cells and protein synthesis,[65] which leads to an improved BIC outcome.[34] However, in vivo studies do not clearly differentiate whether de novo bone formation occurs by means of distance or contact osteogenesis.[3] Histologic studies have shown signs of bone formation directly on implant surfaces; however, 2-dimensional tissue sections cannot reveal the true 3-dimensional features of the BIC.[3] Depending on the dimension of the measured surface features, implant surface roughness can be divided into microroughness, macroroughness, and nanoroughness.[27]

Biological Response to Macrorough Implant Surfaces

Macroroughness is directly related to implant geometry. Threaded screw and macroporous surface treatments range in scale from millimeters to tens of microns (μm). They present a relatively smooth surface and incorporate surface defects, such as grooves, ridges, and marks.[34] Macroroughness enhances mechanical interlocking between the implant surface and surrounding bone, thereby enhancing primary implant fixation and long-term mechanical stability.[66,67] Macrorough features include implant body shape (parallel and tapered) and various geometric thread patterns.[68,69] In an attempt to preserve crestal bone, implants were designed with a tapered apex and larger cervical diameter (Nobel Speedy Groovy implants). However, tapered implants have greater crestal bone loss compared with parallel implants.[68] Thread geometry affects the distribution of stress forces around the implant.[70] **Table 2** summarizes the effects and the clinical relevance of various macrorough geometric thread patterns.

Osteoblastic cells grow along the grooves on macrorough surfaces, therefore requiring a longer waiting time between surgery and implant loading (3–6 months).[27] Long-term clinical outcomes demonstrate enhanced bone quality when implants with macrorough surfaces are used; however, lower success rates are seen in areas of low bone density.[27]

Biological Response to Microrough Implant Surfaces

Microroughness is defined as being in the range of 1 to 100 μm, and is accomplished by different manufacturing techniques including machining, acid-etching, anodization, sandblasting, grit-blasting, or other coating procedures. These processes increase surface area due to the formation of pits, grooves, and protrusions.[27] Most implants have a surface roughness of 1 to 2 μm, which provides an optimal degree of roughness to promote OI.[72]

Microroughness induces platelets to secrete biological mediators that attract differentiating osteogenic cells and promote adhesion and stabilization of the blood clot, including the formation of the fibrin matrix.[35] The fibrin matrix acts as an osteoconductive scaffold for the migration of osteogenic cells, leading to bone formation on the implant surface.[35] The microtopography alters the growth, metabolism, and migration of these osteogenic cells. The alteration allows for the induction and regulation of the expression of specific osteoblastic integrin subunits that are in contact with the implant. In turn, bone matrix proteins interact with these integrins mediating osteoblast activity.[48,73] In addition to microroughness enhancing mechanical stability, incremental increases of bone along with increased levels of BIC have been demonstrated

Table 2
Effects and clinical relevance of macrorough geometric thread patterns

Irnplants Geometry	Definition	Effects	Clinical Relevance
Thread shape	Thread shapes available for screw-retained implants include square shape, V-shape, and buttress and reverse buttress threads, which are defined by the thread thickness and face angle.[71]	Thread shape plays an important role in stress transfer between the implant and the surrounding tissue and determines the primary stability of the implant.	Effective insertion and force transmission.
Thread pitch	The distance between 2 neighboring threads, measured on the same side of the axis. Also includes the number of threads per unit length.	Has a significant effect because of the available surface area (SA) for BIC. With lower pitch, the number of threads increases, which in turn gives higher SA and BIC and leads to a more favorable stress distribution.	For primary stability and stress production.
Face angle	The angle between the face of a thread and a plane perpendicular to the long axis of the implant.	Shear forces increase as the face angle of the thread increases.	V-shaped thread shows more stability and less stress.
Thread depth (height) and thickness (width)	Thread depth is the distance from the outermost tip to the innermost body of the thread, the difference between the outer/major diameter and the inner/minor diameter of the implant. Thread width is the distance between the superior-most and inferior-most tip of a single thread measured axially.	Deep threads increase the functional SA at the BIC, which can improve primary stability in low bone density or in areas with high occlusal load.	Thread depth and width clinically influence implant insertion and SA. The shallower the thread depth, the easier the implantation procedure, especially in high bone density. It may eliminate the need for tapping during surgery.
Helix angle (lead)	Lead is the distance within the same thread between before and after 1 complete rotation in the axial direction. In a single threaded screw, lead is the same as pitch. In a double or triple threaded screw, lead is double and triple the pitch, respectively.	Lead indicates the distance that an implant would move after 1 turn. It plays an important role in determining the speed of implant insertion.	Lead is clinically significant due to its effect on SA and insertion speed.
Crestal module	Crest module refers to the neck portion of the implant.	Having retentive elements, such as microthreads, results in less marginal bone loss compared with smooth necked implants.[69]	Implant neck configurations can be critical for minimizing marginal bone loss.

(thereby maximizing the interlocking between mineralized bone and implant surface).[8,35,67]

Biological Response to Nanorough Implant Surfaces

Implants with nanoscale modifications ranging in size between 1 and 100 nm have shown higher BIC contact with increased torque removal values after 1 month of placement compared with implants with microrough surfaces.[5] Nanoroughness enhances wound healing by increasing the wettability of the surface to blood, fibrin, matrix proteins, growth, and differentiation factors.[5] Micrometer and nanometer peaks and valleys of nanorough surfaces direct the differentiation of mesenchymal cells toward an osteogenic lineage, and affect the interaction of osteogenic cells with the ECM. This leads to the organization of the cytoskeleton and intracellular transduction signaling pathways, which triggers alterations in cell shape by interacting with cellular filopodia.[74] This influences cell differentiation and the further directive differentiation of already present osteoprogenitor cells toward an osteoblastic phenotype.[74,75] Furthermore, this is associated with increased levels of gene expression, which promote high levels of insulin growth factor 2, BMP2, and BMP6 expression by adherent human MSCs, indicating rapid osteoblastic differentiation.[76]

The interaction between integrins and their ligands on ECM proteins or biomaterials are affected by nanorough surfaces.[77] Cell adhesion is altered by indirect (protein-surface interactions) and direct (cell-surface interactions) mechanisms. During these protein-surface interactions, adherent proteins are interposed with cell integrins. Direct cell to surface interactions allow for integrin receptors to react with the surface and transmit signals to control adhesion, spreading, and motility.[77] This leads to modulation of cell activity, including adhesion, migration, proliferation, and differentiation of osteoblastic cells, thereby influencing the secondary integration of implants, that is, bone growth, turnover, and remodeling.[5]

It is still unknown, however, whether nanostructural topography is directly responsible for the above osteogenic effects, or whether these effects are indirectly a result of the selective adsorption of serum and local tissue fluid proteins. It may also be as a result of the nanostructure-induced increase in surface energy/wettability, whereby all the above mechanisms operate synergistically in bringing about an osteogenic effect.[74] Nanometer-scale topography alone may not be sufficient to assure robust OI. However, micron-level roughness may be additionally needed for OI to incorporate the interlocking of forming tissues with microroughness surfaces.[78]

OVERVIEW OF IMPLANT SYSTEM TOPOGRAPHY

Implant manufacturers have evaluated the roughness of surfaces using the average roughness over a surface in 3-dimensional height (Sa) and the surface height and spatial roughness parameter (Sdr) values.[64,79] See **Table 3**.

Table 3
Sa and Sdr values for commercially available implant surfaces

Implant Surface	Sa (μm)	Sdr (%)
Brånemark implant cp Ti grade 1	0.9	34
TiUnite Nobel Biocare	1.1	37
Sandblasted surface with a large grit and the acid-etched (SLA) Straumann	1.75	143
OsseoSpeed Astra Tech	1.4	37

A systematic review, which evaluated 7711 implants from well-documented implant systems, reported a mean success rate of 89.7% (34.4%–100%) over a mean follow-up time of 13.4 years (10–20 years).[80] Cumulative mean values for the survival rates and marginal bone resorption values were reported to be 94.6% and 1.3 mm, respectively. It was concluded that osseointegrated implants are safe and present a high survival rate with minimal marginal bone resorption in the long term.[80]

SUMMARY

Implant surface topography has an influential effect on the process and rate of OI,[81] as well as on the amount of BIC.[82] However, biocompatibility, surgical technique, status of the host bed, and loading conditions are also contributing factors for successful OI.[83] Implant surfaces with micro-features or nano-features are beneficial for accelerated OI; however, the long-term success is debatable because there is a higher risk of peri-implantitis due to a higher affinity to plaque accumulation.[82] The quality and quantity of newly formed bone on contaminated different implant surfaces still need to be determined.[79]

Although implant surfaces and their composition have been enhanced, no optimal implant surface has yet been identified. However, choosing an implant system should be determined by the individual patient's biological, psychological, and physiologic conditions, as well as the clinician's skills.[79] Further randomized controlled clinical trials are needed to compare various implant systems and surfaces in identically healthy individuals, as well as those with local and systemic risk factors.

REFERENCES

1. Bruschi M, Steinmüller-Nethl D, Goriwoda W, et al. Composition and modifications of dental implant surfaces. J Oral Implants 2015. https://doi.org/10.1155/2015/527426. Article ID 527426.
2. Elias CN, Lima JHC, Valiev R, et al. Biomedical applications of titanium and its alloys. J Miner Met Mater Soc 2008;60:46–9.
3. Bosshardt DD, Chappuis V, Buser D. Osseointegration of titanium, titanium alloy and zirconia dental implants: current knowledge and open questions. Periodontology 2000 2017;73:22–40.
4. Feller L, Jadwat Y, Khammissa RAG, et al. Cellular responses evoked by different surface characteristics of intra osseous titanium implants. Biomed Res Int 2015. https://doi.org/10.1155/2015/171945.
5. Dohan Ehrenfest MD, Coelho PG, Kang B-S, et al. Classification of osseointegrated implant surfaces: materials, chemistry and topography. Trends Biotechnol 2010;28:198–206.
6. Wennerberg A, Albrektsson T. Effects of titanium surface topography on bone integration: a systematic review. Clin Oral Implants Res 2009;20:172–84.
7. Le Guéhennec L, Soueidan A, Layrolle P, et al. Surface treatments of titanium dental implants for rapid osseointegration. Dent Mater 2007;23:844–54.
8. Junker R, Dimakis A, Thoneick M, et al. Effects of implant surface coatings and composition on bone integration: a systematic review. Clin Oral Impl Res 2009; 20(Suppl. 4):185–206.
9. Weber HP, Morton D, Gallucci GO, et al. Consensus statements and recommended clinical procedures regarding loading protocols. Int J Oral Maxillofac Implants 2009;24:180–3.
10. Novaco AB Jr, de Souza SLC, de Barros RPM, et al. Influence of implant surfaces on osseointegration. Braz Dent J 2010;21:471–81.

11. Hisbergues M, Vendeville S, Vendeville P. Zirconia: established facts and per-spectives for a biomaterial in dental implantology. J Biomed Mater Res B Appl Biomater 2009;88:519–29.

12. Josset Y, Oum'Hamed Z, Zarrinpour A, et al. In vitro reactions of human osteo-blasts in culture with zirconia and alumina ceramics. J Biomed Mater Res 1999;47:481–93.

13. Ogle OE. Implant surface material, design, and osseointegration. Dent Clin N Am 2015;59:505–20.

14. Elias CN, Oshida Y, Lima JHC, et al. Relationship between surface properties (roughness, wettability and morphology) of titanium and dental implant removal torque. J Mech Behav Biomed Mater 2008;1:234–42.

15. Johansson CB, Han CH, Wennerberg A, et al. Quantitative comparison of machined commercially pure Ti and Ti-6Al-4V implant in rabbit. J Oral Maxillofac Implants 1998;13:315–21.

16. Cadosch D, Al-Mushaiqri MS, Gautschi OP, et al. Biocorrosion and uptake of tita-nium by human osteoclasts. J Biomed Mater Res A 2010;95A:1004–10.

17. Morais LS, Serra GG, Muller CA, et al. Titanium alloy mini-implants for orthodontic anchorage: Immediate loading and metal ion release. Acta Biomater 2007;3: 331–9.

18. Grandin HM, Berner S, Dard M. A review of titanium zirconium (TiZr) alloys for use in endosseous dental implants. Materials 2012;5:1348–60.

19. Abd El-Ghany OS, Sherief AH. Zirconia based ceramics, some clinical and bio-logical aspects: review. Future Dental J 2016;2:55–64.

20. Pieralli S, Kohal RJ, Jung RE, et al. Clinical outcomes of zirconia dental Implants: a systematic review. J Dent Res 2017;96:38–46.

21. Güngör MB, Aydın C, Yılmaz H, et al. An overview of zirconia dental implants: basic properties and clinical application of three cases. J Oral Implant 2014; 40:485–94.

22. Warashina H, Sakano S, Kitamura S, et al. Biological reaction to alumina, zirconia, titanium and polyethylene particles implanted onto murine calvaria. Biomaterials 2003;24:3655–61.

23. Ved VP, Sequeira VV, Shah DH, et al. Mechanism of osseous healing in zirconia dental implants - a short review. Int J Biol Environ Eng 2018;1:9–12.

24. Özkurt Z, Kazazoglu E. Zirconia dental implants: a literature review. J Oral Implant 2011;37:367–76.

25. Puleo DA, Thomas MV. Implant surfaces. Dent Clin North Am 2006;50:323–38.

26. Terheyden H, Lang NP, Bierbaum S, et al. Osseointegration—communication of cells. Clin Oral Impl Res 2012;23:1127–35.

27. Smeets R, Stadlinger B, Schwarz F, et al. Impact of dental implant surface mod-ifications on osseointegration [review article]. Biomed Res Int 2016;2016. https://doi.org/10.1155/2016/6285620.

28. Dhir S. Biofilm and dental implant: the microbial link. J Indian Soc Periodontol 2013;17:5–11.

29. Gittens RA, Scheideler L, Rupp F, et al. A review on the wettability of dental implant surfaces II: Biological and clinical aspects. Acta Biomater 2014;10: 2907–18.

30. Kim I-H, Kwon T-Y, Kim K-H. Wetting behavior of dental implants, wetting and wettability. IntechOpen 2015. https://doi.org/10.5772/61098.

31. Rupp F, Scheideler L, Eichler M, et al. Wetting behavior of dental implants. Int J Oral Maxillofac Implants 2011;26:1256–66.

32. Kilpadi DV, Lemons JE. Surface-energy characterization of unalloyed titanium implants. J Biomed Mater Res 1994;28:1419–25.

33. Spijker HT, Graaff R, Boonstra PW, et al. On the influence of flow conditions and wettability on blood material interactions. Biomaterials 2003;24:4717–27.

34. Patil PS, Bhongade ML. Dental implant surface modifications: a review. IOSR-JDMS. 2016;15:132–41.

35. Feller L, Chandran R, Khammissa RAG, et al. Osseointegration: biological events in relation to characteristics of the implant surface. SADJ 2014;69:112–7.

36. Zhao G, Schwartz Z, Wieland M, et al. High surface energy enhances cell response to titanium substrate microstructure. J Biomed Mater Res A 2005;74: 49–58.

37. Keselowsky BG, Bridges AW, Burns KL, et al. Role of plasma fibronectin in the foreign body response to biomaterials. Biomaterials 2007;28:3626–31.

38. Salasznyk RM, Williams WA, Boskey A, et al. Adhesion to vitronectin and collagen I promotes osteogenic differentiation of human mesenchymal stem cells. J Biomed Biotechnol 2004;2004:24–34.

39. Hotchkiss KM, Reddy GB, Hyzy SL, et al. Titanium surface characteristics, including topography and wettability, alter macrophage activation. Acta Biomater 2016;31:425–34.

40. Eriksson C, Nygren H. Polymorphonuclear leukocytes in coagulating whole blood recognize hydrophilic and hydrophobic titanium surfaces by different adhesion receptors and show different patterns of receptor expression. J Lab Clin Med 2001;137:296–302.

41. Hamlet S, Alfarsi M, George R, et al. The effect of hydrophilic titanium surface modification on macrophage inflammatory cytokine gene expression. Clin Oral Implant Res 2012;23:584–90.

42. Kou PM, Schwartz Z, Boyan BD, et al. Dendritic cell responses to surface properties of clinical titanium surfaces. Acta Biomater 2011;7:1354–63.

43. Donath K, Laass M, Gunzl HJ. The histopathology of different foreign-body reactions in oral soft tissue and bone tissue. Virchows Arch A Pathol Anat Histopathol 1992;420:131–7.

44. Wilson CJ, Clegg RE, Leavesley DI, et al. Mediation of biomaterial–cell interactions by adsorbed proteins: a review. Tissue Eng 2005;11:1–18.

45. Albertini M, Fernandez-Yague M, Lázaro P, et al. Advances in surfaces and osseointegration in implantology. Biomimetic surfaces. Med Oral Pathol Oral Cir Bucal 2015;1:316–25.

46. Olivares-Navarrete R, Hyzy SL, Hutton DL, et al. Direct and indirect effects of microstructured titanium substrates on the induction of mesenchymal stem cell differentiation towards the osteoblast lineage. Biomaterials 2010;31:2728–35.

47. Gittens RA, Olivares-Navarrete R, Cheng A, et al. The roles of titanium surface micro/nanotopography and wettability on the differential response of human osteoblast lineage cells. Acta Biomater 2013;9:6268–77.

48. Vlacic-Zischke J, Hamlet SM, Friis T, et al. The influence of surface microroughness and hydrophilicity of titanium on the up-regulation of TGF-ß/BMP signaling in osteoblasts. Biomaterials 2011;32:665–71.

49. An N, Rausch-Fan X, Wieland M, et al. Initial attachment, subsequent cell proliferation/viability and gene expression of epithelial cells related to attachment and wound healing in response to different titanium surfaces. Dent Mater 2012;28: 1207–14.

50. Puckett SD, Lee PP, Ciombor DM, et al. Nanotextured titanium surfaces for enhancing skin growth on transcutaneous osseointegrated devices. Acta Biomater 2010;6:2352–62.
51. Groessner-Schreiber B, Neubert A, Muller WD, et al. Fibroblast growth on surface-modified dental implants: an in vitro study. J Biomed Mater Res A 2003;64:591–9.
52. Zaugg LK, Astasov-Frauenhoffer M, Braissant O, et al. Determinants of biofilm formation and cleanability of titanium surfaces. Clin Oral Impl Res 2017;28: 469–75.
53. John G, Becker J, Schwarz F. Modified implant surface with slower and less initial biofilm formation. Clin Implant Dent Relat Res 2015;17:461–8.
54. Doyle RJ. Contribution of the hydrophobic effect to microbial infection. Microb Infect 2000;2:391–400.
55. Lorenzetti M, Dogša I, Stošicki T, et al. The influence of surface modification on bacterial adhesion to titanium-based substrates. ACS Appl Mater Inter 2015;7: 1644–51.
56. Schwarz F, Sculean A, Wieland M, et al. Effects of hydrophilicity and microtopography of titanium implant surfaces on initial supragingival plaque biofilm formation. A pilot study. Mund Kiefer Gesichts Chir 2007;11:333–8.
57. Rizzello L, Sorce B, Sabella S, et al. Impact of nanoscale topography on genomics and proteomics of adherent bacteria. ACS Nano 2011;5:1865–76.
58. Renvert S, Lindahl C, Renvert H. Clinical and microbiological analysis of subjects treated with Branemark or Astratech implants: a 7 year follow up study. Clin Oral Implants Res 2008;19:342–7.
59. Keselowsky BG, Collard DM, Garcia AJ. Surface chemistry modulates fibronectin conformation and directs integrin binding and specificity to control cell adhesion. J Biomed Mater Res A 2003;66A:247–59.
60. MacKintosh EE, Patel JD, Marchant RE, et al. Effects of biomaterial surface chemistry on the adhesion and biofilm formation of *Staphylococcus epidermidis* in vitro. J Biomed Mater Res 2006;78:836–42.
61. Mediaswanti K. Influence of physicochemical aspects of substratum nanosurface on bacterial attachment for bone implant applications. J Nanotechnol 2016;2016. https://doi.org/10.1155/2016/5026184.
62. Eriksson C, Nygren H, Ohlson K. Implantation of hydrophilic and hydrophobic titanium discs in rat tibia: cellular reactions on the surfaces during the first 3 weeks in bone. Biomaterials 2004;25:4759–66.
63. Lang NP, Salvi GE, Huynh-Ba G, et al. Early osseointegration to hydrophilic and hydrophobic implant surfaces in humans. Clin Oral Implants Res 2011;22: 349–56.
64. Wennerberg A, Albrektsson T. On implant surfaces: a review of current knowledge and opinions. Int J Oral Maxillofac Implants 2010;25:63–74.
65. Zhao G, Zinger O, Schwartz Z, et al. Osteoblast like cells are sensitive to submicron-scale surface structure. Clin Oral Implants Res 2006;17:258–64.
66. Wennerberg A, Albrektsson T, Andersson B. Bone tissue response to commercially pure titanium implants blasted with fine and coarse particles of aluminum oxide. Int J Oral Maxillofac Implants 1996;11:38–45.
67. Shalabi MM, Gortemaker A, Van't Hof MA, et al. Implant surface roughness and bone healing: a systematic review. J Dent Res 2006;85:496–500.
68. Dagorne C, Malet J, Bizouard G, et al. Clinical evaluation of two dental implant macrostructures on peri-implant bone loss: a comparative, retrospective study. Clin Oral Implants Res 2014;26:307–13.

69. Abuhussein H, Pagni G, Rebaudi A, et al. The effect of thread pattern upon implant osseointegration. Clin Oral Implants Res 2010;21:129–36.
70. Al-Thobity AM, Kutkut A, Almas K. Micro threaded implants and crestal bone loss: a systematic review. J Oral Implantol 2017;43:157–66.
71. Boggan RS, Strong JT, Misch CE, et al. Influence of hex geometry and prosthetic table width on static and fatigue strength of dental implants. J Prosthet Dent 1999;82:436–40.
72. Albrektsson T, Wennerberg A. Part 1–review focusing on topographic and chemical properties of different surfaces and in vivo responses to them. Int J Prosthodont 2004;17:536–43.
73. Zhao G, Raines AL, Wieland M, et al. Requirement for both micron- and submicron scale structure for synergistic responses of osteoblasts to substrate surface energy and topography. Biomaterials 2007;28:2821–9.
74. de Oliveira PT, Zalzal SF, Beloti MM, et al. Enhancement of in vitro osteogenesis on titanium by chemically produced nanotopography. J Biomed Mater Res A 2007;80:554–64.
75. Bucci-Sabattini V, Cassinelli C, Coelho PG, et al. Effect of titanium implant surface nanoroughness and calcium phosphate low impregnation on bone cell activity in vitro. Oral Surg Oral Med Oral Pathol Oral Radiol Endod 2010;109:217–24.
76. Guo J, Padilla RJ, Ambrose W, et al. Modification of TiO2 grit blasted titanium implants by hydrofluoric acid treatment alters adherent osteoblast gene expression in vitro and in vivo. Biomaterials 2007;28:5418–25.
77. Mendonça G, Mendonça DBS, Aragão FJL, et al. Advancing dental implant surface technology—from micron- to nanotopography. Biomaterials 2008;29:3822–35.
78. Davies JE. Understanding peri-implant endosseous healing. J Dent Educ 2003;67:932–49.
79. Lee J, Ku Y. What is an ideal implant surface? Indian J Dent Res 2016;27:341–2.
80. Moraschini V, Poubel LA, Ferreira VF, et al. Evaluation of survival and success rates of dental implants reported in longitudinal studies with a follow-up period of at least 10 years: a systematic review. Int J Oral Maxillofac Surg 2015;44:377–88.
81. Albrektsson T, Zarb GA, Worthington P, et al. The long term efficacy of current used dental implants: a review and proposed criteria of success. Int J Oral Maxillofac Implants 1986;1:11–25.
82. Parlar A, Bosshardt DD, Cetiner D, et al. Effects of decontamination and implant surface characteristics on re-osseointegration following treatment of peri-implantitis. Clin Oral Implants Res 2009;20:391–9.
83. Esposito M, Coulthard P, Thomsen P, et al. Interventions for replacing missing teeth: different types of dental implants. Cochrane Database Syst Rev 2005;(25):CD003815.

Can Osseointegration Be Achieved Without Primary Stability?

Mohanad Al-Sabbagh, DDS, MS[a],*, Walied Eldomiaty, BDS[b],
Yasser Khabbaz, DDS, MS[c]

KEYWORDS

- Primary stability • Secondary stability • Osseointegration • Bone density
- Insertion torque • Resonance frequency analysis • Bone-to-implant contact (BIC)

KEY POINTS

- Factors influencing primary stability include implant design, bone density, and surgical techniques used.
- Implant primary stability is not an absolute prerequisite to osseointegration; however, it has an effect on the implant survival rate.
- Resonance Frequency analysis is the most frequent method used by clinician to assess both primary and secondary stability.

INTRODUCTION

The term osseointegration was coined and first defined in 1977 as a direct structural and functional connection between living bone and the surface of a load-carrying implant.[1] Histologically, osseointegration can be identified by the presence of regenerated bone at the implant-bone interface. For dental implant osseointegration to occur, adherence of cells to the surface of the biomaterial is a critical factor. The implant surface characteristics can modulate the adsorption of proteins, lipids, sugar, and ions present in the tissue fluids. Accordingly, several factors[2] have been determined to influence these interactions at the implant-host interface (**Fig. 1**).

PRIMARY STABILITY

In the Branemark paradigm, implant immobility during the first 6 months of healing is a perquisite for osseointegration to occur. Primary stability is defined as the biometric

[a] Division of Periodontology, Department of Oral Health Practice, University of Kentucky, College of Dentistry, D-438 Chandler Medical Center, 800 Rose Street, Lexington, KY 40536-0927, USA; [b] Division of Periodontology, Department of Oral Health Practice, University of Kentucky, College of Dentistry, Lexington, KY 40536, USA; [c] Ambulatory healthcare services -SEHA-, Muroor Street, Po box 111355, Abu Dhabi, United Arab Emirates
* Corresponding author.
E-mail address: malsa2@email.uky.edu

Dent Clin N Am 63 (2019) 461–473
https://doi.org/10.1016/j.cden.2019.02.001
0011-8532/19/© 2019 Elsevier Inc. All rights reserved.

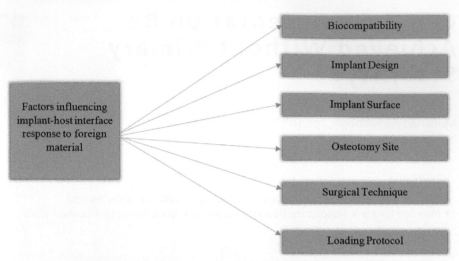

Fig. 1. Factors affecting implant-host interface response with foreign body.

stability immediately following the insertion of an implant and is a direct result of the mechanical engagement of an implant with the surrounding bone. Primary stability has been widely referenced in the literature as a requirement for the osseointegration of dental implant and the long-term success.[3,4] This "mechanical stability" gradually decreases during the early stages of healing due to bone remodeling. As new bone is formed along the implant surface, secondary stability is established, which is the direct result of the osseointegration corresponding to both mechanical and biological features[5] (**Fig. 2**).

Micromotion of dental implants is the minimal displacement of an implant body from the surrounding bone, which is not visible to the naked eye.[6] It has been suggested that micromotion between implant and surrounding bone must not exceed a threshold value of 150 μm for a successful implant healing.[7] Any movement even at the micrometer range can induce stress and strain that may hinder the recruitment of new cells

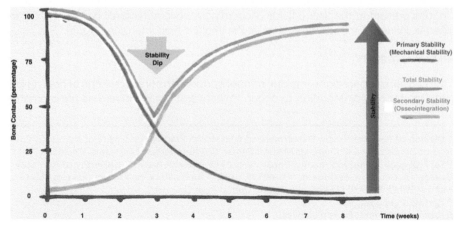

Fig. 2. Implant stability curve study. (*Adapted from* Raghavendra S, Wood MC, Taylor TD. Early wound healing around endosseous implants: a review of the literature. Int J Oral Maxillofac Implants 2005;20(3):430; with permission.)

and negatively influence osseointegration and bone remodeling leading to forming fibrous tissues.[8]

FACTORS INFLUENCING PRIMARY STABILITY

Primary stability is influenced by multiple factors, including implant design (length/diameter, microscopic/macroscopic morphology of implant), bone condition (quality/quantity), and the surgical protocol specific for each implant system (**Fig. 3**).

Implant Design (Macro/Microstructure)

The 3-dimensional structural design of an implant plays a vital role in attaining primary stability.[9,10] The threaded design increases the surface area of the implant in contact with bone, thereby offering a higher percentage of bone-to-implant contact (BIC) in comparison to implants with cylindrical design. Tapered implants were later introduced to provide a degree of compression of the cortical bone in an implant site with inadequate bone.[11,12]

Several implant surface modifications have been developed to modulate and enhance biological response to improve osseointegration and primary stability (**Fig. 4**). Studies have shown that surface topography and roughness increases the surface area of the implant and allows a firmer mechanical link to the surrounding tissues, thus enhancing primary stability.[13]

Veis and colleagues[14] showed that implants with acid-etched surfaces can achieve a significantly higher BIC and primary stability in poor bone quality sites in comparison to implants with machined surface. Schätzle and colleagues[15] compared a chemically modified sandblasted/acid-etched titanium surface (modSLA) with a standard SLA

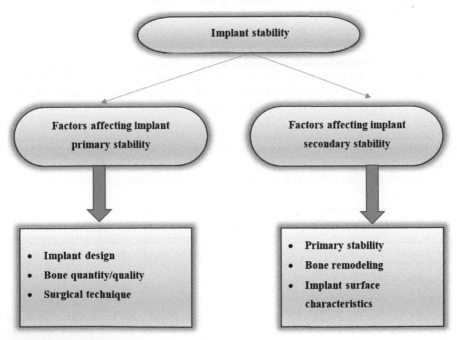

Fig. 3. Factors influencing implant stability.

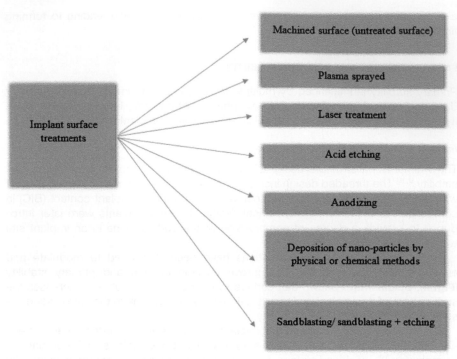

Fig. 4. Types of implant surface treatments.

surface and found higher implant stability quotient (ISQ) values at 12 weeks in the (modSLA) group versus SLA group.

Bone Density and Quality

Clinical studies have reported that dental implants in the mandible have higher survival rates compared with those in the maxilla, especially the posterior region.[16] The distribution and percentage of both the cancellous and cortical bone in the implant site play a crucial role in determining the insertion resistance of an implant during placement.[17–19]

A balance between the cancellous and cortical part of the bone is always desired. Type I cortical bone will lead to highly insertion torques with possible negative bone resorption.[12] On the other hand, type IV bone with no cortical bone provides minimal or no primary stability, which in turn may result in no osseointegration due to implant micromotion.[12,20,21]

Turkyilmaz and colleagues[22] observed a significance correlation between mean voxel values (gray scale) (751 ± 257) and ISQ values (70.5 ± 7) at implant placement. In a similar study, Fuster-Torres and colleagues[23] found a significance relationship between mean voxel values (623 ± 209) and ISQ values (62.4 ± 8).

Surgical Techniques

Several modalities of osteotomy preparation techniques have been proposed to optimize a high degree of implant stability. Among these techniques are using undersized drilling protocol, osteotomes to laterally condense the bone, and counter-clock wise rotational surgical drills.

It is worth mentioning that drilling into the implant bed not only incurs mechanical damage to the bone but also increases the temperature of the bone directly adjacent to implant surface. Bone cell necrosis occurs when the temperature exceeds 47°C for 1 min. Mechanical and thermal damage to the surrounding tissue around the implant surface can have a destructive effect on the initial state of the osteotomy housing the implant.[24]

Even though primary stability is always desired, it may not be achievable either from patient specific reasons, for an example bone quality, or from operator related factors, such as overpreparing the implant osteotomy.[25] However, it has been reported in the literature that implants that lacked or had low primary stability have comparable survival rates to those with high primary stability.[3,18,26–28]

MEASURING PRIMARY STABILITY

Although primary stability is widely discussed in the literature, there is no simple and clear method to quantify or measure it rather than unreliable clinicians' hand tactile sensation. Several investigators presented techniques and methods to quantify implant stability in general and primary stability in particular.[29]

Cutting Torque Resistance Analysis

Cutting torque resistance analysis (CRA) was developed by Friberg and colleagues[30] in 1995. This method measures the required current needed in an electric motor to cut off a unit volume of bone during the low-speed threading of implant osteotomy site. The measured energy is significantly correlated to the bone density because it identifies areas with soft, cancellous bone.[30,31] The technique consists of incorporating a torque gauge within the drilling unit to measure implant insertion torque in newton centimeter (Ncm) to be converted to J/mm^3. The major limitation of the CRA technique is that it does not give any information on bone quality until the osteotomy site is prepared. CRA also fails to provide a clear lower cutting torque threshold to indicate the risk of implant failure.[32]

Insertion Torque

Clinically, insertional torque (IT) is more widely used in assessing primary stability than CRA.[33,34] However, torque measurement can only be recorded at the time of implant placement and does not assess any changes that happens after implant placement. Ottoni and colleagues[35] investigated the relation between IT and implant survival in single implants. The recommendation of this study to achieve osseointegration was a minimum IT value of 20 Ncm and an optimal torque of 32 Ncm. A high IT value maybe an indication of good primary stability; however, maximum insertion torque can be deceiving; direct pressure of the implant on the dense cortical bone without adequate BTI contact at the rest of implant surface can produce high IT.

IT and resonance frequency analysis (RFA) are the most widely used methods to measure primary stability so their relationship has been extensively analyzed by numerous researchers and yet remains controversial. Lages and colleagues,[36] in a recent systematic review, concluded that insertion torque and RFA are independent and incomparable methods to measure primary stability.

Periotest

Periotest (Siemens A, Benshein, Germany) has been considered a reliable method to measure primary stability.[37,38] It was originally developed by Schulte to test natural tooth mobility using a metallic rod that applies an electronically controlled tapping force to the object (tooth or an implant). The response time to this "controlled tapping" is measured by a sensor on the handpiece and converted into a value called periotest value (PTV). This value represents the damping characteristics of the surrounding tissues around the tooth or implant. PTV ranges from −8 (low mobility) to +50 (high mobility). Olive and colleagues[39] found that a normal PTV of an osseointegrated implant falls in a relatively narrow zone (−5 to +5). Other studies[40,41] found that PTVs of osseointegrated implants falls within a narrower zone (−4 to −2 or −4 to +2).

Many investigators presumed that PTV precisely reflects the condition of BIC.[40,42] However, the prognostic accuracy of PTV for implant stability has been criticized for poor sensitivity, difficulty of application in posterior region, and susceptibility to operator variables.[43,44]

Resonance Frequency Analysis

RFA suggested by Meredith in 1998 has recently gained popularity as a noninvasive diagnostic method to measure both primary and secondary implant stability.[45] It uses an L-shaped transducer that is inserted into the implant or abutment containing a vibrating element and a receptor. The vibrating element applies a sinusoidal wave or an impact force wave and the receptor measures the resonance signal from the implant-bone component that has shown to measure implant stability.[29] It represents a measurement of the axial stiffness between implant and bone.

Currently, 2 machines are available in the market that measures implant stability via RFA: Osstell (Integration diagnostics) and Implomates (Bio TechOne). Osstell is a more widely used device and combines the transducer, computerized analysis, and vibration source into one device. Initially, Hertz was used as a measurement unit; then ISQ was developed as a measurement unit by Osstell. The ISQ value ranges from 0 to 100, of which the higher value referring to more implant stability.[29] The Implomates device applies an impact force instead of the sinusoidal effect to trigger the resonance of the implant and a receptor measures in range from 2 to 20 kilohertz. More research has been conducted on the application and efficacy of the Osstell device compared with the Implomates.

IMPLANT BED PREPARATION

The goal of improving primary stability has been a constant objective ever since the development of the early endosseous implants. The concept of placing a longer, wider implant suitable for an implant site is the most commonly cited method to improve primary stability. However, the development of tapered implant with aggressive thread design challenged such a concept.[11,12]

The quality and dimension of implant site can be assessed through cone beam computed tomography to customize the surgical protocol in sites where softer type III or IV bone is present.[46]

Summers Osteotome Technique

After using the pilot drill, a series of osteotomes can be tapped into the implant site to laterally compact the cancellous bone, which results in better dense bone allowing for better implant primary stability.[47] Markovic and colleagues obtained significantly higher implant stability values using lateral bone condensation versus conventional bone drilling techniques, both immediately after implant placement surgery (74.03 ± 3.53 vs 61.2 ± 1.63 ISQ) and at 6 weeks following the surgery (70.3 ± 1.21 vs 65.23 ± 0.43 ISQ).

Undersized Drilling Technique

Several studies[48–50] have proved that when dental implants are inserted in underprepared osteotomy sites using smaller diameter drills, maximum bone volume preservation and enhanced bone density are achieved. Furthermore, underpreparation of osteotomy sites will allow translocation of osteogenic bone fragments along the implant surface, which will contribute to bone healing and remodeling.[51]

In the presence of soft trabecular bone, experienced clinicians may choose to underprepare the osteotomy by not using the last drill of the implant system surgical protocol.[50] Degidi and colleagues[52] compared primary stability parameters (insertion torque and RFA) of 3 study groups of implants placed in poor-quality fresh bovine bone where standard osteotomy preparation (control group), 10% undersized preparation, and 25% undersized preparation were performed. They found improved primary stability with 10% undersized preparation group; however, 25% undersized group did not provide an added benefit to stability.

Osseodensification Technique (VERSAH)

Unlike traditional drilling techniques, osseodensification does not excavate and subtract bone tissue. During the drilling process, bone tissue in this technique is simultaneously compacted and autografted in an outward expanding direction from the osteotomy, resembling somewhat a traditional hammered osteotome technique, but without the trauma. When a Densah Bur is rotated at high speed in a reversed, noncutting direction with steady external irrigation, a strong and dense layer of bone tissue is formed along the walls and the base of the osteotomy.[53]

Bicortical Fixation

Bicortical fixation has historically been implemented to increase the primary stability of implants. The technique entails the use of long implant to engage 2 layers of cortical bone: the cervical crest and the sinus or nasal floor cortex or lower border of anterior mandibular cortex. In a study by Hsu and colleagues,[54] they used a stopper drill and self-threading implants to firmly engage the sinus floor cortex to improve implant stability in one group, an indirect vertical sinus floor lift in a second group, and unicortical fixation in a third group. They found that primary and secondary implant stabilities of bicortical fixation did not differ significantly from those of unicortical fixation and indirect sinus elevation. However, bicortical fixation technique is simpler and more economical than indirect sinus elevation. In contrast, Ivanoff and colleagues[55] found that bicortically anchored implants failed nearly 4 times more often than the monocortical ones. Bicortical fixation is currently not widely used. Further studies are needed to validate the outcomes of this concept.

RESONANCE FREQUENCY ANALYSIS AND LACK OF PRIMARY STABILITY

Lack of primary stability does not have a clear definition in the literature. Rodrigo and colleagues[26] classified lack of primary stability into 4 categories according to the perception of rotation: (1) No rotation, (2) light rotation with a feeling of resistance, (3) rotation with no resistance, and (4) rotation and lateral oscillation. Second, third, and fourth groups were categorized as having no primary stability. Other investigators identified lack of primary stability as low insertion torque of less than 10 Ncm and slight lateral mobility,[56] implants without rotational primary stability,[57] and implants without apical or rotational primary stability that can be rotated or depressed with gentle force.[25,58]

Multiple studies have correlated ISQ values (obtained by RFA) with primary stability and future implant survival rates.[59–61] However, most of the studies did not investigate RFA in implants that lacked primary stability with exception of few.[26,62] Rodrigo and colleagues[26] collected ISQ values from 542 implants (42 out of 542 were grouped as unstable implants) at time of insertion and restoration. The results showed significant association between the degree of the implant initial stability and the corresponding RFA values taken at implant insertion. However, low RFA values at time of insertion were not correlated with implant failure. Only low secondary stability RFA values (>60 ISQ) taken at the time of restoration predicted implant failure. In a similar fashion, Nedir and colleagues[62] investigated whether primary stability assessed by RFA can predict osseointegration. They concluded that RFA is not a reliable method for assessing mobile implants. However, it was a reliable method to determine implant stability at the time of placement with a subsequent successful osseointegration if ISQ greater than or equal to 47.

Turkyilmaz and colleagues[50] investigated the difference in insertion torque and RFA values for implants placed in the posterior region of maxilla following a modified surgical protocol using thinner drills in the test implant sites. They found strong correlation between insertion torque measurements and RFA values. This was in agreement with other study findings.[19,34,61]

The clinician tactile assessment (lack of resistance to rotation and/or presence of lateral or depressible mobility to gently hand forces) of an implant at insertion seems to be a more reliable method identifying the implants with minimal or no primary stability.

OSSEOINTEGRATION PREDICTABILITY OF IMPLANTS WITH NO OR LOW PRIMARY STABILITY

Clinical studies that evaluated osseointegration of implants with no primary stability at the time of placement are scarce and are mostly conducted on animal model.[63,64] Orenstein and colleagues[58] followed 2770 implants of 6 different designs for 3 years following placement, and among those, 89 implants were mobile at placement. The implants were mainly split into 2 groups: hydroxyapatite (HA)-coated and non-HA–coated (Titanium alloy) groups. Implants were placed in a 2-stage protocol and were left submerged for 4 to 6 months in the mandible and 6 to 8 months in the maxilla before uncovering. The cumulative survival rate at 3 years of mobile implants was 79.8% (71 out of 89) compared with 93.4% for the stable implants. When the survival rate was broken down by the implant surface coating of the mobile implant group, the difference was very significant with 91.8% in the HA-coated group (56/61) compared with 53.6% survival (15/28) for the non-HA–coated (Ti alloy) group. The conclusion of the study was that implant primary stability is not an absolute prerequisite to osseointegration; however, it significantly affects the implant survival rate.

An advancement in the treatment of implant surface has been introduced to enhance primary stability and accelerate osseointegration. Current implants have modified macro/micro design when compared with the older machined surface and HA-coated implants. It is thought that an improved survival rate exists when those modified implant surfaces are inserted even when primary stability is not achieved.

In a retrospective analysis, Balshi and colleagues[57] found that implants (total 88) with apical but no rotational primary stability have a cumulative survival rate of 82%. Survival rate of implants with smooth machined surface (20 out of 44) and titanium oxide rough surface (20 out of 44) is 70% and 91.7%, respectively. This is in agreement with the Orenstein and colleagues' study that showed implants with rough surface may have a more predictable outcome when primary stability is not achieved at the time of implant placemat.[25,58] In a prospective study, Rodrigo and colleagues (2010) evaluated 4114 SLA Straumann implants.[26] The survival rate of implants with primary stability was 99.1% compared with 97.2% in implants with no primary stability. The investigators concluded that the high (97%) survival rate of nonstable implants clearly shows that primary stability is not a prerequisite for osseointegration. This is in agreement with a more recent report by Verardi and colleagues.[56] He reported a 100% survival rate for 11 implants that had less than 10 Ncm insertion torque and slight mobility to lateral force of 250 g at the time of placement.

In conclusion, early literature suggested a low survival rate for machined surface implants[25,57,58]; however, osseointegration of rough surface implants with no primary stability at placement is predictable and is similar to implants with primary stability at time of placement.[18,26,57]

RECOMMENDATIONS FOR MANAGING IMPLANTS WITH NO PRIMARY STABILITY

1. *Planning and execution*: the clinician should properly assess the implant site before and during the osteotomy preparation. Osteotomy preparation protocol can be modified with the use of osteotome, undersized implant bed preparation, or osseodensification to improve the quality of bone and achieve adequate primary stability.
2. *Implant design*: in the presence of soft trabecular bone, tapered implant with aggressive thread design is recommended to engage bone and enhance primary stability.
3. *Rescue implant*: if the planned implant used did not achieve proper primary stability, a rescue implant (longer/wider implant) can be considered to further engage available bone.
4. *Bone graft:* in case of the mobility of an implant due to overpreparation of the osteotomy or the presence of a jumping distance in an immediate implant following extraction, adding bone graft particles within the osteotomy may help create a wedging effect of the implant, thus minimizing any micromovement during healing.
5. *Two-stage protocol:* an implant with no primary stability should be submerged and the flap should be repositioned with primary closure to minimize micromotions and disturbances of the nonstable implants during the healing time until secondary stability is achieved. Caution should be followed to eliminate any forces on the nonstable implants during healing. For example, the intaglio of the denture corresponding to implant site needs to be relieved.
6. *Prolonged healing period:* extra healing time is needed before loading to assure adequate osseointegration, especially in less dense bone.
7. *Abort implant placement:* the golden rule of prosthetically driven implant placement should always be applied. If the abovementioned recommendations cannot be attained in nonstable implant with crown-down position, then the implant placement should be aborted.

SUMMARY

It is essential to aim for primary stability; preoperative assessment of bone quality, an appropriate implant size and design, and osteotomy preparation technique modification for those sites with suspected poor bone quality need to be considered. However, even with all measures taken, clinicians may experience cases where the implant has no primary stability. A decision must be made to keep that implant, replace it with a longer/wider implant, graft around the implant, or simply abort implant placement all together. From the few studies discussing this topic along with the investigators' personal experience, keeping the implant with no primary stability has a high chance of integrating similar to the ones with good primary stability.

The current titanium surface treatments along with a more engaging implant geometry seem to have a major role in a high survival rate of mobile implants at the time of insertion. More studies with larger sample sizes and with different implant systems are warranted to develop a standard management protocol for implants that have no primary stability or are mobile at the time of placement.

REFERENCES

1. Branemark PI, Hansson BO, Adell R, et al. Osseointegrated implants in the treatment of the edentulous jaw. Experience from a 10-year period. Scand J Plast Reconstr Surg Suppl 1977;16:1–132.
2. Albrektsson T, Albrektsson B. Osseointegration of bone implants. A review of an alternative mode of fixation. Acta Orthop Scand 1987;58(5):567–77.
3. Albrektsson T. Direct bone anchorage of dental implants. J Prosthet Dent 1983; 50(2):255–61.
4. Rabel A, Kohler SG, Schmidt-Westhausen AM. Clinical study on the primary stability of two dental implant systems with resonance frequency analysis. Clin Oral Investig 2007;11(3):257–65.
5. Raghavendra S, Wood MC, Taylor TD. Early wound healing around endosseous implants: a review of the literature. Int J Oral Maxillofac Implants 2005;20(3): 425–31.
6. Laney WR. Glossary of oral and maxillofacial implants. Int J Oral Maxillofac Implants 2017;32(4). Gi–G200.
7. Szmukler-Moncler S, Salama H, Reingewirtz Y, et al. Timing of loading and effect of micromotion on bone-dental implant interface: review of experimental literature. J Biomed Mater Res 1998;43(2):192–203.
8. Brunski JB. Avoid pitfalls of overloading and micromotion of intraosseous implants. Dent Implantol Update 1993;4(10):77–81.
9. Chong L, Khocht A, Suzuki JB, et al. Effect of implant design on initial stability of tapered implants. J Oral Implantol 2009;35(3):130–5.
10. Romanos G, et al. Dental implant design and primary stability. A histomorphometric evaluation. in 42nd annual meeting, International Association of Dental Research meeting Continental European Division. Thessaloniki, 2008.
11. Shapoff CA. Clinical advantages of tapered root form dental implants. Compend Contin Educ Dent 2002;23(1):42–4, 46, 48 passim.
12. O'Sullivan D, Sennerby L, Meredith N. Influence of implant taper on the primary and secondary stability of osseointegrated titanium implants. Clin Oral Implants Res 2004;15(4):474–80.
13. Davies J. Mechanisms of endosseous integration. Int J Prosthodont 1998;11(5).
14. Veis AA, Papadimitriou S, Trisi P, et al. Osseointegration of Osseotite® and machined-surfaced titanium implants in membrane-covered critical-sized defects: a histologic and histometric study in dogs. Clin Oral Implants Res 2007; 18(2):153–60.
15. Schätzle M, Männchen R, Balbach U, et al. Stability change of chemically modified sandblasted/acid-etched titanium palatal implants. A randomized-controlled clinical trial. Clin Oral Implants Res 2009;20(5):489–95.
16. Jemt T, Stenport V. Implant treatment with fixed prostheses in the edentulous maxilla. Part 2: prosthetic technique and clinical maintenance in two patient

cohorts restored between 1986 and 1987 and 15 years later. Int J Prosthodont 2011;24(4):356–62.

17. Miyamoto I, Tsuboi Y, Wada E, et al. Influence of cortical bone thickness and implant length on implant stability at the time of surgery–clinical, prospective, biomechanical, and imaging study. Bone 2005;37(6):776–80.

18. Norton MR. The influence of low insertion torque on primary stability, implant survival, and maintenance of marginal bone levels: a closed-cohort prospective study. Int J Oral Maxillofac Implants 2017;32(4):849–57.

19. Trisi P, De Benedittis S, Perfetti G, et al. Primary stability, insertion torque and bone density of cylindric implant ad modum Branemark: is there a relationship? An in vitro study. Clin Oral Implants Res 2011;22(5):567–70.

20. Fugazzotto PA, Vlassis J, Butler B. ITI implant use in private practice: clinical results with 5,526 implants followed up to 72+ months in function. Int J Oral Maxillofac Implants 2004;19(3):408–12.

21. Jaffin RA, Berman CL. The excessive loss of Branemark fixtures in type IV bone: a 5-year analysis. J Periodontol 1991;62(1):2–4.

22. Turkyilmaz I, Tumer C, Ozbek EN, et al. Relations between the bone density values from computerized tomography, and implant stability parameters: a clinical study of 230 regular platform implants. J Clin Periodontol 2007;34(8):716–22.

23. Fuster-Torres MÁ, Peñarrocha-Diago M, Peñarrocha-Oltra D, et al. Relationships between bone density values from cone beam computed tomography, maximum insertion torque, and resonance frequency analysis at implant placement: a pilot study. Int J Oral Maxillofac Implants 2011;26(5):1051–6.

24. Anitua E, Carda C, Andia I. A novel drilling procedure and subsequent bone autograft preparation: a technical note. Int J Oral Maxillofac Implants 2007;22(1):138.

25. Orenstein IH, Tarnow DP, Morris HF, et al. Factors affecting implant mobility at placement and integration of mobile implants at uncovering. J Periodontol 1998;69(12):1404–12.

26. Rodrigo D, Aracil L, Martin C, et al. Diagnosis of implant stability and its impact on implant survival: a prospective case series study. Clin Oral Implants Res 2010; 21(3):255–61.

27. Trisi P, Berardini M, Falco A, et al. Effect of implant thread geometry on secondary stability, bone density, and bone-to-implant contact: a biomechanical and histological analysis. Implant Dent 2015;24(4):384–91.

28. Degidi M, Daprile G, Piattelli A. Implants inserted with low insertion torque values for intraoral welded full-arch prosthesis: 1-year follow-up. Clin Implant Dent Relat Res 2012;14:e39–40.

29. Atsumi M, Park SH, Wang HL. Methods used to assess implant stability: current status. Int J Oral Maxillofac Implants 2007;22(5):743–54.

30. Friberg B, Sennerby L, Roos J, et al. Evaluation of bone density using cutting resistance measurements and microradiography: an in vitro study in pig ribs. Clin Oral Implants Res 1995;6(3):164–71.

31. Friberg B, Sennerby L, Roos J, et al. Identification of bone quality in conjunction with insertion of titanium implants. A pilot study in jaw autopsy specimens. Clin Oral Implants Res 1995;6(4):213–9.

32. Friberg B, Sennerby L, Gröndahl K, et al. On cutting torque measurements during implant placement: a 3-year clinical prospective study. Clin Implant Dent Relat Res 1999;1(2):75–83.

33. Makary C, Rebaudi A, Mokbel N, et al. Peak insertion torque correlated to histologically and clinically evaluated bone density. Implant Dent 2011;20(3):182–91.

34. Turkyilmaz I. A comparison between insertion torque and resonance frequency in the assessment of torque capacity and primary stability of Branemark system implants. J Oral Rehabil 2006;33(10):754–9.

35. Ottoni JM, Oliveira ZF, Mansini R, et al. Correlation between placement torque and survival of single-tooth implants. Int J Oral Maxillofac Implants 2005;20(5): 769–76.

36. Lages FS, Douglas-de Oliveira DW, Costa FO. Relationship between implant stability measurements obtained by insertion torque and resonance frequency analysis: A systematic review. Clin Implant Dent Relat Res 2018;20(1):26–33.

37. Romanos GE, Nentwig G-H. Immediate functional loading in the maxilla using implants with platform switching: five-year results. Int J Oral Maxillofac Implants 2009;24(6):1106–12.

38. Romanos GE, Nentwig G-H. Immediate versus delayed functional loading of implants in the posterior mandible: a 2-year prospective clinical study of 12 consecutive cases. Int J Periodontics Restorative Dent 2006;26(5):459–69.

39. Olive J, Aparicio C. Periotest method as a measure of osseointegrated oral implant stability. Int J Oral Maxillofac Implants 1990;5(4):390–400.

40. Morris HE, Ochi S, Crum P, et al. Bone density: its influence on implant stability after uncovering. J Oral Implantol 2003;29(6):263–9.

41. Teerlinck J, Quirynen M, Darius P, et al. Periotest: an objective clinical diagnosis of bone apposition toward implants. Int J Oral Maxillofac Implants 1991;6(1): 55–61.

42. Hurzeler MB, Quiñones CR, Schüpbach P, et al. Influence of the suprastructure on the peri-implant tissues in beagle dogs. Clin Oral Implants Res 1995;6(3): 139–48.

43. Meredith N. Assessment of implant stability as a prognostic determinant. Int J Prosthodont 1998;11(5):491–501.

44. Salvi GE, Lang NP. Diagnostic parameters for monitoring peri-implant conditions. Int J Oral Maxillofac Implants 2004;19(Suppl):116–27.

45. Aparicio C, Lang NP, Rangert B. Validity and clinical significance of biomechanical testing of implant/bone interface. Clin Oral Implants Res 2006;17(S2):2–7.

46. Schwarz MS, Rothman SL, Rhodes ML, et al. Computed tomography: Part II. Preoperative assessment of the maxilla for endosseous implant surgery. Int J Oral Maxillofac Implants 1987;2(3):143–8.

47. Summers RB. A new concept in maxillary implant surgery: the osteotome technique. Compendium 1994;15(2):152, 154–6, 158 passim; quiz 162.

48. Friberg B, Ekestubbe A, Mellström D, et al. Brånemark implants and osteoporosis: a clinical exploratory study. Clin Implant Dent Relat Res 2001;3(1):50–6.

49. Friberg B, Ekestubbe A, Sennerby L. Clinical outcome of Brånemark system implants of various diameters: a retrospective study. Int J Oral Maxillofac Implants 2002;17(5):671–7.

50. Turkyilmaz I, Aksoy U, McGlumphy EA. Two alternative surgical techniques for enhancing primary implant stability in the posterior maxilla: a clinical study including bone density, insertion torque, and resonance frequency analysis data. Clin Implant Dent Relat Res 2008;10(4):231–7.

51. Tabassum A, Meijer GJ, Wolke JG, et al. Influence of surgical technique and surface roughness on the primary stability of an implant in artificial bone with different cortical thickness: a laboratory study. Clin Oral Implants Res 2010, 21(2):213–20.

52. Degidi M, Daprile G, Piattelli A. Influence of underpreparation on primary stability of implants inserted in poor quality bone sites: an in vitro study. J Oral Maxillofac Surg 2015;73(6):1084–8.
53. Huwais S, Meyer EG. A novel osseous densification approach in implant osteotomy preparation to increase biomechanical primary stability, bone mineral density, and bone-to-implant contact. Int J Oral Maxillofac Implants 2017;32(1): 27–36.
54. Hsu A, Seong WJ, Wolff R, et al. Comparison of initial implant stability of implants placed using bicortical fixation, indirect sinus elevation, and unicortical fixation. Int J Oral Maxillofac Implants 2016;31(2):459–68.
55. Ivanoff CJ, Gröndahl K, Bergström C, et al. Influence of bicortical or monocortical anchorage on maxillary implant stability: a 15-year retrospective study of Branemark System implants. Int J Oral Maxillofac Implants 2000;15(1):103–10.
56. Verardi S, Swoboda J, Rebaudi F, et al. Osteointegration of tissue-level implants with very low insertion torque in soft bone: a clinical study on SLA surface treatment. Implant Dent 2018;27(1):5–9.
57. Balshi SF, Wolfinger GJ, Balshi TJ. A retrospective analysis of 44 implants with no rotational primary stability used for fixed prosthesis anchorage. Int J Oral Maxillofac Implants 2007;22(3):467–71.
58. Orenstein IH, Tarnow DP, Morris HF, et al. Three-year post-placement survival of implants mobile at placement. Ann Periodontol 2000;5(1):32–41.
59. da Cunha HA, Francischone CE, Filho HN, et al. A comparison between cutting torque and resonance frequency in the assessment of primary stability and final torque capacity of standard and TiUnite single-tooth implants under immediate loading. Int J Oral Maxillofac Implants 2004;19(4):578–85.
60. Friberg B, Sennerby L, Linden B, et al. Stability measurements of one-stage Branemark implants during healing in mandibles. A clinical resonance frequency analysis study. Int J Oral Maxillofac Surg 1999;28(4):266–72.
61. Makary C, Rebaudi A, Sammartino G, et al. Implant primary stability determined by resonance frequency analysis: correlation with insertion torque, histologic bone volume, and torsional stability at 6 weeks. Implant Dent 2012;21(6):474–80.
62. Nedir R, Bischof M, Szmukler-Moncler S, et al. Predicting osseointegration by means of implant primary stability. Clin Oral Implants Res 2004;15(5):520–8.
63. Ivanoff CJ, Sennerby L, Lekholm U. Influence of initial implant mobility on the integration of titanium implants. An experimental study in rabbits. Clin Oral Implants Res 1996;7(2):120–7.
64. Sivolella S, Bressan E, Salata LA, et al. Osteogenesis at implants without primary bone contact - an experimental study in dogs. Clin Oral Implants Res 2012;23(5): 542–9.

Are There Alternatives to Invasive Site Development for Dental Implants? Part I

Vaughan J. Hoefler, DDS, MBA[a],*, Mohanad Al-Sabbagh, DDS, MS[b]

KEYWORDS

- Dental implants • Bone augmentation • Bone grafting • Implant site
- Short dental implants • Narrow diameter implants

KEY POINTS

- Alternatives to invasive site development for dental implant therapy include the use of short dental implants and narrow diameter implants.
- These alternatives have the advantages of reduced morbidity, fewer complications, shorter treatment time, lower costs, and better patient acceptance.
- Short dental implants may provide comparable outcomes to standard length implants in vertically augmented sites.
- Narrow diameter implants can be a valid alternative to standard diameter implants in horizontally grafted bone.

INTRODUCTION

Dental implant therapy is a widely accepted, long-term treatment option to restore edentulous sites.[1-4] However, the most favorable outcomes have been reported in sites with adequate native bone or with minor bone regenerative procedures.[5,6] Placement of longer and wider implants was initially preferred to improve bone-to-implant contact, primary stability, crown-to-implant ratio,[7] esthetics, hygiene, and restoration support.[8,9] However, edentulous sites are often characterized by inadequate bone quality and quantity.[10-12]

Implant sites with deficient bone often have to be augmented laterally, vertically, or a combination of both to achieve ideal 3-dimensional implant positioning that is prosthetically driven.[13,14] However, bone grafting increases the cost, time, and morbidity

Disclosure: The authors have nothing to disclose.
[a] Department of Oral Health Practice, Division of Prosthodontics, University of Kentucky College of Dentistry, D630 UK Chandler Hospital, 800 Rose Street, Lexington, KY 40536-0297, USA;
[b] Division of Periodontology, Department of Oral Health Practice, University of Kentucky College of Dentistry, D-438 Chandler Medical Center, 800 Rose Street, Lexington, KY 40536-0927, USA
* Corresponding author.
E-mail address: vaughan.hoefler@uky.edu

Dent Clin N Am 63 (2019) 475–487
https://doi.org/10.1016/j.cden.2019.02.011
0011-8532/19/© 2019 Elsevier Inc. All rights reserved.

dental.theclinics.com

of treatment.[15] Tooth loss and edentulism also disproportionately afflict low-income populations, for which the cost of both bone augmentation and restoration of edentulous sites with dental implants may be prohibitive.[16] This finding has led to the search for less invasive treatment options with greater patient acceptance.[6,17]

The broader use of 3-dimensional imaging techniques and computer-aided guided surgery, as well as the introduction of stronger implant alloys with improved surface structures, has led to the development of alternative treatment protocols. These alternatives include the use of shorter, narrower, and tilted implants to avoid bone grafting, as well as fewer implants to restore edentulous arches.

In Part I, we investigate the following questions: (1) Are short dental implants (SDIs) a reasonable alternative to vertically augmented bone with standard length implants? (2) Are narrow diameter implants (NDIs) a valid alternative to laterally augmented bone with standard diameter implants? The use of tilted and fewer implants as an alternative to conventional treatment protocols will be discussed in Part II.

ARE SHORT DENTAL IMPLANTS A REASONABLE ALTERNATIVE TO VERTICALLY AUGMENTED BONE WITH STANDARD LENGTH IMPLANTS?

When an implant site is completely devoid of bone, missing bone volume must be surgically regained before implant placement. However, there are times when a site has insufficient alveolar ridge height for standard length implants, but is otherwise adequate for SDIs. The use of SDIs is controversial. Higher failure rates have been associated with the use of SDIs in some studies,[18–24] whereas other reports indicate similar outcomes regardless of implant length.[25–32] Factors that explain these conflicting outcomes include a lack of standardized definitions for SDIs, and implant primary stability and surgical protocols. The skill and experience level of the clinician, implant surface characteristics, and bone quality are additional contributing factors that influence the predictability of SDIs.[7,33–36]

Short Dental Implant Definition

The maximum length of an SDI in the published literature remains controversial, with proposals ranging from 5 to 11 mm.[26,36–40] The length of the implant has been defined as the distance from the platform to the apex.[8] However, the intrabony length (ie, the distance from the apex to the most coronal bone-to-implant contact) has a greater relevance. Intrabony length represents the height of the implant that is anchored in bone and determines how external forces are transmitted to surrounding bone.[35,41]

The first European Association of Osseointegration consensus conference in 2006 defined SDI as an implant fixture with an intrabony length of 8 mm or less.[39] This SDI definition is used in this article because it is gaining acceptance and been adopted in a number of recent studies and reviews.[30–32,42]

Surgical Protocol and Primary Stability

Some studies that reported lower survival rate of SDI used a standard surgical protocol regardless of bone density.[21,43,44] Such protocols, often using tapping and countersinking, may have resulted in implants with reduced primary stability. Other publications reported favorable clinical outcomes for SDIs when modified surgical protocols that ensured greater primary stability in sites with lower bone quality were used.[45,46]

Clinician Experience

The clinician's skill and experience have been postulated to be factors affecting SDI outcomes.[7,39,47] A systematic review compared survival and complications for implant-supported prostheses of current studies (studies completed after 2000) with studies published in 2000 or prior years.[48] Higher implant survival rates and lower reported technical, biological, and esthetic complications were found in the more current studies. The authors concluded that the learning curve has a positive impact on implant clinical outcomes.

As an example, a retrospective study reported an 88% implant cumulative survival rate (CSR) over 5 years for 17 patients treated with SDI-retained overdentures from 1989 to 1993.[10] The identical clinical protocol was followed by the same authors via a randomized, controlled trial in 2003. They reported a 100% CSR at 12 months.[41] Although there was a difference in the duration of the reporting period between these 2 studies, the outcomes are comparable, because 7 of the 8 failures in the earlier study occurred in the initial healing period, before prosthetic loading.

Short Dental Implant Surface Structure

Rough textured implant surfaces have been recommended by some authors because they provide greater bone-to-implant contact and higher removal torque.[49,50] A recent systematic review reported a higher CSR for SDIs with rough surfaces.[33] In contrast, studies documenting increased numbers of SDI failures used machined surface implants.[19,21,24,51–53] Several studies indicated that the implant length did not influence survival when SDIs with textured surfaces were used.[54–57] This finding suggests that SDIs with a more favorable surface topography may have greater success than implants with machined surfaces.[58]

Bone Quality

Poor bone quality as well as low bone volume are risk factors for implant failure, particularly with SDIs.[34,43] Of the 2 factors, bone quality has a greater impact on SDI survival than bone quantity.[59] Short implants are mostly used in the posterior regions,[33] and the posterior maxilla in particular has the poorest quality of bone.[40] A study compared the implant survival of SDIs and standard implants in poor quality bone. SDIs had failure rates of 78%, whereas standard length implants had a failure rate of 0% in the most unfavorable quality and shape of bone.[51] Although the difference was not significant owing to low patient enrollment, SDIs were used in disproportionately high numbers in this study in sites with low volumes of poor quality bone.

Short Dental Implant Outcomes for Fixed Dental Prostheses

A multicenter, randomized, controlled trial compared SDIs with standard length implants placed in vertically augmented bone of the posterior maxilla and restored with single crowns.[60,61] At 3 years, there were no reported differences between the 2 groups with respect to implant survival or periimplant bone loss.[61]

Another research group compared SDIs with standard length implants placed in vertically augmented bone in posterior sites of both arches.[31,55,56,62] Significantly more complications occurred with grafts in mandibular sites, and greater periimplant marginal bone loss (MBL) was associated with longer implants in grafted sites in both arches compared with SDIs.[56,62] Although these reported outcomes suggest a therapeutic advantage for SDIs, the weaknesses of these studies include short follow-up periods ($\leq$5 years), small sample sizes, and procedures that were performed by a single, highly skilled and experienced clinical research group. These limitations should be considered before forming a generalized conclusion regarding the use of SDIs (Fig. 1).

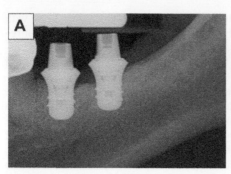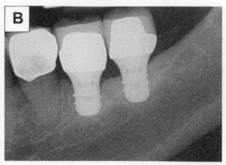

Fig. 1. (A) SDIs (6 mm) placed in the posterior mandible to avoid vertical augmentation and placement of standard length implants. (B) Adequate crestal bone stability present after 5 years of function.

Short Dental Implant as Abutments for Mandibular Implant Overdentures

The 2-implant retained overdenture is the standard of care for the edentulous mandible.[63] In contrast, maxillary implant-assisted overdentures are associated with lower rates of implant survival and a greater frequency of prosthetic complications.[64,65] In a prospective cohort study, 19 functionally dependent elderly adults with conventional dentures received 2 SDIs in the canine regions of their edentulous mandibles.[66] After 6 to 8 weeks of healing, the SDIs received Locator attachments (Zest Dental Solutions, Carlsbad, CA) which were retrofitted to the mandibular complete dentures. Implant survival was 94.7% at 5 years, with acceptable periimplant bone loss and other soft tissue biological parameters. The limitations of this study included a small study cohort, high levels of dropouts, and the lack of a comparison group. However, it demonstrates that cognitive decline and the inability to provide self-care may not be contraindications or risk factors for SDIs. A 10-year study followed 49 patients with severely atrophic mandibles that were restored with fixed or removable full-arch prostheses retained by 260 SDIs.[67] Seventeen implants failed over the study period with a CSR of 92.3%.

Short Dental Implants Outcomes for Full-Arch Fixed Dental Prostheses

Studies comparing SDIs with longer implants in vertically augmented bone for the support of full arch fixed dental prostheses are lacking. One retrospective study reported outcomes for 43 patients with edentulous maxillae rehabilitated with fixed prostheses supported by 172 short and long implants following the all-on-4 treatment concept.[68] After an average observation period of 3 years, 3 short and 3 long implants were lost with a CSR of 95.7% and 95.4% for short and all implants, respectively. MBL for short implants at 3 years was 1.25 mm, with no significant differences in bone loss between the groups. The limitations of this study included the use of outcomes from an individual clinical center as well as a short follow-up periods. In addition, SDIs were splinted to standard and longer length implants in the same arch in many patients. These factors should be considered before generalizing conclusions to full arch fixed dental prostheses supported entirely by SDIs.

ARE NARROW DIAMETER IMPLANTS A VALID ALTERNATIVE TO LATERALLY AUGMENTED BONE WITH STANDARD DIAMETER IMPLANTS?

Owing to volumetric bone loss after tooth extraction, lateral ridge augmentation is often performed before or simultaneously with implant placement. Although bone grafting is a common and a predictable treatment, it is associated with higher levels of complications and increased expense. Therefore, NDIs have been used as a less invasive alternative to laterally augmented sites with standard implant diameters.

Implant diameter is the maximum cross-sectional dimension within the intrabony length of an implant. It is measured from the peak of the widest thread to the same point on the opposite side of the implant.[8] Each implant system has its own inventory of diameters and lengths, with most manufacturers offering narrow, standard, and wide diameter implants.[69]

Implant diameter selection should be steered by site-specific surgical and prosthetic requirements. Surgical considerations include the location of the surgical site, the volume of residual bone, the level of primary stability, and the proximity to adjacent teeth and surrounding vital structures. The implant should engage as much crestal and buccolingual cortical bone as possible,[70] with at least 1 mm of residual bone adjacent to the implant surface.[9,71,72] Prosthetic factors include the planned occlusion, gingival esthetics, emergence profile, and the prosthesis design such as the size of the tooth or teeth to be replaced.[9,73]

Narrow Diameter Implant Definition

Implants with diameters of 3.75 mm and larger are widely regarded as standard or regular diameter implants.[9,70,71,74] However, the definition of an NDI remains controversial. The terms reduced diameter, narrow diameter, small diameter, microimplants, and miniimplants are used interchangeably with overlap in their definitions across studies.[72,75–80] A lower narrow diameter threshold of less than 3.0 mm has been proposed in systematic reviews by some authors,[79,81] whereas others agree with 3.5 mm or less as the upper diameter limit.[72,81,82] For this reason, implants with diameters that fall within the range of 3.0 to 3.5 mm are gaining acceptance for meeting the NDI criteria.[81]

Narrow Diameter Implant Limitations

Several factors should be considered before selecting an NDI. NDIs have biomechanical limitations relative to implants with wider diameters.[71] Although NDIs are significantly narrower than implants with standard diameters, they are subject to the same stresses under loading. For this reason, the material and design of NDIs must fulfill similar demands for strength and stability.[83] The thin fixture wall around the abutment or screw, resulting from the decreased implant diameter, can increase the risk for fixture or screw fracture.[84] In addition, NDI abutments have decreased surface areas relative to standard designs. This characteristic may result in greater numbers of prosthetic complications such as retention loss and screw loosening.[78] Finally, NDIs purportedly are at greater risk for fatigue failure than standard and wide diameter implants, particularly in posterior areas subject to high occlusal loads.[70,77,84]

NDIs were originally designed for the replacement of teeth with small cervical diameters, such as maxillary lateral and mandibular central and lateral incisors, as well as for implant sites with limited interdental space[78,84,85] (**Fig. 2**). It is recommended that the diameter of the implant should be slightly less than that of the crown for single tooth restorations.[9] A single mandibular incisor has a cervical diameter of 3.5 mm, which is ideally suited for an NDI.[71] However, maxillary and mandibular premolars and molars have diameters that exceed twice those of NDIs.[71] The nonjudicious use of NDIs for these situations can result in unsightly, overcontoured restorations with large gingival embrasures that lead to plaque accumulation, food impaction, periimplant soft tissue inflammation, and gingival recession, all of which can contribute to decreased implant survival.[86]

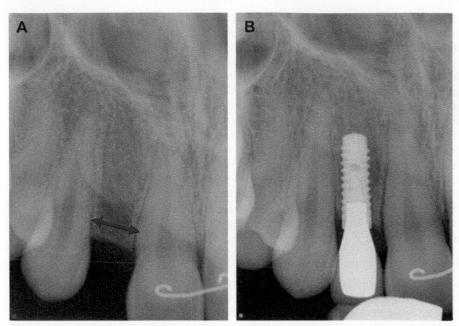

Fig. 2. (*A*) Limited mesiodistal space (5-mm interradicular distance at narrowest dimension) after comprehensive orthodontic treatment. (*B*) Narrow diameter Straumann implant at site after 1 year of function.

Narrow Diameter Implant and Anterior Full-Arch Fixed Dental Prostheses

Anterior NDI-supported fixed dental prostheses must be able to withstand the functional forces of mastication and occlusion, as well as meeting esthetic requirements. This means that the implant restoration is expected to provide appropriate protrusive and lateral guidance for the patient without fracture or displacement.

In a prospective, single-arm study on NDIs that replaced missing maxillary lateral and mandibular incisors with single implant crowns,[87,88] a 95.9% implant survival rate form the time of placement to the time of loading and 100% implant survival rate from the time of loading up to a 5-year follow-up was reported. The mean change in MBL from the day of the surgery to 5 years was −0.15 mm. Although 8.43% of the implants lost more than 1 mm of crestal bone, there was no measurable bone loss for 50.6% of the implants after 5 years. A number of technical complications were reported in this study. Seven implants in 7 patients experienced abutment fracture, and retention loss of 6 crowns occurred for 6 patients. In some cases, patients lost the crowns more than once.

A second prospective, single-arm study reported similar outcomes for NDIs that replaced congenitally missing maxillary lateral and mandibular incisors.[89] An overall 96.8% CSR at 36 months was reported, and none of the implants were lost after loading. Gingival recession was negligible, and the mean change in MBL from implant insertion to 36 months was a loss of 0.21 mm. Technical complications were also similar, with 5 fractured abutments, 1 loose abutment screw, and 8 crowns that needed to be recemented.

Despite these reported complications, the investigators in both previous studies demonstrated acceptable biological outcomes and implant survival over a period of 3 to 5 years when NDIs were used to restore maxillary lateral and mandibular incisor sites.[87-89] Although prosthetic complications were reported in the 2 studies cited, a direct comparison between NDIs and anterior single crowns supported by standard diameter implants in similar sites was not possible owing to the lack of comparison groups.

A longitudinal study used 20 NDIs at the maxillary lateral incisor sites of 10 patients to support 4-unit partial fixed dental prostheses replacing numbers 7 to 10.[90] After 5 years, no implants were lost and there were no reported technical or biological complications. Marginal bone levels were stable over 5 years for all implants, gingival recession was negligible, and overall patient satisfaction was 96.9%. Although the results of this study illustrate the usefulness of NDIs in multiunit fixed applications, the expertise and clinical skills of this research group should be given consideration before adopting this treatment concept.

Narrow Diameter Implants and Posterior Full-Arch Fixed Dental Prostheses

Posterior natural teeth have cervical diameters much greater than the diameters of NDIs. The occlusal load from the cantilever created by the increased occlusal surface diameter relative to the NDI diameter increases the risk for overload on abutments, abutment screws, and fixtures.[70,91]

A retrospective study on 247 NDIs in posterior sites (follow-up of ≤11 years) reported a CSR of 95.1%.[83] This study did not report prosthetic complications. A second retrospective study on 98 NDIs placed in premolar and molar sites and restored with single crowns and short span multiunit fixed dental prostheses reported a 96.9% implant CSR at 8 years.[86] There were no implant fractures or abutment screw loosening or fracture. The most common mechanical complication was ceramic veneer chipping (18.4%) and retention loss (5 single crowns). Although 84.6% of the patients were satisfied with restorative function, the main reason for dissatisfaction was gingival recession and food impaction around the restorations. A third study reported the 5- to 10-year outcomes on NDIs placed in anterior as well as posterior sites.[92] An overall CSR of 92.3% was reported at 124 months. In this study, posterior sites demonstrated increased risk for failure and retention loss was the most common prosthetic complication.

Narrow Diameter Implants as Overdenture Abutments

The mandibular edentulous arch is often severely resorbed and characterized by narrow crestal bone. A 2-implant overdenture using standard diameter implants may require either surgically reducing the height of the ridge to a level of adequate buccolingual width, or lateral bone augmentation followed by implant surgery. In addition, patients requesting this treatment are often elderly, under the care of a physician, and have limited self-care capability.[66] Two-implant overdentures retained by NDIs can be the most conservative treatment alternative for these patients.

A longitudinal study reported implant and prosthesis outcomes at 3 and 5 years.[92,93] The majority of implant sites showed minimal change in crestal bone and an implant CSR of 97.8%. Complications requiring intervention included prosthesis fracture, peri-implant inflammation and infection, and replacement of the retentive matrix.[92] A second NDI study that included 24 two- and four-implant overdentures reported an implant CSR of 92.3% at 124 months.[94] Another study investigating immediate versus delayed loading of mandibular NDI overdentures reported 98% implant CSR and very few prosthesis complications at 12 months.[95]

The lack of studies using a comparison group make it difficult to directly compare 2-implant mandibular overdentures retained by NDIs to overdentures retained by standard diameter implants. However, reported clinical outcomes for NDIs are acceptable, and the minimally invasive treatment approach makes this option particularly suitable for patients who are at higher surgical risk with limited economic means.

SUMMARY

Short and narrow implants have proven to be successful within certain applications. However, they still require a minimum volume and quality of bone to succeed. Questions regarding the long-term effects of MBL and fatigue on SDIs and NDIs success and survival remain unanswered.

There are clear indications for surgical site development, including gross bone deficiencies in the esthetic zone, severe alveolar ridge resorption resulting from prolonged periods of edentulism, and congenital or acquired defects that prevent proper 3-dimensional implant positioning. To this end, considerable effort has been directed toward developing methods for ridge augmentation. Despite progress in regenerating lost bone, augmentation procedures are expensive, invasive, technically demanding, and accompanied by greater morbidity and longer treatment times. Furthermore, although bone regeneration is predictable over the short term, the long-term volumetric stability of grafted bone is not well-documented. For these reasons, alternatives to invasive site development should always be considered when planning implant care.

REFERENCES

1. Hjalmarsson L, Gheisarifar M, Jemt T. A systematic review of survival of single implants as presented in longitudinal studies with a follow-up of at least 10 years. Eur J Oral Implantol 2016;9(Suppl 1):S155–62.
2. Wyatt CC, Zarb GA. Treatment outcomes of patients with implant-supported fixed partial prostheses. Int J Oral Maxillofac Implants 1998;13(2):204–11.
3. Chrcanovic BR, Kisch J, Albrektsson T, et al. A retrospective study on clinical and radiological outcomes of oral implants in patients followed up for a minimum of 20 years. Clin Implant Dent Relat Res 2018;20(2):199–207.
4. Goodacre BJ, Goodacre S, Goodacre CJ. Prosthetic complications with implant prostheses (2001-2017). Eur J Oral Implantol 2018;11(Suppl 1):S27–36.
5. Albrektsson T, Zarb G, Worthington P, et al. The long-term efficacy of currently used dental implants: a review and proposed criteria for success. Int J Oral Maxillofac Implants 1986;1(1):11–25.
6. Thoma DS, Cha JK, Jung UW. Treatment concepts for the posterior maxilla and mandible: short implants versus long implants in augmented bone. J Periodontal Implant Sci 2017;47(1):2–12.
7. Nisand D, Renouard F. Short dental implant in limited bone volume. Periodontol 2000 2014;66(1):72–96.
8. Lee JH, Frias V, Lee KW, et al. Effect of implant size and shape on implant success rates: a literature review. J Prosthet Dent 2005;94(4):377–81.
9. Lazzara RJ. Criteria for implant selection: surgical and prosthetic considerations. Pract Periodontics Aesthet Dent 1994;6(9):55–62.
10. Stellingsma C, Meijer HJ, Raghoebar GM. Use of short endosseous implants and an overdenture in the extremely resorbed mandible: a five-year retrospective study. J Oral Maxillofac Surg 2000;58(4):382–7 [discussion: 387–8].
11. Chiapasco M, Zaniboni M, Boisco M. Augmentation procedures for the rehabilitation of deficient edentulous ridges with oral implants. Clin Oral Implants Res 2006;17(Suppl 2):136–59.

12. Fortin Y, Sullivan RM, Rangert BR. The Marius implant bridge: surgical and prosthetic rehabilitation for the completely edentulous upper jaw with moderate to severe resorption: a 5-year retrospective clinical study. Clin Implant Dent Relat Res 2002;4(2):69–77.

13. Aghaloo TL, Moy PK. Which hard tissue augmentation techniques are the most successful in furnishing bony support for implant placement? Int J Oral Maxillofac Implants 2007;22(Suppl):49–70 [Erratum appears in Int J Oral Maxillofac Implants 2008;23(1):56].

14. Aloy-Prósper A, Peñarrocha-Oltra D, Peñarrocha-Diago M, et al. The outcome of intraoral onlay block bone grafts on alveolar ridge augmentations: a systematic review. Med Oral Patol Oral Cir Bucal 2015;20(2):e251–8.

15. Thoma DS, Haas R, Tutak M, et al. Randomized controlled multicenter study comparing short dental implants (6 mm) versus longer dental implants (11-15 mm) in combination with sinus floor elevation procedures. Part 1: demographics and patient-oriented outcomes at 1 year of loading. J Clin Periodontol 2015;42(1):72–80.

16. Henshaw MM, Garcia RI, Weintraub JA. Oral health disparities across the life span. Dent Clin North Am 2018;62(2):177–93.

17. Pommer B, Mailath-Pokorny G, Haas R, et al. Patients' preferences towards minimally invasive treatment alternatives for implant rehabilitation of edentulous jaws. Eur J Oral Implantol 2014;7(Suppl 2):S91–109.

18. Andersson B, Odman P, Carlsson GE. A study of 184 consecutive patients referred for single-tooth replacement. Clin Oral Implants Res 1995;6(4):232–7.

19. Friberg B, Jemt T, Lekholm U. Early failures in 4,641 consecutively placed Brånemark dental implants: a study from stage 1 surgery to the connection of completed prostheses. Int J Oral Maxillofac Implants 1991;6(2):142–6.

20. Queiroz TP, Aguiar SC, Margonar R, et al. Clinical study of survival rate of short implants placed in posterior mandibular region: resonance frequency analysis. Clin Oral Implants Res 2015;26(9):1036–42.

21. Weng D, Jacobson Z, Tarnow D, et al. A prospective multicenter clinical trial of 3i machined-surface implants: results after 6 years of follow-up. Int J Oral Maxillofac Implants 2003;18(3):417–23.

22. Goodacre CJ, Kan JY, Rungcharassaeng K. Clinical complications of osseointegrated implants. J Prosthet Dent 1999;81(5):537–52.

23. Naenni N, Sahrmann P, Schmidlin PR, et al. Five-year survival of short single-tooth implants (6 mm): a randomized controlled clinical trial. J Dent Res 2018;97(8):887–92.

24. Winkler S, Morris HF, Ochi S. Implant survival to 36 months as related to length and diameter. Ann Periodontol 2000;5(1):22–31.

25. Lai HC, Si MS, Zhuang LF, et al. Long-term outcomes of short dental implants supporting single crowns in posterior region: a clinical retrospective study of 5-10 years. Clin Oral Implants Res 2013;24(2):230–7.

26. Perelli M, Abundo R, Corrente G, et al. Short (5 to 7 mm long) porous implant in the posterior atrophic mandible: a 5-year report of a prospective study. Eur J Oral Implantol 2011;4(4):363–8.

27. Stellingsma K, Bouma J, Stegenga B, et al. Satisfaction and psychosocial aspects of patients with an extremely resorbed mandible treated with implant-retained overdentures. A prospective, comparative study. Clin Oral Implants Res 2003;14(2):166–72.

28. Bechara S, Kubilius R, Veronesi G, et al. Short (6-mm) dental implants versus sinus floor elevation and placement of longer (>10-mm) dental implants: a

randomized controlled trial with 3-year follow-up. Clin Oral Implants Res 2017; 28(9):1097–107.

29. Esposito M, Cannizzaro G, Soardi E, et al. Posterior atrophic jaws rehabilitated with prostheses supported by 6 mm-long, 4 mm-wide implants or by longer implants in augmented bone. Preliminary results from a pilot randomized controlled trial. Eur J Oral Implantol 2012;5(1):19–33.

30. Fan T, Li Y, Deng WW, et al. Short implants (5 to 8 mm) versus longer implants (>8 mm) with sinus lifting in atrophic posterior maxilla: a meta-analysis of RCTs. Clin Implant Dent Relat Res 2017;19(1):207–15.

31. Felice P, Cannizzaro G, Barausse C, et al. Short implants versus longer implants in vertically augmented posterior mandibles: a randomized controlled trial with 5-year after loading follow-up. Eur J Oral Implantol 2014;7(4):359–69.

32. Nisand D, Picard N, Rocchietta I. Short implants compared to implants in vertically augmented bone: a systematic review. Clin Oral Implants Res 2015; 26(Suppl 11):170–9.

33. Annibali S, Cristalli MP, Dell'Aquila D, et al. Short dental Implants: a systematic review. J Dent Res 2012;91(1):25–32.

34. Das Neves FD, Fones D, Bernardes SR, et al. Short implants—an analysis of longitudinal studies. Int J Oral Maxillofac Implants 2006;21(1):86–93.

35. Neldam CA, Pinholt EM. State of the art of short dental implants: a systematic review of the literature. Clin Implant Dent Relat Res 2012;14(4):622–32.

36. Olate S, Lyrio MC, de Moraes M, et al. Influence of diameter and length of implant on early dental implant failure. J Oral Maxillofac Surg 2010;68(2):414–9.

37. Misch CE, Steignga J, Barboza E, et al. Short dental implants in posterior partial edentulism: a multicenter retrospective 6-year case series study. J Periodontol 2006;77(8):1340–7.

38. Stellingsma K, Raghoebar GM, Visser A, et al. The extremely resorbed mandible, 10-year results of a randomized control trial on 3 treatment strategies. Clin Oral Implants Res 2014;25:926–32.

39. Renouard F, Nisand D. Impact of implant length and diameter on survival rates. Clin Oral Implants Res 2006;17(Suppl 2):35–51.

40. Telleman G, Raghoebar GM, Vissink A, et al. A systematic review of short (<10 mm) dental implants placed in the partially edentulous patient. J Clin Periodontol 2011;38(7):667–76.

41. Qian L, Todo M, Matsushita Y, et al. Effects of implant diameter, insertion depth, and loading angle on stress/strain fields in implant/jawbone systems: finite element analysis. Int J Oral Maxillofac Implants 2009;24(5):877–86.

42. Thoma DS, Zeltner M, Hüsler J, et al. EAO supplement working group 4 - EAO CC 2015 Short implants versus sinus lifting with longer implants to restore posterior maxilla: a systematic review. Clin Oral Implants Res 2015;26(Suppl 11):154–69.

43. Jemt T, Lekholm U. Implant treatment in edentulous maxillae: a 5-year follow-up report on patients with different degrees of jaw resorption. Int J Oral Maxillofac Implants 1995;10(3):303–11.

44. Naert I, Koutsikakis G, Duyck J, et al. Biological outcome of implant-supported restorations in the treatment of partial edentulism. Part 1: a longitudinal clinical evaluation. Clin Oral Implants Res 2002;13(4):381–9.

45. Maló P, Nobre MD, Lopes A. Short dental implants in posterior jaws. A prospective 1-year study. Eur J Oral Implantol 2011;4(1):47–53.

46. Renouard F, Nisand D. Short dental implants in the severely resorbed maxilla: a 2-year retrospective clinical study. Clin Implant Dent Relat Res 2005;7(Suppl 1): S104–10.

47. Fugazzotto PA, Beagle JR, Ganeles J, et al. Success and failure rates of 9 mm or shorter implants in the replacement of missing maxillary molars when restored with individual crowns: preliminary results 0 to 84 months in function. A retrospective study. J Periodontol 2004;75(2):327–32.

48. Pjetursson BE, Asgeirsson AG, Zwahlen M, et al. Improvements in implant dentistry over the last decade: comparison of survival and complication rates in older and newer publications. Int J Oral Maxillofac Implants 2014;29(Suppl): 308–24.

49. Buser D, Schenk RK, Steinemann S, et al. Influence of surface characteristics on bone integration of titanium implants. A Histomorphic study in miniature pigs. J Biomed Mater Res 1991;25(7):889–902.

50. Sullivan DY, Sherwood RL, Mai TN. Preliminary results of a multicenter study evaluating a chemically enhanced surface for machined commercially pure titanium implants. J Prosthet Dent 1997;78(4):379–86.

51. Herrmann I, Lekholm U, Holm S, et al. Evaluation of patient and implant characteristics as potential prognostic factors for oral implant failures. Int J Oral Maxillofac Implants 2005;20(2):220–30.

52. Jemt T. Failures and complications in 391 consecutively inserted fixed prostheses supported by Brånemark implants in edentulous jaws: a study of treatment from the time of prosthesis placement to the first annual checkup. Int J Oral Maxillofac Implants 1991;6(3):270–6.

53. Lekholm U, Gunne J, Henry P, et al. Survival of the Brånemark implant in partially edentulous jaws: a 10-year prospective multicenter study. Int J Oral Maxillofac Implants 1999;14(5):639–45.

54. Buser D, Mericske-Stern R, Bernard JP, et al. Long-term evaluation of non-submerged ITI implants. Part 1: 8-year life table analysis of a prospective multi-center study with 2359 implants. Clin Oral Implants Res 1997;8(3):161–72.

55. Esposito M, Pistilli R, Barausse C, et al. Three-year results from a randomized controlled trial comparing prostheses supported by 5-mm long implants or by longer implants in augmented bone in posterior atrophic edentulous jaws. Eur J Oral Implantol 2014;7(4):383–95.

56. Gastaldi G, Felice P, Pistilli V, et al. Posterior atrophic jaws rehabilitated with prostheses supported by 5 X 5 mm implants with a nanostructured calcium-incorporated titanium surface or by longer implants in augmented bone. 3-year results from a randomized controlled trial. Eur J Oral Implantol 2018;11(1):49–61.

57. Romeo E, Storelli S, Casano G, et al. Six-mm versus 10-mm long implants in the rehabilitation of posterior edentulous jaws: a 5-year follow-up of a randomized controlled trial. Eur J Oral Implantol 2014;7(4):371–81.

58. ten Bruggenkate CM, Asikainen P, Foitzik C, et al. Short (6-mm) nonsubmerged dental implants: results of a multicenter clinical trial of 1 to 7 years. Int J Oral Maxillofac Implants 1998;13(6):791–8.

59. Tawil G, Younan R. Clinical evaluation of short, machined-surface implants followed for 12 to 92 months. Int J Oral Maxillofac Implants 2003;18(6):894–901.

60. Schincaglia GP, Thoma DS, Haas R, et al. Randomized controlled multicenter study comparing short dental implants (6 mm) versus longer dental implants (11-15 mm) in combination with sinus floor elevation procedures. Part 2: clinical and radiographic outcomes at 1 year of loading. J Clin Periodontol 2015;42(11):1042–51.

61. Pohl V, Thoma DS, Sporniak-Tutak K, et al. Short dental implants (6 mm) versus long dental implants (11-15 mm) in combination with sinus floor elevation procedures: 3-year results from a multicenter, randomized controlled clinical trial. J Clin Periodontol 2017;44(4):438–45.

62. Felice P, Barausse C, Pistilli V, et al. Posterior atrophic jaws rehabilitated with prostheses supported by 6 mm long X 4 mm wide implants or by longer implants in augmented bone. 3-year post-loading results from a randomized controlled trial. Eur J Oral Implantol 2018;11(2):175–87.

63. Feine JS, Carlsson GE, Awad MA, et al. The McGill consensus statement on overdentures. Mandibular two-implant overdentures as first choice standard of care for edentulous patients. Gerodontology 2002;19(1):3–4.

64. Jemt T, Chai J, Harnett J, et al. A 5-year prospective multicenter follow-up report on overdentures supported by osseointegrated implants. Int J Oral Maxillofac Implants 1996;11(3):291–8.

65. Andreiotelli M, Att W, Strub JR. Prosthodontic complications with implant overdentures: a systematic literature review. Int J Prosthodont 2010;23(3):195–203.

66. Maniewicz S, Buser R, Duvernay E, et al. Short dental implants retaining two-implant mandibular overdentures in very old, dependent patients: radiologic and clinical observations up to 5 years. Int J Oral Maxillofac Implants 2017; 32(2):415–22.

67. Friberg B, Gröndahl K, Lekholm U, et al. Long-term follow-up of severely atrophic edentulous mandibles reconstructed with short Brånemark implants. Clin Implant Dent Relat Res 2000;2(4):184–9.

68. Maló P, de Araújo Nobre MA, Lopes AV, et al. Immediate loading short implants inserted on low bone quantity for the rehabilitation of the edentulous maxilla using an all-on-4 design. J Oral Rehabil 2015;42(8):615–23.

69. Al-Johany SS, Al Amri MD, Alsaeed S, et al. Dental implant length and diameter: a proposed classification scheme. J Prosthodont 2017;26(3):252–60.

70. Lee JS, Kim HM, Kim CS, et al. Long-term retrospective study of narrow implants for fixed dental prostheses. Clin Oral Implants Res 2013;24(8):847–52.

71. Davarpanah M, Martinez H, Tecucianu JF, et al. Small diameter implants: indications and contraindications. J Esthet Dent 2000;12(4):186–94.

72. Klein MO, Schiegnitz E, Al-Nawas B. Systematic review on success of narrow-diameter dental implants. Int J Oral Maxillofac Implants 2014;29(Suppl):43–54.

73. Degidi M, Piattelli A, Carinci F. Clinical outcome of narrow diameter implants: a retrospective study of 510 implants. J Periodontol 2008;79(1):49–54.

74. Mendonça JA, Senna PM, Francischone CE, et al. Influence of the diameter of dental implants replacing single molars: 3- to 6-year follow-up. Int J Oral Maxillofac Implants 2017;32(5):1111–5.

75. Hallman M. A prospective study of treatment of severely resorbed maxillae with narrow nonsubmerged implants: results after 1 year of loading. Int J Oral Maxillofac Implants 2001;16(5):731–6.

76. Sohrabi K, Mushantat A, Esfandiari S, et al. How successful are small-diameter implants? A literature review. Clin Oral Implants Res 2012;23(5):515–25.

77. Zinsli B, Sägesser T, Mericske E, et al. Clinical evaluation of small-diameter ITI implants: a prospective study. Int J Oral Maxillofac Implants 2004;19(1):92–9.

78. Pieri F, Forlivesi C, Caselli E, et al. Narrow- (3.0 mm) versus standard-diameter (4.0 and 4.5 mm) implants for splinted partial fixed restoration of posterior mandibular and maxillary jaws: a 5-year retrospective cohort study. J Periodontol 2017;88(4):338–47.

79. Bidra AS, Almas K. Mini implants for definitive prosthodontic treatment: a systematic review. J Prosthet Dent 2013;109(3):156–64.

80. Morneburg TR, Pröschel PA. Success rates of microimplants in edentulous patients with residual ridge resorption. Int J Oral Maxillofac Implants 2008;23(3):270–6.

81. Marcello-Machado RM, Faot F, Schuster AJ, et al. Mini-implants and narrow diameter implants as mandibular overdenture retainers: a systematic review and meta-analysis of clinical and radiographic outcomes. J Oral Rehabil 2018;45(2): 161–83.
82. Cinel S, Celik E, Sagirkaya E, et al. Experimental evaluation of stress distribution with narrow diameter implants: a finite element analysis. J Prosthet Dent 2018; 119(3):417–25.
83. Maló P, de Araújo Nobre MA. Implants (3.3 mm diameter) for the rehabilitation of edentulous posterior regions: a retrospective clinical study with up to 11 years of follow-up. Clin Implant Dent Relat Res 2011;13(2):95–103.
84. Quek CE, Tan KB, Nicholls JI. Load fatigue performance of a single-tooth implant abutment system: effect of diameter. Int J Oral Maxillofac Implants 2006;21(6): 929–36.
85. Andersen E, Saxegaard E, Knutsen BM, et al. A prospective study evaluating the safety and effectiveness of narrow-diameter threaded implants in the anterior region of the maxilla. Int J Oral Maxillofac Implants 2001;16(2):217–24.
86. Shi JY, Xu FY, Zhuang LF, et al. Long-term outcomes of narrow diameter implants in posterior jaws: a retrospective study with at least 8-year follow-up. Clin Oral Implants Res 2018;29(1):76–81.
87. Maiorana C, King P, Quaas S, et al. Clinical and radiographic evaluation of early loaded narrow-diameter implants: 3 years follow-up. Clin Oral Implants Res 2015; 26(1):77–82.
88. Galindo-Moreno P, Nilsson P, King P, et al. Clinical and radiographic evaluation of early loaded narrow-diameter implants: 5-year follow-up of a multicenter prospective clinical study. Clin Oral Implants Res 2017;28(12):1584–91.
89. King P, Maiorana C, Luthardt RG, et al. Clinical and radiographic evaluation of a small-diameter dental implant used for the restoration of patients with permanent tooth agenesis (hypodontia) in the maxillary lateral incisor and mandibular incisor regions: a 36-month follow-up. Int J Prosthodont 2016;29(2):147–53.
90. Moráguez O, Vailati F, Grütter L, et al. Four-unit fixed dental prostheses replacing maxillary incisors supported by two narrow-diameter implants-a five-year case series. Clin Oral Implants Res 2017;28(7):887–92.
91. Jemt T, Albrektsson T. Do long-term followed-up Branemark implants commonly show evidence of pathological bone breakdown? A review based on recently published data. Periodontol 2000 2008;47:133–42.
92. Quirynen M, Al-Nawas B, Meijer HJ, et al. Small-diameter titanium grade IV and titanium-zirconium implants in edentulous mandibles: three-year results from a double-blind, randomized controlled trial. Clin Oral Implants Res 2015;26(7): 831–40.
93. Müller F, Al-Nawas B, Storelli S, et al. Small-diameter titanium grade IV and titanium-zirconium implants in edentulous mandibles: five-year results from a double-blind, randomized controlled trial. BMC Oral Health 2015;15(1):123.
94. Arisan V, Bölükbasi N, Ersanli S, et al. Evaluation of 316 narrow diameter implants followed for 5-10 years: a clinical and radiographic retrospective study. Clin Oral Implants Res 2010;21(3):296–307.
95. Giannakopoulos NN, Ariaans K, Eberhard L, et al. Immediate and delayed loading of two-piece reduced-diameter implants with locator-analog attachments in edentulous mandibles: one-year results from a randomized clinical trial examining clinical outcomes and patient expectations. Clin Implant Dent Relat Res 2017;19(4):643–53.

Are There Alternatives to Invasive Site Development for Dental Implants? Part II

Vaughan J. Hoefler, DDS, MBA[a],*, Mohanad Al-Sabbagh, DDS, MS[b]

KEYWORDS

- Tilted implant - All-on-4 - Atrophic ridge - Site development - Zygomatic implant

KEY POINTS

- Alternatives to invasive site development for dental implant therapy include the use of tilted dental implants, zygomatic implants, and fewer numbers of implants. These alternatives have the advantages of reduced morbidity, fewer complications, shorter treatment time, lower costs, and better patient acceptance.
- Tilted implants often eliminate the need for bone grafting.
- Use of tilted and upright implants in combination allows clinicians to predictably rehabilitate edentulous arches with a fixed prosthesis supported by as few as 4 dental implants.
- Zygomatic implants, either alone or in combination with upright and tilted maxillary implants, can provide a graftless solution to restore the atrophic edentulous maxilla when there is inadequate bone for conventional or all-on-4 treatment.

INTRODUCTION

Edentulous sites are often characterized by moderate or advanced ridge resorption and irregular crestal bone topography, which compromises proper 3-dimensional implant positioning. If a given site cannot be functionally or esthetically restored with a dental implant, bone grafting is often needed.[1–3] Bone grafting often prolongs treatment time and increases morbidity and expense. For these reasons, patients prefer less invasive treatment alternatives.[4–6]

One alternative to bone grafting is the use of tilted implants that engage native bone with adequate volume, density, and structure to support a fixed restoration. For the

Disclosure: The authors have nothing to disclose.
[a] Department of Oral Health Practice, Division of Prosthodontics, University of Kentucky, College of Dentistry, UK Chandler Hospital, D630, 800 Rose Street, Lexington, KY 40536-0297, USA; [b] Division of Periodontology, Department of Oral Health Practice, University of Kentucky College of Dentistry, D-438 Chandler Medical Center, 800 Rose Street, Lexington, KY 40536-0927, USA
* Corresponding author.
E-mail address: vaughan.hoefler@uky.edu

Dent Clin N Am 63 (2019) 489–498
https://doi.org/10.1016/j.cden.2019.02.012
0011-8532/19/© 2019 Elsevier Inc. All rights reserved.

dental.theclinics.com

edentulous arch, a second alternative is to use a combination of four or fewer tilted and upright implants to support full-arch fixed dental prostheses (FAFDPs). This chapter will address three questions: (1) Are tilted implants a sound alternative to axially loaded implants placed in grafted edentulous sites? (2) Are 4 or fewer axially loaded and tilted implants adequate to support a cross-arch fixed prosthesis? (3) Are zygomatic implants a viable alternative to invasive bone grafting of severely atrophic edentulous maxillary ridges?

Are Tilted Implants a Sound Alternative to Axially Loaded Implants Placed in Grafted Sites in Edentulous Arches?

Historically, the use of upright implants (implants placed perpendicular to the plane of occlusion) was the standard procedure for the rehabilitation of completely edentulous arches with implant-supported fixed prostheses.[7,8] However, this is often not achievable without extensive bone grafting and avoiding vital anatomic structures (eg, the inferior alveolar nerve, the maxillary sinus, and the nasal cavity).[8] The use of tilted implants is an alternative to upright implant placement in grafted bone. Tilted implants engage the maximum available residual bone in remote sites for enhanced anchorage and stability.

Guidelines and history

Tilted implants allows fixtures to be placed in any direction targeting native bone.[9] For the edentulous maxilla, these sites include the anterior and posterior walls of the maxillary sinus, the nasal floor, the nasal spine, the pterygoid process, and the maxillary tuberosity.[10,11] The use of tilted implants to avoid bone grafting in the edentulous maxilla was first described by Mattson et al.[10] This study utilized 86 axial and tilted implants to treat 15 patients who needed bone grafting for conventional axial implant placement. In the edentulous mandible, a combination of axially loaded and tilted implants can be placed in the interforaminal region to avoid bone grafting in the posterior region. In addition, angulated implants can optimize anchorage, minimize cantilever length, and maximize interimplant distance.[8,12] Maló et al[12] restored the edentulous mandibles of 44 patients with FAFDPs supported by 176 axially and distally inclined Brånemark implants.[12] Maló et al called this the "all-on-4" treatment concept.[12]

Advantages of tilted implants

Implant angulations, lengths, and diameters are generally selected to fit within the boundaries of available bone. A minimum angulation that defines a tilted implant has not been established. However, a range of 15° to 45° off the vertical axis has been used to describe tilted implants by several authors.[8,12–15] Longer implants are generally preferred to improve primary stability and engage as much residual bone as possible.[14,15] Most tilted implant diameters fall within the range of 3.3 to 5.0 mm.[12,14,16]

For implant rehabilitation of edentulous arches with inadequate bone volume, tilted implants have several advantages over axially loaded implants. The use of longer fixtures improves primary stability by engaging more bone.[15] The increased distance between the anterior and posterior restorative platforms created by tilting implants reduces cantilever length and improves load distribution.[8,9] Tilted implants are placed in residual native bone, eliminating the need for nerve lateralization and bone grafting, thereby reducing morbidity, expense and treatment time.[8,10,11] Finally, tilted implants with good primary stability and cross-arch distribution can generally be immediately loaded with a fixed interim prosthesis, while allowing fewer numbers of implants to be used (**Figs. 1–4**).[12–14]

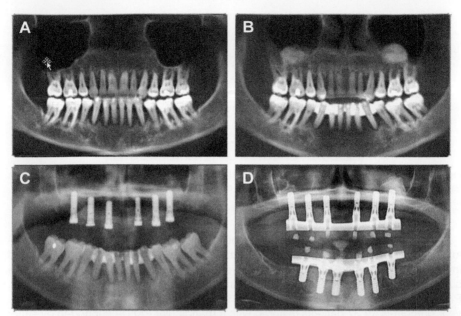

Fig. 1. Full arch implant rehabilitation using axially loaded implants to support FAFDP. (*A*) Teeth were diagnosed with severe periodontitis. (*B*) Bilateral maxillary sinus grafting was performed before extraction of teeth. (*C*) All maxillary teeth were extracted, and 6 parallel implants were placed perpendicular to the occlusal plane and distributed to minimize cantilevers and optimize load distribution. (*D*) Final maxillary and mandibular FAFDPs after 5 years in function.

Outcomes for tilted versus upright implants

There is a scarcity of randomized controlled trials (RCTs) comparing outcomes for patients treated with upright implants placed in grafted sites with similar groups restored with tilted implants in nongrafted sites. One of the first forays into this area was by Widmark et al., who reported that in the maxilla, implants placed in native bone had a higher success rate after five years (87%) than implants placed in grafted sites (74%).[17] A limitation of this study is that although trial implants were positioned to avoid bone grafting, not all were tilted.[17,18]

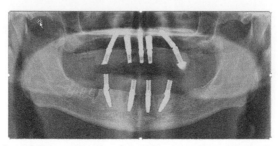

Fig. 2. Rehabilitation of the maxillary and mandibular arches with implant supported fixed prostheses using tilted implants. The use of tilted implants allows for longer implants to engage more native bone. This promotes primary stability and eliminates the need for onlay, interpositional block grafts, or maxillary sinus grafting. Additional advantages include reduced treatment time and decreased numbers of implants to support an FAFDP.

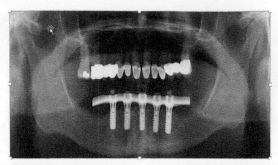

Fig. 3. Full-arch fixed dental mandibular prosthesis with 5 implants. The mandibular arch is square, and the interforaminal area is wide enough to accommodate 5 well-distributed, axially loaded implants.

Another early study restored maxillary posterior quadrants of 25 partially-edentulous patients with partial fixed dental prosthesis (PFDP) using 101 upright and tilted implants in nongrafted sites.[11] After five years, investigators reported a cumulative survival rate (CSR) of 95.2% for 42 tilted implants and 91.3% for 59 axial implants. Prosthesis survival at five years was 100%. A more recent study reported three-year outcomes for 37 patients restored with a mandibular FAFDP supported by either four upright implants, or two upright anterior and two tilted posterior implants.[16] There were no reported differences in outcomes between the 2 groups with respect to implant survival, prosthesis complications, marginal bone loss (MBL), or periodontal probing depth. Recent systematic reviews pooling data from a number of clinical studies using tilted implants reported similar findings.[9,14,15,19]

In summary, tilted implants, placed in tandem or in combination with upright implants, can reduce or eliminate the need for bone grafting, reduce complication risk, and result in high levels of patient satisfaction when used to restore partially and fully edentulous jaws.[6,9,11,14]

Are Four or Fewer Implants Adequate to Support a Full Arch Fixed Prosthesis?

An implant load analysis investigation concluded that as few as four implants may be adequate for a full-arch fixed prosthesis when the implants are properly positioned.[20] An early application of this finding was the introduction of the all-on-4

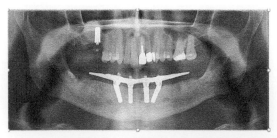

Fig. 4. Full-arch fixed dental mandibular prosthesis with 4 implants. The mandibular arch is V-shaped, and the interforaminal area is narrow. Posterior implants were tilted to avoid the mental foramina and increase the anteroposterior spread. Four implants (2 axially loaded implants in the anterior segment of the mandible and 2 tilted implants mesial to the mental foramina) were adequate to support full a 12-unit FAFDP.

immediate-function treatment concept for the mandible in 2003,[12] and the maxilla in 2005.[12,21] The all-on-4 immediate-function treatment concept consists of 3 principles: the use of a combination of upright and tilted implants to avoid bone grafting, 4 implants in each edentulous jaw to support a fixed prosthesis, and immediate loading.

The all-on-4 treatment protocol uses four upright and tilted implants in the anterior edentulous jaw to support an immediately loaded, cross-arch fixed prosthesis. Two anterior implants are axially oriented and placed in the incisor region, while posterior implants are tilted distally with the implant platform in the second premolar/first molar area.[12,13,21] The goal is to create a large inter-implant distance that minimizes cantilever length. To facilitate immediate loading, a modified surgical protocol can be followed which achieves an adequate minimum insertion torque depending on the quality and volume of available bone.[12,21]

All-on-4 treatment outcomes
Studies comparing the effectiveness of the all-on-4 treatment concept to 5 or more upright implants in grafted bone are lacking. One retrospective study reported outcomes for 380 patients restored with 482 immediately loaded FAFDPs supported by 4, 5, and 6 upright and tilted implants.[22] The 7-year CSR for the 2081 implants was 97.0%. Implant survival rates for restorations supported by 4, 5, and 6 implants were 96.5%, 96.6%, and 99.7%, respectively. However, the study protocol dictated that if an insertion torque of ≥30 Ncm was achieved for 4 implants, no additional implants were placed. This suggests that when five or six implants were placed they may have been used in arches with lower bone volume or quality.

Two systematic reviews reported favorable all-on-4 treatment outcomes,[13,23] although some of the included studies were of limited quality and short duration. A long-term clinical study followed 245 patients with edentulous mandibles treated with the all-on-4 protocol for 10 years.[24] The 10-year implant CSR was 94.8%, with a prosthesis survival rate of 99.2%. Another clinical research group treated 200 maxillary and mandibular arches with 800 implants following the all-on-4 treatment protocol.[25] After five-years, an, implant CSR of 97.3% was reported for both axial and tilted implants. The prosthetic survival rate was 99.0%. Similar outcomes were reported in another study where 111 patients were treated and followed for up to 7 years.[26] The 7-year implant CSR was 94.5%, while prosthetic survival rate was 97.8%. The average MBL at 5 years was 1.27 mm for tilted implants and 1.34 mm for axial implants. A study that followed 12 patients for 7 years reported 100% implant and prosthetic survival rates, but documented several prosthetic complications.[27] These complications included tooth fracture (6.25%), loosening of prosthetic and abutments screws (18.75%), and replacement of denture teeth (18.75%)

Full-arch fixed dental prostheses with 2 or 3 implants
Recent preliminary investigations report 6- and 12-month outcomes for FAFDPs supported by 2 (fixed-on-2) or 3 (fixed-on-3) implants in the mandible and maxilla, respectively.[28,29] A 6-month cohort study placed machined surface implants as parallel as possible using a flapless surgical approach to treat 25 patients.[28] If a minimum insertion torque could be achieved, an immediate, interim fixed prosthesis was placed. Investigators reported 100% implant and prosthesis survival for both arches after 6 months of loading.

Another 12-month study followed a similar treatment protocol (fixed-on-2 for the mandible, fixed-on-3 for the maxilla), with 40 patients randomly assigned to 1 of 2 treatment arms.[29] Group 1 received machined surface implants, while the other received rough surface implants. For the mandible, implants were placed in both canine/first premolar positions, while in the maxillae, the 2 distal implants were placed as far posteriorly on each side of the arch as bone volume allowed. The third implant site was placed as centrally as possible, preferably in the central incisor region but, wherever bone volume allowed. Two implants were lost during the reporting period. Only minor prosthetic complications were reported, including several functional or esthetic complaints associated with the shortened dental arch prosthesis. Otherwise, significant differences were not detected between the two treatment groups.

Advantages of these treatment protocols include the ability to simultaneously treat both jaws in a single, relatively short surgical session, the comparative ease of fabricating prosthesis frameworks that precisely and passively seat on fewer numbers of implants, and lower expense associated with fewer implants. However, while these results suggest that an immediately loaded cross-arch fixed prosthesis can be supported by only 2 mandibular and 3 maxillary dental implants, it must be emphasized that this treatment approach has not been validated. For this reason, it should be considered preliminary and highly experimental at this time.

It remains unclear as to the optimal minimal number of implants needed to support a partial or cross-arch fixed prosthesis at this time. Two well-constructed recent reviews independently concluded that successful outcomes after 5 years and beyond should be expected for FAFDPs supported by 4 to 6 implants.[30,31] However, the number of teeth replaced by an implant-supported FAFDP can be variable, making it difficult to make direct comparisons across studies. Since FAFDPs generally replace 10 to 12 teeth,[22,29,30] the implant-to-replaced-units ratio may be a more reliable metric for reporting implant and prosthetic survival outcomes in the future.[30]

Are Zygomatic Implants a Viable Alternative to Invasive Bone Grafting Severely Atrophic Edentulous Maxillary Ridges?

Planning the restoration of the edentulous maxilla with an implant-supported FAFDP can sometimes require addressing profound anatomic challenges. The combination of a severely atrophic maxillary ridge and large pneumatized maxillary sinus can lead to inadequate bone volume for vertical or tilted implants.[32] In 1998, Branemark introduced zygomatic implants as an alternative anchorage solution for cancer patients who had undergone maxillectomy.[33] Zygomatic implants are self-tapping, screw-shaped fixtures that engage the zygomatic buttress to gain primary stability and anchorage.

Zygomatic implants can be used to restore the severely atrophic edentulous maxilla without bone grafting and in reduced treatment time.[34–36] Zygomatic implants can be used independently, or in combination with vertical and tilted implants placed in the anterior and posterior maxilla.[34–36] A limitation of zygomatic implants is the surgical parameters dictated by the anatomy of zygomatic bone.[37] Zygomatic implants have also been associated with increased sinusitis and peri-implant bleeding due to oral hygiene difficulties.[38]

Zygomatic implants are available in 8 different lengths starting from 30 mm to 52.5 mm. They have a 45° angulated head to create a restorative platform that is accessible to the restorative dentist and parallel to the platforms of vertically placed implants.[36] The apical section, which engages the zygomatic bone, is threaded with a diameter of 4 mm, while the head of the fixture, which engages the maxillary residual alveolar ridge, has a diameter of 4.5 mm.

General guidelines for zygomatic implants

Patient selection is determined following a detailed prosthetic and surgical evaluation.[35] Bedrossian et al divided the maxilla into three zones, the anterior teeth (zone 1), the premolars (zone 2), and the molars (zone 3).[35,36] The treatment concept is based on the volume of available bone in each of the 3 zones. If adequate bone is available in zones 1, 2, and 3 for axially loaded implants, a traditional approach can be followed using upright implants in the anterior and posterior maxilla.[36] If adequate bone is only available in zones 1 and 2, the all-on-4 treatment concept can be implemented.[36] The zygomatic implant concept was developed for patients with insufficient bone in zones 2 and 3, or lacking bone in all 3 zones. In cases where bone is only available in zone 1, prosthesis support can be derived from a minimum of 4 implants, 2 premaxillary implants and 2 zygomatic implants.[36,37] The angulation of the head of the zygomatic implant allows the restorative platform of all implants to be in the same plane.[36] Anterior and zygomatic fixtures can then be splinted to support a screw-retained fixed prosthesis. In situations whereby bone is lacking in all 3 zones, 4 zygomatic implants (quad zygoma), 2 in each buttress, can be used to support an FAFDP.[36,37]

In summary, when posterior bone is unilaterally or bilaterally lacking in zones 2 and 3 for proper prosthesis support, zygomatic implants can complement upright or tilted conventional implants. It is also provides a graftless solution when all 3 zones are deficient in bone.

Treatment outcomes with zygomatic implants

A recent systematic review[38] investigated the survival and complications of zygomatic implants over 12 years. The survival rate of zygomatic implants was 95.21%. Implant failure was only detected in the first six months following surgery, with sinusitis the main complication at a rate of 2.4%. In three additional reports, zygoma quad and two zygoma implants coupled with maxillary anterior axial implants have been shown to have similar survival rates.[39-41]

SUMMARY

At this time, the literature does not report greater risk for implant loss, MBL, and peri-implant soft tissue complications for tilted implants compared to upright implants placed in grafted bone. Moreover, tilted implants create several advantages when used in combination with upright implants to support FAFDPS. Tilted implants reduce, and in many cases eliminate, the need for vital structure navigation and complex bone regenerative procedures. Tilted implants also allow greater spacing between their restorative platforms relative to upright implants, optimizing load distribution and allowing prosthesis designs with reduced distal cantilevers. Tilted implants in many cases allow the use of fewer implants to replace missing teeth in edentulous jaws restored with FAFDPs.

While the all-on-4 treatment concept appears to provide a predictable long-term outcome when used to restore edentulous jaws with FAFDPs, there is no evidence at this time that similar results should be expected with fixed-on-2 or fixed-on 3 protocols. Properly designed controlled trials comparing different numbers and distributions of implants are needed before adopting these protocols.

Finally, for the severely atrophic maxilla with pneumatized maxillary sinuses, the use of zygomatic implants can be the treatment of choice as an alternative to an invasive bony ridge augmentation and/or maxillary sinus elevation procedure. Long-term RCTs comparing diverse populations of patients treated with zygomatic implants to similar groups treated with upright and tilted implants placed in grafted maxillary sites are not available at this time.

REFERENCES

1. Chiapasco M, Zaniboni M, Boisco M. Augmentation procedures for the rehabilitation of deficient edentulous ridges with oral implants. Clin Oral Implants Res 2006;17(Suppl 2):136–59.
2. Aghaloo TL, Moy PK. Which hard tissue augmentation techniques are the most successful in furnishing bony support for implant placement? Int J Oral Maxillofac Implants 2007;22(Suppl):49–70 [Erratum in Int J Oral Maxillofac Implants 2008;23(1):56].
3. Aloy-Prósper A, Peñarrocha-Oltra D, Peñarrocha-Diago M, et al. The outcome of intraoral onlay block bone grafts on alveolar ridge augmentations: a systematic review. Med Oral Patol Oral Cir Bucal 2015;20(2):e251–8.
4. Thoma DS, Haas R, Tutak M, et al. Randomized controlled multicenter study comparing short dental implants (6 mm) versus longer dental implants (11-15 mm) in combination with sinus floor elevation procedures. Part 1: demographics and patient-oriented outcomes at 1 year of loading. J Clin Periodontol 2015;42(1):72–80.
5. Felice P, Barausse C, Pistilli V, et al. Posterior atrophic jaws rehabilitated with prostheses supported by 6 mm long X 4 mm wide implants or by longer implants in augmented bone. 3-year post-loading results from a randomized controlled trial. Eur J Oral Implantol 2018;11(2):175–87.
6. Pommer B, Mailath-Pokorny G, Haas R, et al. Patients' preferences towards minimally invasive treatment alternatives for implant rehabilitation of edentulous jaws. Eur J Oral Implantol 2014;7(Suppl 2):S91–109.
7. Block MS, Widner JS. Method for insuring parallelism of implants placed simultaneously with maxillary sinus bone grafts. J Oral Maxillofac Surg 1991;49(4): 435–7.
8. Krekmanov L, Kahn M, Rangert B, et al. Tilting of posterior mandibular and maxillary implants for improved prosthesis support. Int J Oral Maxillofac Implants 2000;15(3):405–14.
9. Peñarrocha-Oltra D, Candel-Marti E, Ata-Ali J, et al. Rehabilitation of the atrophic maxilla with tilted implants: review of the literature. J Oral Implantol 2013;39(5): 625–32.
10. Mattson T, Köndell PA, Gynther GW, et al. Implant treatment without bone grafting in severely resorbed edentulous maxillae. J Oral Maxillofac Surg 1999;57(3): 281–7.
11. Aparicio C, Perales P, Rangert B. Tilted implants as an alternative to maxillary sinus grafting: a clinical, radiologic, and periotest study. Clin Implant Dent Relat Res 2001;3(1):39–49.
12. Maló P, Rangert B, Nobre M. "All-on-Four": immediate-function concept with Brånemark System implants for completely edentulous mandibles: a retrospective clinical study. Clin Implant Dent Relat Res 2003;5(Suppl 1):2–9.
13. Patzelt SB, Bahat O, Reynolds MA, et al. The all-on-four treatment concept: a systematic review. Clin Implant Dent Relat Res 2014;16(6):836–55.
14. Del Fabbro M, Bellini CM, Romeo D, et al. Tilted implants for the rehabilitation of edentulous jaws. a systematic review. Clin Implant Dent Relat Res 2012;14(4): 612–21.

15. Chrcanovic BR, Albrektsson T, Wennerberg A. Tilted versus axially placed dental implants: a meta-analysis. J Dent 2015;43(2):149–70.
16. Krennmair S, Weinländer M, Malek M, et al. Mandibular full-arch fixed prostheses supported on 4 implants with either axial or tilted distal implants: a 3-year prospective study. Clin Implant Dent Relat Res 2016;18(6):1119–33.
17. Widmark G, Andersson B, Carlsson GE, et al. Rehabilitation of patients with severely resorbed maxillae by means of implants with or without bone grafts: a 3- to 5-year follow-up clinical report. Int J Oral Maxillofac Implants 2001;16(1): 73–9.
18. Widmark G, Andersson B, Andrup B, et al. Rehabilitation of patients with severely resorbed maxillae by means of implants with or without bone grafts. A 1-year follow-up study. Int J Oral Maxillofac Implants 1998;13(4):474–82.
19. Menini M, Signori A, Tealdo T, et al. Tilted implants in the immediate loading rehabilitation of the maxilla: a systematic review. J Dent Res 2012;91(9):821–7.
20. Duyck J, Van Oosterwyck H, Vander Sloten J, et al. Magnitude and distribution of occlusal forces on oral implants supporting fixed prostheses: an in vivo study. Clin Oral Implants Res 2000;11(5):465–75.
21. Maló P, Rangert B, Nobre M. All-on-Four immediate-function concept with Brånemark System implants for completely edentulous maxillae: a 1-year retrospective clinical study. Clin Implant Dent Relat Res 2005;7(Suppl 1):S88–94.
22. Niedermaier R, Stelzle F, Riemann M, et al. Implant-supported immediately loaded fixed full-arch dentures: evaluation of implant survival rates in a case cohort of up to 7 years. Clin Implant Dent Relat Res 2017;19(1):4–19.
23. Soto-Penaloza D, Zaragozi-Alonso R, Penarrocha-Diago M, et al. The all-on-four treatment concept: systematic review. J Clin Exp Dent 2017;9(3):e474–88.
24. Malo P, de Araújo Nobre M, Lopes A, et al. A longitudinal study of the survival of All-on-4 implants in the mandible with up to 10 years of follow-up. J Am Dent Assoc 2011;142(3):310–20.
25. Balshi TJ, Wolfinger GJ, Slauch RW, et al. A retrospective analysis of 800 Brånemark System implants following the All-on-Four protocol. J Prosthodont 2014; 23(2):83–8.
26. Lopes A, Maló P, de Araújo Nobre M, et al. The NobelGuide® All-on-4® treatment concept for rehabilitation of edentulous jaws: a retrospective report on the 7-years clinical and 5-years radiographic outcomes. Clin Implant Dent Relat Res 2017;19(2):233–44.
27. Ayub KV, Ayub EA, Lins do Valle A, et al. Seven-year follow-up of full-arch prostheses supported by four implants: a prospective study. Int J Oral Maxillofac Implants 2017;32(6):1351–8.
28. Cannizzaro G, Felice P, Loi I, et al. Immediately loading of bimaxillary total fixed prostheses supported by five flapless-placed implants with machined surfaces: a 6-month follow-up prospective single cohort study. Eur J Oral Implantol 2016; 9(1):67–74.
29. Cannizzaro G, Gastaldi G, Gherlone E, et al. Two or three machined vs roughened surface dental implants loaded immediately supporting total fixed prostheses: 1-year results from a randomized controlled trial. Eur J Oral Implantol 2017; 10(3):279–91.
30. Heydecke G, Zwahlen M, Nicol A, et al. What is the optimal number of implants for fixed reconstructions: a systematic review. Clin Oral Implants Res 2012; 23(Suppl 6):217–28.
31. Mericske-Stern R, Worni A. Optimal number of oral implants for fixed reconstructions: a review of the literature. Eur J Oral Implantol 2014;7(Suppl 2):S133–53.

32. Higuchi KW. The zygomaticus fixture: an alternative approach for implant anchorage in the posterior maxilla. Ann R Australas Coll Dent Surg 2000;15: 28–33.

33. Brånemark P. Surgery and fixture installation. Zygomaticus Fixture Clinical Procedures. Göteborg (Sweden): Nobel Biocare; 1998. p. 1.

34. Branemark PI, Gröndahl K, Ohrnell LO, et al. Zygoma fixture in the management of advanced atrophy of the maxilla: technique and long-term results. Scand J Plast Reconstr Surg Hand Surg 2004;38(2):70–85.

35. Bedrossian E, Sullivan RM, Fortin Y, et al. Fixed-prosthetic implant restoration of the edentulous maxilla: a systematic pretreatment evaluation method. J Oral Maxillofac Surg 2008;66:112–22.

36. Bedrossiasn E. Rescue implant concept: the expanded use of the zygoma implant in the graftless solution. Dent Clin North Am 2011;55(4):745–77.

37. Aparicio C, Manresa C, Francisco K, et al. Zygomatic implants: indications, techniques and outcomes, and the zygomatic success codes. Periodontol 2000 2014;66(1):41–58.

38. Chrcanovic BR, Albrektsson T, Wennerberg A. Survival and Complications of Zygomatic Implants: An Updated Systematic Review. J Oral Maxillofac Surg 2016;74(10):1949–64.

39. Balshi TJ, Wolfinger GJ, Petropoulos VC. Quadruple zygomatic implant support for retreatment of resorbed iliac crest bone graft transplant. Implant Dent 2003; 12(1):47–53.

40. Davo R, Malevez C, Rojas J, et al. Clinical outcome of 42 patients treated with 81 immediately loaded zygomatic implants: a 12- to 42-month retrospective study. Eur J Oral Implantol 2008;9. Suppl 1(2):141–50.

41. Aboul-Hosn Centenero S, Lázaro A, Giralt-Hernando M, et al. Zygoma quad compared with 2 zygomatic implants: a systematic review and meta-analysis. Implant Dent 2018. [Epub ahead of print].

Zygoma Implants or Sinus Lift for the Atrophic Maxilla with a Dentate Mandible
Which is the Better Option?

Enif A. Dominguez, DDS[a],*, Cesar Guerrero, DDS[b,c,d],
Ehab Shehata, DDS, MD, MSc (GS), PhD[a,e], Joseph E. Van Sickels, DDS[a]

KEYWORDS

- Tilted implants • Immediate loading • Delayed loading • Maxillary sinus grafting
- Zygoma implant

KEY POINTS

- "Teeth-in-a-day" in atrophic maxilla is achieved by immediate loading of zygomatic implants following the concept of cross-arch stabilization.
- Placement of zygomatic implant is technique sensitive and requires knowledge of the local anatomy. However, it reduces the treatment time before the prosthetic reconstruction.
- In cases of severe maxillary anatomic constraints, zygomatic implant to rehabilitate maxillary atrophy is considered a valid alternative treatment to maxillary sinus graft or alveolar ridge bone augmentation.
- Zygomatic implant is performed in atrophic maxilla with dentate mandible. Restoration varies depending on the residual maxillary anatomy.

INTRODUCTION

Maxillary atrophy represents a challenge for surgeons and restorative providers. Ideally, prosthetic restoration should restore mastication, comfort, and phonation, allowing for an improved quality of life.[1–4] Autogenous bone graft is considered the

Disclosure: The authors have nothing to disclose.
[a] Division of Oral and Maxillofacial Surgery, Department of Oral Health Science, University of Kentucky, College of Dentistry, Albert B. Chandler Hospital, D508, 800 Rose Street, Lexington, KY 40536, USA; [b] Private Practice, Clear Choice Dental Implant Center, 929 Gessner Road, Suite 2050, Houston, TX 77024, USA; [c] The Woodlands Oral & Facial Surgery Center, 10857 Kuykendahl Road. Ste 150, The Woodlands, Tx 77382, USA; [d] Private Practice, Oral and Maxillofacial Surgery, 907 Bay Area Boulevard, Houston, TX 77058, USA; [e] Department of Maxillofacial and Plastic Surgery, College of Dentistry, Alexandria University, Alexandria, Egypt
* Corresponding author.
E-mail address: enif.dominguez@uky.edu

Dent Clin N Am 63 (2019) 499–513
https://doi.org/10.1016/j.cden.2019.02.013
0011-8532/19/© 2019 Elsevier Inc. All rights reserved.

dental.theclinics.com

gold standard technique because of its osteogenic, osteoconductive, and osteoinductive properties.[5–7] Historically, restoration of the severely atrophic maxilla involved obtaining bone graft from the iliac crest for onlay or interpositional techniques. Such surgical procedures required multiple surgical sites, prolonged hospital stays, and possible donor site morbidities.[4,8] Potential complications encountered include sinusitis, graft exposure or resorption, infection, neurosensory deficits, and insufficient bone quantity or quality. In addition, failure and unpredictable outcome of such autogenous grafting techniques often reduced patient acceptance.[4,8,9]

To avoid the disadvantages of autogenous bone grafting, bone substitutes and biologics (bone morphogenetic proteins, membranes, platelet-rich plasma, platelet-rich fibrin) are commonly used. However, they remain inferior to clinical outcomes achieved by using autogenous bone grafts.[5–7]

Sinus Augmentation

Maxillary sinus augmentation and bone grafting has provided an alternative treatment option to augment maxillary atrophic ridges, allowing for restoration with immediate or delayed implant placement. Primary implant stability requires a minimum of 3 to 5 mm of crestal bone to justify simultaneous implant placement with maxillary sinus lift and bone grafting.[10] When inadequate alveolar bone height is present, a maxillary sinus graft and 4 to 8 months healing time is required before the implant placement. In addition, a third surgical procedure is needed to uncover the implants for the final prosthetic rehabilitation. Three surgical stages is still a common practice in many clinics; however, it prolongs the time before the prosthetic reconstruction.[10–12]

Chin[13] introduced a dental implant stabilization system for simultaneous sinus lift and implant placement when poor primary stability is present that allows the osseointegration to occur in conjunction with bone healing. This technique is applied to single or multiple implants and is combined with temporary implants for immediate provisional prosthetic anchorage.

All-on-X

The introduction of all-on-four by Malo and coworkers[14–17] has changed the clinical protocols emphasizing the use of available bone with predictable bone maintenance and implant success.[18] He demonstrated the use of longer, wider implants with deeper threads and newer implant surfaces. In addition, tilted implants with multiunit abutments placed at different angulations allow the clinician to immediately deliver the provisional prosthesis and avoid additional surgical procedures, such as maxillary sinus and ridge augmentation. The definitive restoration may be delivered after 3 or 4 months of healing.[19] To overcome anatomic limitations to atrophic maxillae, all-on-four is modified to include placement of zygoma implants.

Zygoma Implants

The use of zygoma implants in the posterior maxilla and conventional implants in the anterior zone offers the possibility to provide anchorage for immediate provisional teeth in the upper arch.[20]

This technique eliminates donor site morbidity and reduces the treatment time. Zygoma implants engage multiple cortical walls, allowing for adequate primary stability for immediate loading.[21] Implants are inserted through the crestal bone into the bicortical zygoma with adequate quality and quantity of bone. Even when crestal bone of the maxillary alveolar ridge is not adequate, the implant fixtures allow a minimum of 8 to 10 mm of bone contact within the body of the zygoma for primary stability. The zygomatic implant platform is straight (0°) or angled up to 45° to allow the platforms to be in the same plane as the conventional implants for passive prosthetic insertion.[21–25] Cross-arch distribution of the functional is essential to prevent undesirable forces, osseointegration failure, and prosthetic complications. The prosthesis must be reinforced with a rigid bar for cross-arch stabilization.[25–29]

SURGICAL APPROACHES FOR VARIOUS ANATOMIC PRESENTATIONS

The maxillary anatomy as assessed is divided into three radiographic zones as described by Bedrossian and colleagues.[24] Zone 1 is the maxillary anterior teeth, zone 2 is the premolar region, and zone 3 is at the molar region. We use this classification to stratify our treatment as seen next.

Ideal Bone Morphology

Modified classical implant distribution and immediate loading
When ideal bone quantity and quality are present in all zones of the maxilla, six parallel implants are placed in sites 3, 5, 7, 10, 12, and 14 (wide implants in sites 3 and 14, if possible). After implants are integrated, a fixed prosthesis is installed. Bone reduction may be required to allow room for the prosthetic suprastructure.[10–12]

Large Maxillary Sinus with Moderate Posterior Vertical Bone Deficiency

All-on-X concept (five or six fixtures) with immediate loading
Sinus pneumatization decreases the amount of available vertical bone in the posterior maxilla (zone 3). Two tilted implants (up to 45°) avoiding the sinus floor cavity can be placed in sites 4 and 13. Three or four additional implants are placed anteriorly in sites 6, 8, 9, and 11. Bone reduction (ostectomy) may be required for insertion of a prosthesis. Immediate loading with provisional teeth is often predictable because of the cross-arch stabilization concept (**Fig. 1**).[14–17]

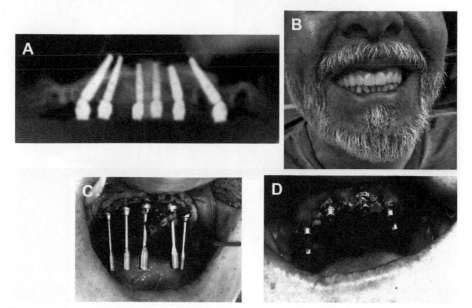

Fig. 1. Implants avoiding the sinus. (*A*) Panoramic view showing angulated implants avoiding the maxillary sinus. (*B*) Immediate temporary dental rehabilitation. (*C*) Verifying parallelism and adjusting the need to move the implant (*arrow*) for passive prosthetic Insertiton. (*D*) Implants placed and wounds sutured with perfect emergence profile.

Large Maxillary Sinus with Severe Posterior Vertical Bone Deficiency

Two- or three-stage surgery (treatment time 24–36 months)
The maxillary sinus graft is completed first, followed by 5 to 6 months of healing time. Next, the implants are placed and an additional 4 to 6 months of healing time is needed for osseointegration of the implants. Temporary implants are placed during the maturation of the bone and osseointegration, allowing immediate provisional prosthesis (**Fig. 2**).[5–8]

Large Maxillary Sinus with Severe Posterior Bone Deficiency

Two surgical stages (treatment time 6–9 months)
When less than 3 to 5 mm of crestal bone is present, simultaneous sinus lift, implant placement and plate stabilization are used for long-term predictability as described by Chin (**Fig. 3**).[6,7,10–13]

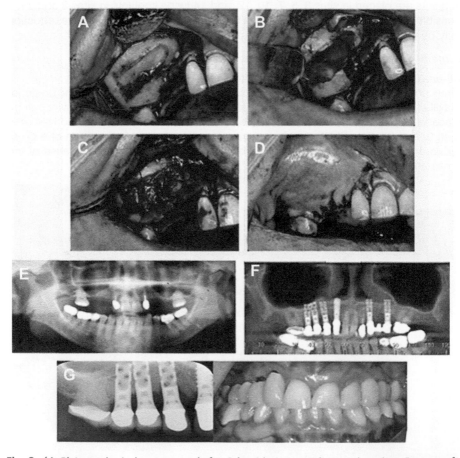

Fig. 2. (*A–D*) Lateral window approach for Schneiderian membrane elevation. Bone graft is placed in the floor of the sinus. Membrane is placed to cover the window and avoid mucosal invagination and flap sutured. Pre and post-op panorex showing (*E*) Severe maxillary sinus pneumatization bilaterally with no room for implant placement (*F*) Long term follow-up with implants and final restorations in place. (14 years F/U). (*G*) Final restorations radiographically and clinically after 14 years of follow-up. (*Courtesy of* Robert Gilbert Triplett, DDS, Dallas, TX.)

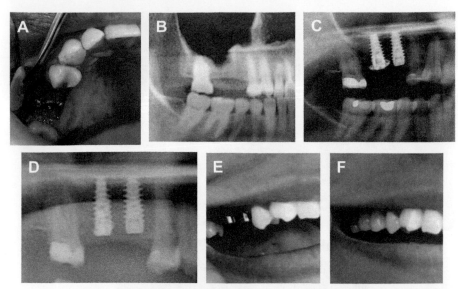

Fig. 3. Martin Chin's protocol. (*A*) Intraoperative view with implant stabilized with a three-hole microplate fixed to buccal and palate and the middle hole is stabilizing the implant by inserting a cover screw through the plate into the implant. (*B*) Preoperative radiograph showing the severe alveolar crest defect with sinus pneumatization. (*C*) Immediate postoperative radiograph to confirm position of the plate and implant. The anterior implant had enough bone for primary stability and did not require sinus lift or plate stabilization. (*D*) Radiographic confirmation of adequate osseointegration of the implants and ready for functional loading. (*E, F*) Intraoral views with healing abutments in place to guide soft tissue healing and final rehabilitation.

Moderate to Severe Generalized Maxillary Atrophy

All-on-X concept with immediate loading

When generalized maxillary atrophy is present (zones 1, 2, and 3), all-on-X is accomplished by placing implants in sites 4, 6, 11, and 13. Long implants placed in the piriform rims are preferred coupled with a wide short implant in the maxillary midline. If inadequate bone is present in sites 4 and 13, an alternative option is placement of angled implants in the tuberosity/pterygoid plate. The stability of these implants is obtained from the pterygoid plate. The wide anteroposterior distribution of implants allows immediate loading (**Fig. 4**).[14–17]

Extremely Severe Generalized Maxillary Atrophy

Multiple zygoma implants with immediate loading

Patients with severe maxillary atrophy, poor alveolar bone quality, or excessive masticatory load have the highest failure rate of maxillary implants.[20–27] Placement of implant should take into consideration the load distribution to follow a short cantilever principle. Three-dimensional placement of anterior and posterior zygoma implants is considered. Other options are used and are described later in the surgical procedure section.

SURGICAL PROTOCOLS

The pattern of implant placement varies with the anatomy present and some are discussed in more detail later in the surgical section (**Fig. 5**).

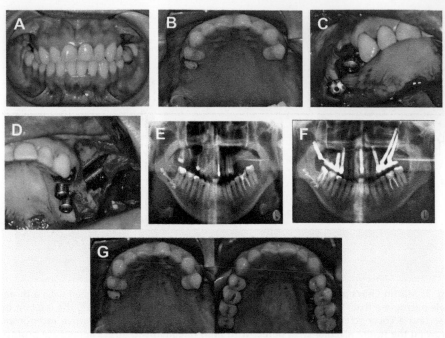

Fig. 4. This case was treated with combined techniques: Angled implants to avoid the maxillary sinus on the right side and unilateral zygoma implants on the left. (*A, B*) Intraoral and occlusal views showing the posterior edentulism. (*C, D*) Right tuberosity implant with two conventional anterior implants. Left; two zygoma implants and one conventional anterior. (*E, F*) Pre and post-op Panoramic radiographs showing right side sinus pneumatization and final restoration with tuberosity and two anterior conventional implants and left side with severe maxillary sinus pneumatization and the final restoration with two unilateral zygoma and one anterior conventional implants. (*G*) Occlusal views showing the failed dentition and edentulous sites and final rehabilitation.

ORIGINAL SURGICAL TECHNIQUE OF ZYGOMA IMPLANT

1. Incision and dissection: A 2.5-cm lateral maxillary vestibular incision,[30] similar to Le Fort approach, with full thickness mucoperiosteal flap is elevated, exposing the lateral wall of the maxilla.[20,21,31] A bony window is created to access the maxillary sinus membrane. Dissection is then carried out superiorly and posteriorly to visualize the infraorbital nerve. The fibers of the masseter muscle are transected as close to the periosteum as possible with Dean scissors. Piezo surgery or conventional round bur are used to create the antrostomy and expose the maxillary sinus membrane. This window is transpositioned superiorly, while still attached to the membrane, or removed to have direct visualization of the antral floor.[1]

2. Retraction of the membrane: Once the membrane has been exposed, a folded wet gauze aids in displacing the membrane medially and superiorly. This technique allows the direct visualization of the drilling protocol avoiding injury to anatomically important structures.

3. Sequential drilling: Under copious irrigation and using the zygoma retractor, a 703-fissure bur is used to create a groove for orientation at the alveolar crest and zygomatic buttress region. Only two twist drills (2.9 and 3.5 mm) are used

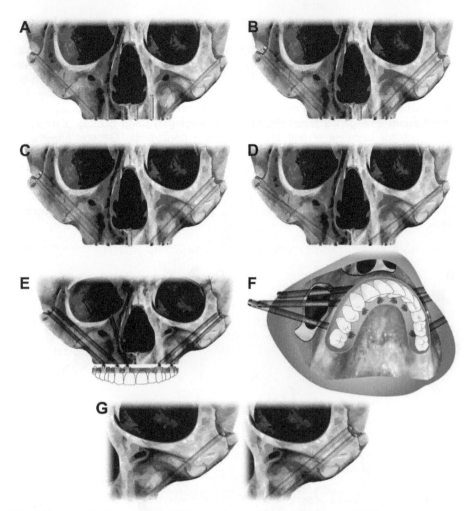

Fig. 5. Zygoma implant design. (*A*) Conventional design by Brånemark with two zygoma implants and four conventional in anterior zone. (*B*) Quadrangular design zygomas with two posterior zygoma implants on each side and two anterior conventional implants. (*C*) Quadrangular design zygomas with two posterior zygoma implants on each side and one anterior conventional implant in the midline area. (*D*) Quadrangular design zygomas with two posterior zygoma implants on each side that are not parallel to avoid rotational forces. (*E*) Pentagonal design with two posterior zygoma implants on each side and one anterior zygoma implant anchored to infraorbital rim. (*F*) Hexagonal design; six zygoma implants sites 3, 5, 7, 10, 12, and 14 for class III patients of severe bruxism, especially with complete mandibular dentition. (*G*) Unilateral zygoma design; unilateral severe atrophy or cleft patients.

for the zygoma implant site preparation. The zygoma drill guard protects the commissure from injury while using the drills at insertion. Double irrigation should be used to avoid overheating of the bone at the crestal and zygoma levels.The path of insertion for zygomatic implants extends from the alveolar crest, through the maxillary sinus, and enters the body of the zygoma anchored to solid bone. The technique is sensitive and requires knowledge of the local anatomy. The presence of a dentate mandible decreases the amount of space available to insert the greater than 50-mm drill bits, making placement challenging and difficult. The presence of mandibular teeth should not be a contraindication for the placement of zygoma implants.The hand piece is positioned on the contralateral side at the level of the commissure with long drills, mandating maximal opening of the mouth be maintained. The drilling sequence starts at the alveolar crest, passing through the maxillary sinus, and the drill is advanced to reach the body of the zygoma to the desired emergence level. The most challenging zygoma fixtures placed are the posterior because of soft and hard tissue constraints. General anesthesia may be required to improve maximum opening.

4. Depth measurement: Final measurement is taken with the depth gauge to confirm adequate implant selection.

5. Implant placement: To ensure adequate cortical anchorage and primary stability, the tip of the zygoma implant should extend 2 mm beyond the body of the zygoma (**Fig. 6**).

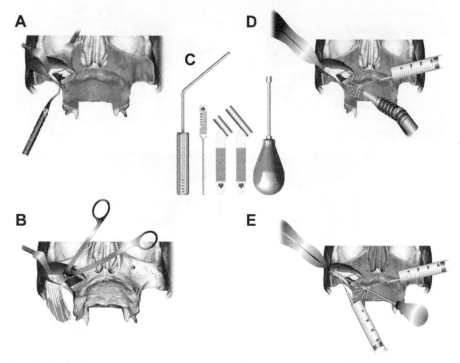

Fig. 6. Surgical steps and armamentarium. (*A, B*) Incision and flap elevation: the lateral maxillary walls are exposed bilaterally and once the masseter fibers are visualized, Dean scissors are used to dissect them from the inferior border of the zygomatic arch to allow for an easier flap retraction. (*C*) Depth gauges, zygoma drill guard (to protect the commissure), and onion (implant manual driver). (*D*) Antrostomy: with piezo surgery or electrical Hall drill, a window in the lateral sinus wall is removed and the maxillary sinus membrane is elevated superiorly and medially with curettes. Brånemark retractor in the zygoma bone for proper visualization and initial drilling with single irrigation with 703 fissure bur at the alveolar ridge and to countersink in the zygoma body to create vector of insertion if extrasinus approach is desired. (*E*) Depth gauge to confirm size of zygoma implant and finally implant insertion with the use of double irrigation.

PROSTHETIC CONSIDERATIONS

Prosthetic restorations (teeth and infrastructure) usually require at least 15 mm of interocclusal space. The recent development of virtual surgical planning allows fabrications of a bone reduction guide before surgery to be used by the surgeon for alveolar crest reduction as needed.[31,32] Multiple zygoma implants with wide distribution avoiding large cantilevers are recommended to restore patients with severe posterior maxillary bone atrophy (**Fig. 7**).[26,31–37]

A. Anteroposterior cantilever: Anterior implants should emerge within the crestal bone at the level of incisors, whereas posterior implants should be positioned to emerge distal to first molars.
B. Vertical cantilever: By placing the implant in the alveolar ridge, the vertical cantilever is less than that seen with one placed more palatal.
C. Transverse cantilever: The posterior implants should emerge in the alveolar crest area to avoid transverse cantilever. Ideal placement of the implants should be following the extrasinus technique. This implies covering the implant with buccal fat pad for closure to avoid exposure to the oral cavity.

MODIFIED PROTOCOLS

1. Pentagonal design: Five maxillary-zygomatic implants are placed at distal of 4, distal of 6, mesial of 7, distal of 11, and distal of 13. The implant stability is based on the body of the zygoma and piriform rim (**Figs. 8 and 9**).[26,31,32,36]
2. Hexagonal design: An additional anterior zygoma implant is placed in the contralateral piriform rim to increase bone anchorage, decrease interdental gap, and to

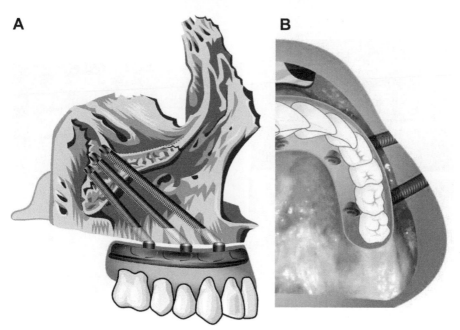

A   **B**

Fig. 7. Medial illustration showing the importance of short cantilevers of the prosthetic restorations to the implants in three dimensions. (*A*) Anteroposterior and vertical. (*B*) Transversal.

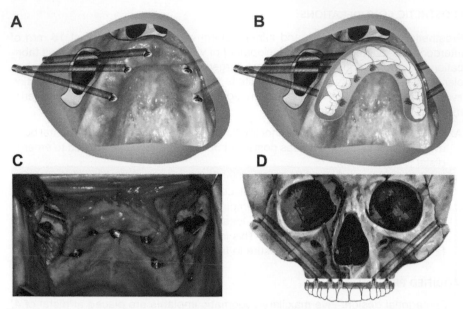

Fig. 8. Medial illustrations demonstrating the pentagonal design. (*A*) Zygoma implants placed posteriorly and anteriorly for load distribution. (*B*) Dental prosthesis with ideal distribution and short transversal cantilevers. (*C*) Intraoperative view with the 5 zygoma implants in place. (*D*) Medical schematic representations for anterior zygoma implant anchored in the infraorbital rim.

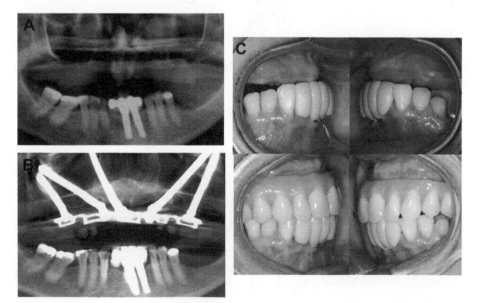

Fig. 9. Pentagonal design of zygoma implant. (*A, B*) Panoramic radiographs showing the severe maxillary atrophy with no bone for conventional implant placement and postoperative with implants and dental prosthesis. (*C*) Intraoral views preoperative and postoperative.

minimize the anteroposterior cantilever. This design is recommended for patients with class III malocclusions, poor zygoma size, and/or severe bruxism habits (**Fig. 10**).[32]

3. Unilateral design: Zygoma implants can also be placed when severe maxillary posterior atrophy is present unilaterally. In these cases, two posterior zygoma implants are placed and rigidly fixated to an anterior conventional implant (**Fig. 11**).[32]

MODIFIED SURGICAL TECHNIQUES

1. Sinus slot: To improve the emergence profile and avoid maxillary sinus window osteotomy, Stella and Warner modified the soft tissue approach and bony engagement points. They used a mucoperiosteal elevation similar to a traditional Le Fort I extending the palatal dissection to reach the crestal bone. Using a fissure bur, marks are made at the crest and zygomatic buttresses, orienting the surgeon during the sequential drilling.[31,32,35,38,39,40]

2. Extrasinus technique: Aparicio described implant placement outside the sinus wall in patients with pronounced buccal concavities. Implants were placed at the level of the alveolar crest achieving ideal emergence profile. A standard drilling sequence was used without violating the integrity of the maxillary sinus membrane. The buccal fat pad must be used to cover the lateral aspect of the implant to avoid exposure to oral cavity (**Fig. 12**).[31,32,35,38,39]

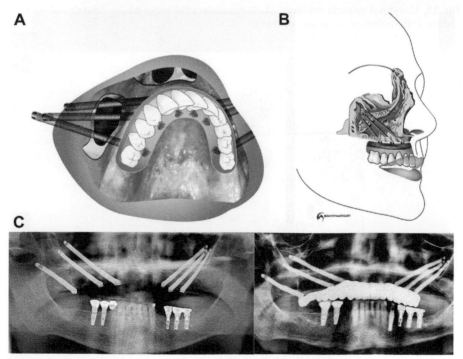

A

B

C

Fig. 10. Hexagonal design of zygoma implant. (*A, B*) Hexagonal design medical illustrations showing six zygoma implants for severely three-dimensional atrophy. Notice there is minimal to no anteroposterior and transverse cantilevers transferred from the implants to the final prosthesis. (*C*) Preoperative and postoperative panorex showing the hexagonal design with six zygoma implants in place immediately after placement.

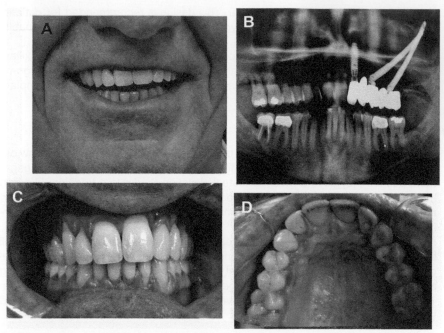

Fig. 11. Unilateral zygoma implants. (*A–D*) Post-operative views of the final dental rehabilitation with unilateral zygoma treatment.

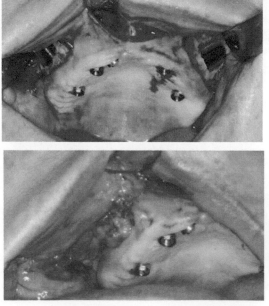

Fig. 12. Buccal fat pad must be used to cover the lateral aspect of the zygoma implants to avoid exposure to the oral cavity.

SUMMARY

This article helps clinicians evaluate different treatment options to rehabilitate maxillary edentulism. The protocols described all have the goal of immediate loading. Patient variables can dictate the ideal procedure in a given situation. Patient variables can include medical comorbidities, the degree of maxillary atrophy, presence or absence of mandibular teeth, and the need for immediate loading. Alternatives for severe atrophy include but are not limited to sinus grafting versus zygoma implants. Sinus grafting requires additional steps and associated bone graft–related morbidities, whereas zygoma implants are placed in one stage but requires specialized skills. It is difficult to tell the reader which is the best technique to use. The ideal technique should be tailored to the individual patient and surgeon experience.

ACKNOWLEDGMENTS

The authors acknowledge the work of colleagues on the cases as shown in the following figures: Joe Shirley, DDS (**Fig. 1**), Rafaelle Pisano, DDS (**Figs. 4** and **9**), Giancarlo Romero, DDS (**Fig. 10**), and Nathan Nussembaum, DDS (**Fig. 11**).

REFERENCES

1. Cawood J, Howell R. Reconstructive preprosthetic surgery. Anatomical considerations. Int J Oral Maxillofac Surg 1991;20:75–82.
2. Brånemark PI, Breine U, Adell R, et al. Intra-osseous anchorage of dental prostheses, I. Experimental studies. Scand J Plast Reconstr Surg 1969;7:321–9.
3. Brånemark P-I. The Brånemark novum protocol for same-day teeth a global perspective. Berlin (Germany): Quintessence; 2001.
4. Barros Saint-Pasteur J. Alveoplasty ridge reconstruction. Acta Odontol Venez 1970;8:168.
5. Chiapasco M, Zaniboni M, Boisco M. Augmentation procedures for the rehabilitation of deficient edentulous ridges with oral implants. Clin Oral Implants Res 2006;17:136.
6. Chiapasco M, Zanibon M. Methods to treat the edentulous posterior maxilla: implants with sinus grafting. J Oral Maxillofac Surg 2009;67:867–71.
7. Choukroun J, Diss A, Simonpieri A, et al. Platelet-rich fibrin (PRF): a second-generation platelet concentrate. Part V: Histologic evaluations of PRF effects on bone allograft maturation in sinus lift. Oral Surg Oral Med Oral Pathol Oral Radiol Endod 2006;101:299–303.
8. Brånemark P-I, Gröndahl K, Worthington P. Osseointegration and autogenous onlay bone grafts: reconstruction of the edentulous atrophic maxilla. Chicago: Quintessence; 2001.
9. Regeev E, Smith RA, Perrot DH, et al. Maxillary sinus complications related to endosseous implants. Int J Oral Maxillofac Implants 1995;10:451–61.
10. Rangert B, Sennerby L, Nilson H. Load factor analysis for implants in the posterior maxilla. In: Jensen T, editor. The sinus bone graft. Chicago: Quintessence; 1999. p. 167–77.
11. Brånemark PI, Svensson B, Van Steenberghe D. Ten- year survival rates of fixed prostheses on four of six implants and modum Brånemark in full edentulism. Clin Oral Implants Res 1995;6:227–331.
12. Schnitman P, Wohrle PS, Rubenstein J, et al. Ten years results for Brånemark implants immediately loaded with fixed prostheses at implant placement. Int J Oral Maxillofac Implants 1997;12:495–503.

13. Chin M. Surgical design for dental reconstruction with implants: a new paradigm. (IL): Quintessence Publishing Co; 2016.
14. Krekmanov L, Kahn M, Rangert B, et al. Tilting of posterior mandibular and maxillary implants for improved prosthesis support. Int J Oral Maxillofac Implants 2000;15:405–14.
15. Malo P, Rangert B, Dvarsater L. Immediate function of Branemark implants in the esthetic zone: a retrospective clinical study with 6 months to 4 years of follow-up. Clin Implant Dent Relat Res 2000;2:138–46.
16. Maló P, Rangert B, Nobre M. All-on-4 immediate- function concept with Brånemark system implants for completely edentulous maxillae: a 1-year retrospective clinical study. Clin Implant Dent Relat Res 2005;7(1):S88–94.
17. Maló P, Araújo M, Nobre M, et al. "All-on-4" immediate-function concept for completely edentulous maxillae: a clinical report on the medium (3 years) and long-term (5 years) outcomes. Clin Implant Dent Relat Res 2012;1:139–50.
18. Hoop M, de Araújo Nobre M, Maló P. Comparison of marginal bone loss and implant success between axial and tilted implants in maxillary All-on-4 treatment concept rehabilitations after 5 years of follow-up. Clin Implant Dent Relat Res 2017;19(5):849–59.
19. Lopes A, Maló P, de Araújo Nobre M, et al. The NobelGUide All-on-4 treatment concept for rehabilitation of edentulous jaws: a prospective report on medium- and long-term outcomes. Clin Implant Dent Relat Res 2015;17(Suppl 2):E406–16.
20. Brånemark PI. Surgery and fixture installation. Zygomaticus fixture clinical procedures. Goteborg (Sweden): Nobel Biocare AB; 1998.
21. Bedrossian E. Implant treatment planning for the edentulous patient: a graftless approach to immediate loading. St. Louis (MO): Mosby Elsevier; 2011.
22. Parel S, Brånemark P, Ohrnell L, et al. Remote implant anchorage for the rehabilitation of maxillary defects. J Prosthet Dent 2001;86:377–81.
23. Bedrossian E, Stumpel L. Immediate stabilization at stage II of zygomatic implants: rationale and technique. J Prosthet Dent 2001;86:10–4.
24. Bedrossian E, Sullivan R, Fortin Y, et al. Fixed-prosthetic implant restoration of the edentulous maxilla: a systematic pretreatment evaluation method. J Oral Maxillofac Surg 2008;66:112–22.
25. Darle C. The zygomaticus fixture minimized treatment for maximal predictability. A new procedure for rehabilitating the severely resorbed maxillar. Gotebörg, (Sweden): Nobel Biocare AB; 2000.
26. Guerrero C, Sabogal A, Dominguez E. Complications. In: Guerrero C, Sabogal A, editors. Zygoma Implants Atlas of surgery and prosthetics. Madrid (Spain): Ripano; 2011. p. 185–200.
27. Guerrero C, Gonzalez M, Henriquez M, et al. Zygomaticus implants: a ten years experience. Oral Surg Oral Med Oral Pathol Oral Radiol Endod 2008;106:508.
28. Guerrero C. Five zygomaticus implants to treat severe maxillary atrophy. Int J Oral Maxillofac Surg 2009;39:505.
29. Mihai A. Nanobiomaterials in dentistry. Cambridge (United Kingdom): Elsevier; 2016 [Chapter and pages].
30. Pisano R. Zygoma implants: surgery and prosthetic evolution. Amazon education 2018.
31. Guerrero C, Sabogal A, Henriquez M, et al. Pentagonal design: five zigomatic implants. In: Guerrero C, Sabogal A, editors. Zygoma Implants Atlas of surgery and prosthetics. Madrid (Spain): Ripano; 2011. p. 144–65.
32. Hirsch J, Öhrnell L, Henry P, et al. A clinical evaluation of the zygoma fixture: one year of follow-up at 16 clinics. J Oral Maxillofac Surg 2004;62:22–9.

33. Block M, Haggerty C, Fisher R. Nongrafting implant options for restoration of the edentulous maxilla. J Oral Maxillofac Surg 2009;67:872–88.
34. Davo R, Malevez C, Rojas J. Immediate function in the atrophic maxilla using zygoma implants: a preliminary study. J Prosthet Dent 2007;97(6 Suppl):544–51.
35. Ferrara E, Stella J. Restoration of the edentulous maxilla: the case for the zygomatic implants. J Oral Maxillofac Surg 2004;62:1418–22.
36. Guerrero C. New possibilities for zygoma implant. J Oral Maxillofac Surg 2010;67: 1503.
37. Kahnberg K, Henry P, Hirsch J, et al. Clinical evaluation of the zygoma implant: 3-year follow-up at 16 clinics. J Oral Maxillofac Surg 2007;65:2033–8.
38. Stella JP, Warner MR. Sinus slot technique for simplification and improved orientation of zygomaticues dental implant: a technical note. Int J Oral Maxillofac Implants 2000;14:197–209.
39. Aparicio C, Ouazzani W, Aparicio A, et al. Extrasinus zygomatic implants: three year experience from a new surgical approach for patients with pronounced buccal concavities in the edentulous maxilla. Clin Implant Dent Relat Res 2010; 12:55–61.

What is the Optimal Material for Implant Prosthesis?

Fadi Al Farawati, DDS, MS, MClinDent, MFDS RCSEd[a],*,
Pranai Nakaparksin, DDS, MSD, FACP, FRCD(c)[b]

KEYWORDS

- Implant prosthesis • Dental implants
- Computer-aided design, computer-aided manufacturing • Titanium • Zirconia
- Cobalt-chromium

KEY POINTS

- With the multiple choices to restore dental implants in single, partial edentulous, and fully edentulous cases, the clinician should be aware of all necessary specifications in the restoring material to achieve an ideal outcome.
- The common materials used in dental implant prostheses are commercially pure titanium, titanium alloys, zirconia, cobalt-chromium alloys, and multiple resin-based immerging materials. The advantages and limitations of these materials are discussed.
- The clinician faces different clinical situations at the dental practice, some of which are complicated and require different techniques or materials to achieve an acceptable outcome. These scenarios are presented with suggested treating protocols.

INTRODUCTION

Over the past 50 years, implant dentistry has evolved to provide a long-term successful and predictable treatment with many biologic and mechanical advantages over conventional fixed and removable treatments.[1] It also has shifted from the surgical placement of implants according to the availability of bone to prosthetically guided implant planning and placement. This shift has influenced the range of available dental materials to restore single crowns and partially and fully edentulous jaws with dental implants.

This article explores the main specifications required for a dental implant prosthesis. It also addresses the commonly used prosthetic materials and different scenarios that may present in a dental practice and the material of choice for each scenario.

Disclosure Statement: The authors have nothing to disclose.
[a] Department of Restorative Sciences, The Dental College of Georgia at Augusta University, 1430 John Wesley Gilbert Drive, GC-4218, Augusta, GA 30912, USA; [b] Mahidol University, 6 Thanon Yothi, Thung Phaya Thai, Ratchathewi, Bangkok 10400, Thailand
* Corresponding author.
E-mail address: falfarawati@augusta.edu

Dent Clin N Am 63 (2019) 515–530
https://doi.org/10.1016/j.cden.2019.02.002
0011-8532/19/© 2019 Elsevier Inc. All rights reserved.

dental.theclinics.com

WHAT IS CONSIDERED AN IDEAL MATERIAL?

Abutments and superstructures for dental implants should ideally possess the following fundamental characteristics:

1. The material should not produce harmful toxicologic or allergic effects to the patient or the operator.
2. The physical and mechanical properties of the material should withstand functional load and the challenging oral environment (eg, fracture resistance, modulus of elasticity, solubility, thermal conduction).
3. The mode of fabrication should be inexpensive and feasible for the dentist and technician.
4. It should enhance the esthetic outcome of color and contour.
5. The connection should fit passively in order not to cause wear at the prosthesis-implant interface.
6. The mode of insertion and removal should be convenient for the dentist to provide maintenance services.
7. The material should promote proper oral hygiene measures and prohibit or eliminate oral plaque accumulation.
8. The material should be reparable when an adverse reaction occurs.
9. Reliable manufacturers should be used to ensure availability of spare parts (abutments, screws, plastic retentive components for bars and single attachments).

WHAT ARE THE COMMONLY USED MATERIALS?
Commercially Pure Titanium, Grade 4 and Titanium Alloy (Ti-6Al-4V)

Titanium and titanium alloys have been used in orthopedic reconstructions for a long time and they have been the materials of choice to fabricate dental implants, abutments, and prosthesis. The durability, corrosion resistance, and biocompatibility are the attractive characteristics that give titanium its importance. Nevertheless, difficulties in porcelain application and casting has motivated the search for other fabrication methods, such as machining, or using monolithic materials, such as ceramics and polymers.

Grade 4 commercially pure titanium and titanium alloys (specifically Ti-6Al-4V) are used to fabricate stock and customized abutments/frameworks to retain or support dental prosthesis. These objects are used during the interim and definitive phases for fixed and removable prosthesis.

Fixed
Implant-supported single crowns or fixed dental prostheses are cement- or screw-retained. Implant prostheses were historically fabricated as screw-retained prostheis.[2] Cement-retained prosthesis has gained popularity because of its cost effectiveness and similarity to tooth-borne restorations. In addition, it has comparable survival rate to screw-retained prostheses.[3] However, there is a shift back to screw retention because more studies showed higher biologic complications associated with cement-retained prosthesis, and because of the retrievability advantage of screw-retained prosthesis.[4]

Abutments Prefabricated (stock) abutments have an emergence profile that was developed to resemble the cross-section of teeth in different oral locations. However, stock abutments often fail to match the patient's anatomy. They are cost-effective and are easily adjusted by laboratory technicians or clinicians. Straight or angled stock abutments (different angulations) with different transgingival heights are commercially available (**Fig. 1**).

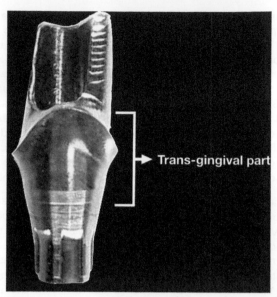

Fig. 1. The transgingival part of the implant abutment.

Hybrid abutments (titanium inserts) (**Fig. 2**) were developed by bonding an individualized monolithic ceramic crown (zirconia or lithium disilicate) to the abutment to protect the implant interface from wear by all-zirconia abutments, which manifest clinically as a titanium tattoo.[5] Titanium inserts have an increased fracture strength of ceramic abutments and crowns and reduced wear of the implant connections.[6]

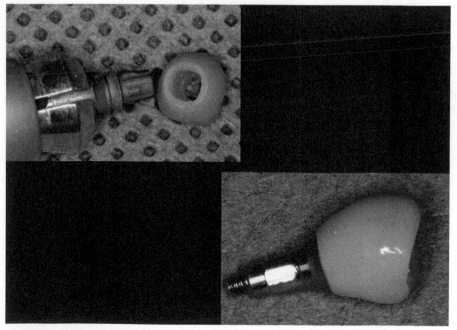

Fig. 2. The titanium insert abutment with the fabricated all-ceramic crown.

Customized implant abutments began with the introduction of the universal clearance limited abutment[7] to bypass the transmucosal cylinders of the Brånemark implant system. This helped in developing a customized emergence profile and allowed restoration of angled implants in the case of limited interocclusal space. However, the abutment did not limit the accumulative error associated with casting. The introduction of computer-aided design/computer-aided manufacturing (CAD/CAM) abutments (**Fig. 3**) helped in overcoming the problems associated with the universal clearance limited abutments, improving the gingival health of the restored implants, and reducing the cost. CAD/CAM abutments show good survival and success rates,[8] provide better soft tissue reaction (less recession),[9] and have less incidence of screw loosening[10] than conventional stock abutments. Custom abutments show comparable, if not better, clinical outcomes when compared with conventional abutments.[8]

Framework Casting titanium frameworks have been popular because of their biocompatibility and corrosion resistance, which is derived from the thin passivating oxide layer.[11] These advantageous properties are attained by undergoing a sensitive casting and finishing processes because titanium has a high melting temperature ($1668°C$) and high rate of oxidation greater than $900°C$. Therefore, it requires special investments and a casting machine with arc-melting capability and cooling cycles.[11] Titanium crystalline structure changes shape at $883°C$, when the alpha-hexagonal phase becomes a beta-cubic phase. This conversion affects the bond between titanium and dental ceramic; therefore, dental ceramics staked on titanium are fired at temperatures less than $800°C$.[12]

The distortion and porosity induced by the classic lost-wax casting technique are eliminated by using CAD-CAM milling (**Fig. 4**). It is logical that larger frameworks with a greater number of implants benefit from the advantages of CAD/CAM technology.[13] The accuracy of CAD/CAM ensures passive fit of frameworks/abutments to limit movement and bacterial leakage.[14] Abduo[13] found that CAD/CAM implant frameworks fabricated with titanium and zirconia have a high level of accuracy with a passive fit that surpasses the one-piece casting or laser-welded frameworks. A systematic review by Kapos and Evans[15] showed the use of CAD/CAM frameworks for implant-supported restorations provides comparable prosthesis survival rate and technical and biologic complications to that of conventional techniques.

Removable
An implant-retained overdenture (IOD) with two nonsplinted implants is the treatment of choice for edentulous mandible, according to McGill consensus.[16] However,

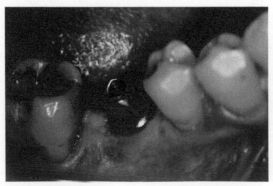

Fig. 3. Customized abutment.

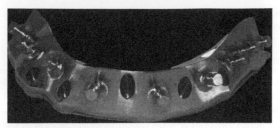

Fig. 4. Milled titanium framework.

splinted anchorage (ie, bar) provided a higher implant survival rate compared with nonsplinted anchorage (ball/locator attachments or telescopic crowns) in implant-supported maxillary overdenture.[17]

Single attachment Single attachments are implant screw-retained abutments that snap into a corresponding secondary housing within the intaglio surface of the IOD. These attachments are divided into resilient and rigid.

The resilient attachments (Ball, locator, and magnets) are usually prefabricated. Locators, which are widely used, offer up to 40° of compensation for nonparallel implants. Prosthesis retained with resilient attachments allows some movement during mastication and requires mucosal support.

Rigid attachments are custom-made abutments that are cast or milled (Atlantis Conus concept, Dentsply Sirona, York, PA).[18] Retention of rigid attachment comes from the metal friction fit between the 5° and 6° tapered abutment and the corresponding metal cap within the prosthesis. Rigid attachments provide support to the IOD preventing any vertical movement during mastication. They also correct implant misalignment.

Locator attachments provide a better access for oral hygiene compared with bars and telescopic crowns on implants. They showed minimal scores of peri-implant health indicators (plaque, gingival, bleeding, and calculus indices) and fewer maintenance appointments over 3 years.[19] Well-designed studies are warranted to explore the advantages of using rigid attachments over resilient ones.

Bar Bar attachments (**Fig. 5**) provide rigid retention and they compensate for implant misalignment. They can provide distal extensions to support an IOD in a class II jaw relation when implants are placed in the anterior maxilla region. However, bars require more interocclusal space (15 mm) compared with locator (8–10 mm) and they are less hygienic. The lack of proper oral hygiene and the negative pressure that forms under a

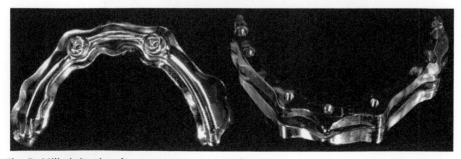

Fig. 5. Milled titanium bar to support an overdenture.

bar-supported IOD predispose to the formation of hyperplastic gingivae, which may require surgical removal.

Zirconia/Zirconium-Alumina

Zirconia is a polycrystalline ceramic and it has mechanical properties advantage over other dental ceramics. These physical properties depend largely on the preparation techniques and the design of the final prosthesis. Color and decreased bacterial plaque adhesion have given zirconia a wide range of applications in dentistry.[20]

Abutment

The gingival architecture around the implant has a major role in esthetic outcome. In addition, color is one of the key esthetic parameters. The undesirable shine-through effect of the underlying metal abutment in thin soft tissue phenotype compromises the peri-implant mucosa shade.[21] Zirconia abutments demonstrate less effect on optical outcomes of peri-implant mucosal tissue when compared with conventional titanium abutments. However, it causes a higher wear rate on the implant connection compared with the titanium abutment.[22] It also has a higher rate of the zirconia abutment fracture.[23] In multiple unit restorations, a higher chance of prosthesis misfit is observed with one-piece zirconia frameworks.[24]

To eliminate the previously mentioned problems with a one-piece zirconia abutment and superstructure, two-piece zirconia abutment (**Fig. 6**) was developed, allowing a customized zirconia abutment to be cemented on top of a prefabricated titanium base. Because of the metal-to-metal contact between the implant internal connection and the titanium base, two-piece zirconia abutments can achieve higher strength than one-piece abatements. A prefabricated titanium abutment provides a passive fit to the internal connection of the implant and minor misfit from the sintering process of zirconia is corrected with resin cement.

Framework

In full arch restoration, traditional acrylic teeth with a metal superstructure require substantial amount of restorative space, which would require significant amount of alveolar bone reduction. In a patient with limited restorative space or the inability to create restorative space, the clinician may consider zirconia as a restorative material (**Fig. 7**) because it has higher strength than titanium alloy or a gold substructure.[25] Zirconia also causes less wear than porcelain, composite, or lithium disilicate on the opposing

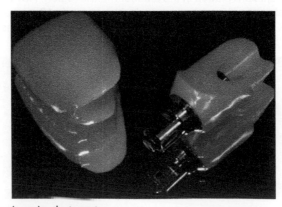

Fig. 6. Two-piece zirconia abutment.

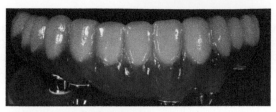

Fig. 7. Full-arch monolithic zirconia prosthesis.

dentition.[26] A 5-year follow-up of 2039 zirconia complete arch fixed implant-supported prostheses showed a cumulative survival rate of 99.3% when zirconia prostheses were used with porcelain veneering limited to the gingival region.[27] Zirconia is a self-healing material that can repair its crystal structure to prevent crack propagation.[28] However, monolithic zirconia has the limitation of high opacity, decreased strength with less bulk, and minimal adjustments. Layered zirconia (**Fig. 8**) was developed to increase the esthetic appearance of the prosthesis. However, extra precaution must be taken when veneering with porcelain on zirconia to minimize the incidence of fracture or chipping.[29]

Cobalt-Chromium Alloys

Cobalt-chromium (Co-Cr) has historically been one of the most highly used alloys in dentistry because of its strength, durability, biocompatibility, corrosion resistance, and bond strength to ceramics. One of the biggest disadvantages in the casting techniques is the effect of the accumulative distortion and porosity and the high labor costs and structural hardness that complicate the finishing process. A retrospective study comparing implant fixed prosthesis made with Co-Cr with grade 3 gold frameworks showed comparable clinical results up to 18 years (average, 10 years).[30]

Most of these disadvantages were eliminated by introducing subtractive and additive technologies to facilitate the fabrication of large frameworks with more precision and accurate fit. Selective laser melting additive technology produces stiffer and harder frameworks than those milled or cast.[31] It also shows better framework fit when compared with the traditional lost-wax casting, milled wax with lost-wax method, or CAD/CAM milled Co-Cr.[32]

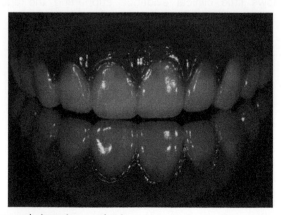

Fig. 8. Full-arch layered zirconia prosthesis.

Fixed

Co-Cr has been used successfully in fixed dental prostheses because of the bond strength of the framework to the porcelain (**Fig. 9**). This bonding results from a combination of chemical bonding (which dominates), van der Waals forces, mechanical interlocking, and compressive bonding.[33] A study comparing bond strengths of ceramics with Co-Cr alloys fabricated by traditional casting, milling, and the additive selective laser melting[33] found that both milling and selective laser melting fabrication result in stronger porcelain adherence when compared with casting.

Removable

One of the most important properties when using a Co-Cr alloy as a removable prosthesis framework is corrosion resistance because this reduces the ions released into the surrounding oral environment, which may affect the physical properties of the framework. High Co-Cr corrosion resistance is improved by using additive and subtractive technologies.[34] Because of the previously mentioned properties, Co-Cr has been widely used for the past 80 years. Removable partial dentures designs have been based on the properties of Co-Cr.[35] However, Keltjens and colleagues[36] found that the most metal clasps were distorted after 8 years of usage and they did not fit the abutment correctly. This fact shows the necessity to search for alternatives to fabricate frameworks for removable dental prosthesis.

Emerging Materials

New materials are emerging in the construction of implant frameworks including: polyaryletherketone (Pekkton), a high-performance thermoplastic polymer material and Trinia, which is a tooth-shade nanohybrid polymer reinforced with multilayered glass fiber. The usage of these metal-free materials has been expanded to overcome the esthetic and mechanical shortcomings in metal frameworks. These lightweight polymers have high elasticity and low solubility. In addition, they are reparable and cost-effective. Their disadvantages include low thermal conductivity, brittleness, weakness when compared with metal based frameworks, low modulus of elasticity, and high cytotoxicity.[35] There are several short-term case reports on the usage of Pekkton frameworks for full mouth rehabilitation[37] and Trinia for full arch fixed prosthesis on four implants.[38] Only a few case reports could be identified concerning these materials, which shows little clinical evidence supporting the adoption of these materials.

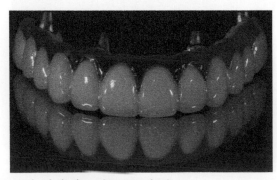

Fig. 9. Full-arch layered cobalt-chromium prosthesis.

SCENARIOS
Straightforward

An implant should be ideally placed in the correct three-dimensional position with adequate restorative space. The clinician should consider esthetics, function, and maintenance when restoring the implant. To ensure long-term predictability and ease of maintenance, the clinician should aim for screw-retained prosthesis with titanium connection. This includes, but is not limited to, two-piece abutments, customized titanium abutments, and screw-cementable crowns. For full mouth superstructure, titanium alloy is commonly used because of its high flexural strength, low cost, and ease of fabrication. However, when bonding porcelain directly to the superstructure is desired, Co-Cr is more favorable over titanium because of the ability to control excessive oxide layer.[33]

Interocclusal Space

The minimum vertical interocclusal space to fabricate the dental prosthesis from the implant/abutment platform to the opposing occlusal table must be ensured during the treatment planning phase. Inadequate interocclusal space can lead to inability to fabricate the prosthesis, loss of retention, screw loosening, and veneering material and framework fractures.

For metal-ceramic single crowns and fixed dental prosthesis, the minimum height for the abutment of a cement-retained restoration must be 4 mm. For smaller spaces, it is advisable to use screw-retained restorations,[39] which eliminate the cement retention factor and the necessity to have a minimum axial wall height. Therefore, the restoring dentist must measure the available vertical space for any metal-ceramic fixed prosthesis and must provide a surgical template that precisely indicates the location of the future gingival zenith of the prosthesis. This allows the surgeon to place the implant platform at the correct vertical location (3–4 mm away from future gingival zenith of the prosthesis), even if this requires the removal or the regeneration of the existing bone.

Removable prosthesis to rehabilitate fully edentulous arches using a splinting bar requires 13 to 14 mm of vertical space,[39] whereas single attachments need 8 to 10 mm of vertical interocclusal clearance. Implant-supported fixed complete dentures (fixed detachable prosthesis) requires a minimal vertical space of 11 to 12 mm because the acrylic tooth and resin requires 3 to 4 mm and the supporting metal framework and prosthetic abutment requires 8 mm (**Fig. 10**). The use of monolithic zirconia or the combination of metal and polymethyl methacrylate to replace the implant-supported fixed complete dentures has been recommended when less vertical space is available because zirconia has a higher strength than titanium alloy.[25] For example, the AccuFrame 360 by Cagenix (Memphis, TN) uses polymethyl methacrylate or Zirconia overlay cemented on a titanium framework. It

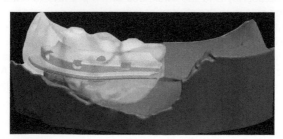

Fig. 10. The CAD designing software, which presents the proposed framework according to the available space.

requires only 8 mm of interarch space for the fixed complete denture prosthesis. The literature provides only case reports regarding these designs and the evidence is still limited.

Implant Position

Misaligned implants have esthetic and functional adverse effects. They cannot be successfully restored and require removal in severely misaligned cases. Proper planning should include presentation of the final prosthesis through a diagnostic wax-up, and fabrication of a radiopaque template to assess the bone envelope where future implants will be placed. This is the only way to fabricate a proper surgical stent (manual or computer guided) to ensure the proper alignment of the executed implants. The industry has recognized the misaligned implant problem and provided options to solve it.

In fixed cases, the restoring clinician can cement-retain the single crown or the fixed dental prosthesis on buccolingual angulated implants using angled abutments. In case of a desired screw-retained option, major implant systems have developed a way to angulate the retaining screw channel (**Fig. 11**). Straumann (Basel, Switzerland) developed the Variobase for angled solution systems, NobelBiocare (Yorba Linda, CA) developed the angled screw channel system, Dentsply Sirona (York, PA) developed the Atlantis CustomBase solution abutment with angulated screw access, and Core3dcentres (Las Vegas, NV) developed Core3d angulation connection (**Fig. 12**). All systems can correct a misalignment of 20° to 25°. It is worth mentioning that angulated screw access requires a screwmentable crown and angled solution provides burnout copings, which help in casting a restoration; otherwise digital fabrication may be used. All systems require special screwdrivers and caution should be taken not to strip the prosthetic screw head by using the improper screwdriver. All systems can restore single crowns and short fixed dental prosthesis. Only Atlantis has developed the same technology (angulated screw access) to be used in long span FDP frameworks or full mouth implant-supported fixed complete denture infrastructures (**Fig. 13**).

If a resilient attachment is to be used in overdenture, the Locator systems can correct a divergence up to 40°. Zest Dental Solutions (Carlsbad, CA) has also developed another system (LOCATOR-RTx removable attachment system) that can correct a divergence of up to 60°. For greater degrees of misalignment, the implant-supported overdenture using the Atlantis Conus system can correct greater misalignment because it uses custom milled abutments. The bar systems can still connect implants with different angulations as long as the final connecting bar can seat passively on the implant/abutment platforms.

Esthetic

The degree of translucency and the thickness of the prosthesis should be taken into consideration when selecting the abutment material in the esthetic zone. Conventional titanium abutments have been shown to have more influence on all-ceramic prosthesis when compared with gold-colored titanium (**Fig. 14**) and zirconia abutments.[40] In certain situation where screw access is placed on the labial surface or incisal edge, an angled screw channel is used to overcome the esthetic problem. An angled screw channel can correct the access hole placement by up to 30° depending on the manufacturer (see **Fig. 12**).

Retrievability

A systematic review conducted by Wittneben and colleagues in 2014[4] to evaluate the clinical performance of cement- and screw-retained fixed implant-supported

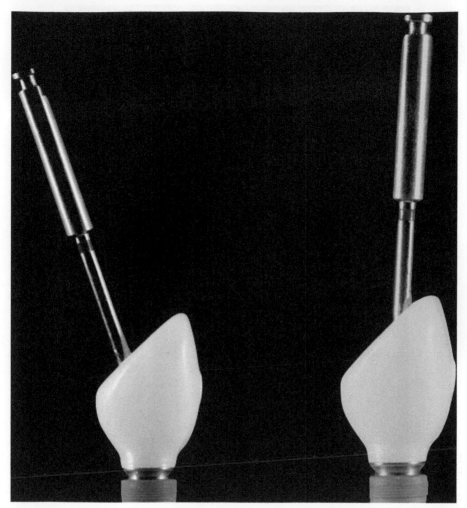

Fig. 11. The difference in screw access angulation after angulating the retaining screw channel.

prosthesis, found comparable overall survival of the prostheses. However, the total percentage of technical and biologic complications were higher when cement-retained prostheses were used.

The following recommendation should be taken into considerations when restoring edentulous arches with fixed implant prostheses (**Fig. 15**). First, it is recommended to construct the restorations at the abutments level using multiunit abutments instead of an implant level reconstruction. This ensures passive fit and keeps complications to the abutment level protecting the endosseous implant. Second, it is recommended to use multiple prostheses instead of one long-span, full-arch reconstruction whenever possible. Third, long-span fixed implant prostheses should be screw-retained for easier maintenance because long-span restorations have a higher complications rate.[41]

Cement-retained prostheses have the advantage of an intact occlusal surface (no screw access hole). They are more economic and allow to restore misaligned implants. However, with the invention of angulated screw channels and the lower

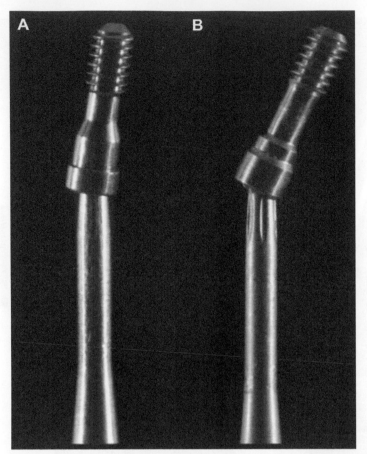

Fig. 12. Different available screw channel angulation systems. (*A*) Core3d screw (Core3dcentres, Las Vegas, NV), (*B*) Atlantis screw (Dentsply Sirona, York, PA).

complications rate and retrievability of screw-retained prostheses, it is recommended to use this retention method whenever feasible.

Implant-supported fixed complete dentures (fixed detachable prosthesis) can be designed to receive individualized crowns (**Fig. 16**). This design helps in replacing

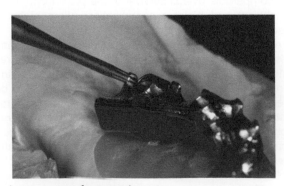

Fig. 13. Angulated screw access framework.

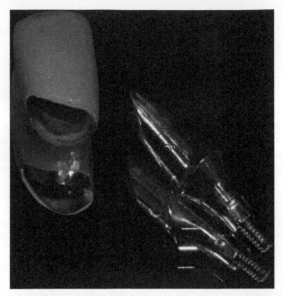

Fig. 14. Gold-colored titanium abutment.

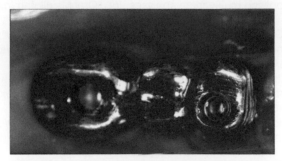

Fig. 15. Cobalt-chromium fixed implant prosthesis framework.

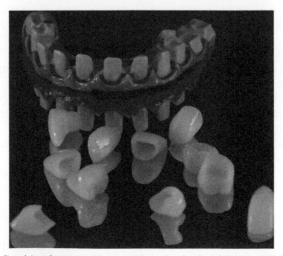

Fig. 16. Full-arch fixed implant prosthesis with individualized lithium disilicate crowns.

these crowns in case of fracture or debonding instead of remaking the complete expensive prosthesis.

SUMMARY

Innovations in implant dental prosthetic materials have enabled the restoration of complicated cases and have solved problems without compromising the function or esthetics outcome. The surgeon and the restorative dentist should always keep a crown-down approach in their minds whenever they are planning for implant-supported/retained prostheses. This review article sheds light on available prosthetic options and the current evidence supporting the discussed treatment modalities.

REFERENCES

1. Buser D, Sennerby L, De Bruyn H. Modern implant dentistry based on osseointegration: 50 years of progress, current trends and open questions. Periodontol 2000 2017;73(1):7–21.
2. Brånemark P-I, Zarb G, Albrektsson T, editors. Tissue-integrated prostheses: osseointegration in clinical dentistry. Chicago: Quintessence Publ Co; 1985.
3. Millen C, Bragger U, Wittneben JG. Influence of prosthesis type and retention mechanism on complications with fixed implant-supported prostheses: a systematic review applying multivariate analyses. Int J Oral Maxillofac Implants 2015;30: 110–24.
4. Wittneben JG, Millen C, Bragger U. Clinical performance of screw- versus cement-retained fixed implant-supported reconstructions: a systematic review. Int J Oral Maxillofac Implants 2014;29(Suppl):84–98.
5. Taylor TD, Klotz MW, Lawton RA. Titanium tattooing associated with zirconia implant abutments: a clinical report of two cases. Int J Oral Maxillofac Implants 2014;29:958–60.
6. Conejo J, Kobayashi T, Anadioti E, et al. Performance of CAD/CAM monolithic ceramic implant supported restorations bonded to titanium inserts: a systematic review. Eur J Oral Implantol 2017;10(Suppl 1):139–46.
7. Lewis S, Beumer J 3rd, Hornburg W, et al. The "UCLA" abutment. Int J Oral Maxillofac Implants 1988;3:183–9.
8. Long L, Alqarni H, Masri R. Influence of implant abutment fabrication method on clinical outcomes: a systematic review. Eur J Oral Implantol 2017;10(Suppl 1): 67–77.
9. Lops D, Bressan E, Parpaiola A, et al. Soft tissues stability of CAD/CAM and stock abutments in anterior regions: 2-year prospective multicentric cohort study. Clin Oral Implants Res 2015;26:1436–42.
10. Korsch M, Walther W. Prefabricated versus customized abutments: a retrospective analysis of loosening of cement-retained fixed implant-supported reconstructions. Int J Prosthodont 2015;28:522–6.
11. Anusavice KJ. Phillips' science of dental materials. 10th edition. Philadelphia: W.B. Saunders Co.; 2013.
12. Jorge JR, Barão VA, Delben JA, et al. Titanium in dentistry: historical development, state of the art and future perspectives. J Indian Prosthodont Soc 2013; 13:71–7.
13. Abduo J. Fit of CAD/CAM implant frameworks: a comprehensive review. J Oral Implantol 2014;40(6):758–66.
14. Karl M, Taylor TD. Parameters determining micromotion at the implant-abutment interface. Int J Oral Maxillofac Implants 2014;29:1338–47.

15. Kapos T, Evans C. CAD/CAM technology for implant abutments, crowns, and superstructures. Int J Oral Maxillofac Implants 2014;29(Suppl):117–36.
16. Thomason JM, Kelly SA, Bendkowski A, et al. Two implant retained overdentures: a review of the literature supporting the McGill and York consensus statements. J Dent 2012;40:22–34.
17. Raghoebar GM, Meijer HJ, Slot W, et al. A systematic review of implant-supported overdentures in the edentulous maxilla, compared to the mandible: how many implants? Eur J Oral Implantol 2014;7:191–201.
18. Alsayed HD, Alqahtani NM, Levon JA, et al. Prosthodontic rehabilitation of an ectodermal dysplasia patient with implant telescopic crown attachments. J Prosthodont 2017;26(7):622–7.
19. Zou D, Wu Y, Huang W, et al. A 3-year prospective clinical study of telescopic crown, bar, and locator attachments for removable four implant-supported maxillary overdentures. Int J Prosthodont 2013;26:566–73.
20. Sailer I, Philipp A, Zembic A, et al. A systematic review of the performance of ceramic and metal implant abutments supporting fixed implant reconstructions. Clin Oral Implants Res 2009;20:4–31.
21. Martinez-Rus F, Prieto M, Salido MP, et al. A clinical study assessing the influence of anodized titanium and zirconium dioxide abutments and peri-implant soft tissue thickness on the optical outcome of implant-supported lithium disilicate single crowns. Int J Oral Maxillofac Implants 2017;32:156–63.
22. Stimmelmayr M, Edelhoff D, Güth J-F, et al. Wear at the titanium–titanium and the titanium–zirconia implant–abutment interface: a comparative in vitro study. Dent Mater 2012;28(12):1215–20.
23. Stimmelmayr M, Sagerer S, Erdelt K, et al. In vitro fatigue and fracture strength testing of one-piece zirconia implant abutments and zirconia implant abutments connected to titanium cores. Int J Oral Maxillofac Implants 2013;28(2):488–93.
24. Papaspyridakos P, Lal K. Computer-assisted design/computer-assisted manufacturing zirconia implant fixed complete prostheses: clinical results and technical complications up to 4 years of function. Clin Oral Implants Res 2013; 24(6):659–65.
25. Chun KY, Lee JY. Comparative study of mechanical properties of dental restorative materials and dental hard tissues in compressive loads. J Dent Biomech 2014;5:1–6.
26. Janyavula S, Lawson N, Lawson N, et al. The wear of polished and glazed zirconia against enamel. J Prosthet Dent 2013;109(1):22–9.
27. Bidra AS, Tischler M, Patch C. Survival of 2039 complete arch fixed implant- supported zirconia prostheses: a retrospective study. J Prosthet Dent 2018;119: 220–4.
28. Vagkopoulou T, Koutayas SO, Koidis P, et al. Zirconia in dentistry: Part 1. Discovering the nature of an upcoming bioceramic. Eur J Esthet Dent 2009;4:130–51.
29. Venezia P, Torsello F, Cavalcanti R, et al. Retrospective analysis of 26 complete-arch implant-supported monolithic zirconia prostheses with feldspathic porcelain veneering limited to the facial surface. J Prosthet Dent 2015;114:506–12.
30. Teigen K, Jokstad A. Dental implant suprastructures using cobalt-chromium alloy compared with gold alloy framework veneered with ceramic or acrylic resin: a retrospective cohort study up to 18 years. Clin Oral Implants Res 2011;23: 853–60.
31. Øilo M, Nesse H, Lundberg OJ, et al. Mechanical properties of cobalt-chromium 3-unit fixed dental prostheses fabricated by casting, milling and additive manufacturing. J Prosthet Dent 2018;120(1):156.e17.

32. Ortorp A, Jonson D, Mouhsen A, et al. The t of cobalt-chromium three unit xed dental prostheses fabricated with 4 different techniques: a comparative in vitro study. Dent Mater J 2011;27:356–63.

33. Li J, Chen C, Liao J, et al. Bond strengths of porcelain to cobalt chromium alloys made by casting, milling, and selective laser melting. J Prosthet Dent 2017; 118(1):69–75.

34. Tuna SH, Ozcicek Pekmez N, Kurkcuoglu I. Corrosion resistance assessment of Co-Cr alloy frameworks fabricated by CAD/CAM milling, laser sintering, and casting methods. J Prosthet Dent 2015;114(5):725–34.

35. Campbell SD, Cooper L, Craddock H, et al. Removable partial dentures: the clinical need for innovation. J Prosthet Dent 2017;118(3):273–80.

36. Keltjens HM, Mulder J, Kayser AF, et al. Fit of direct retainers in removable partial dentures after 8 years of use. J Oral Rehabil 1997;24:138–42.

37. Han KH, Lee JY, Shin SW. Implant-and tooth supported fixed prostheses using a high-performance polymer (Pekkton) framework. Int J Prosthodont 2016;29(5): 451–4.

38. Passareitti A, Petroni G, Miracolo G, et al. Metal free, full arch, fixed prosthesis for edentulous mandible rehabilitation on four implants. J Prosthodont Res 2018; 62(2):264–7.

39. Thalji MB, De Kok IJ, Cooper LF. Prosthodontic management of implant therapy. Dent Clin North Am 2014;58:207–25.

40. Sala L, Bascones-Martínez A, Carrillo-de-Albornoz A. Impact of abutment material on peri-implant soft tissue color. An in vitro study. Clin Oral Investig 2017; 21(7):2221–33.

41. Wittneben J-G, Joda T, Weber H-P, et al. Screw retained vs. cement retained implant-supported fixed dental prosthesis. Periodontol 2000 2017;73:141–51.

What is the Best Available Luting Agent for Implant Prosthesis?

Nehal Almehmadi, BDS[a], Ahmad Kutkut, DDS, MS, FICOI, DICOI[b],
Mohanad Al-Sabbagh, DDS, MS[c],*

KEYWORDS

- Cement-retained • Provisional cements • Permanent cements • Zinc oxide eugenol
- Zinc phosphate • Resin-modified glass ionomer • Resin cement • Retention

KEY POINTS

- A wide variety of dental cements are commercially available to retain an implant-supported prosthesis. Each cement material has certain characteristics and properties.
- Retention of dental cements for implant-supported prosthesis varies from tooth-supported prosthesis. Retention and esthetics are the main factors in cement selection guideline.
- Peri-implant mucositis and peri-implantitis are major concerns when considering cement-retained implant prosthesis. It is customary to use different cementation techniques to minimize excess cement.

INTRODUCTION

Cement-retained implant-supported prostheses (CRISP) have been commonly used because of simplicity and cost effectiveness. Peri-implant health parameters were reported to be similar around screw-retained and cement-retained prosthesis, provided that excess cement is removed.[1] Although the fabrication of cement-retained prostheses is simple and similar to tooth-borne prostheses, the retention of dental cements varies between CRISP and tooth-supported prostheses. A survey by Tarica and colleagues[2] (2010) showed that resin-modified glass ionomer (GI) is the most preferred cement for CRISP in United States dental schools. The second most popular cement is zinc oxide eugenol (ZOE), followed closely by GI. Polycarboxylate (PCB) and acrylic

Disclosure: The authors have nothing to disclose.
[a] Division of Periodontology, Department of Oral Health Practice, College of Dentistry, University of Kentucky, 800 Rose Street, Lexington, KY 40536-7001, USA; [b] Division of Prosthodontics, University of Kentucky, College of Dentistry, D646, 800 Rose Street, Lexington, KY 40536, USA; [c] Division of Periodontology, Department of Oral Health Practice, University of Kentucky College of Dentistry, D-438 Chandler Medical Center, 800 Rose Street, Lexington, KY 40536-0927, USA
* Corresponding author.
E-mail address: malsa2@email.uky.edu

Dent Clin N Am 63 (2019) 531–545
https://doi.org/10.1016/j.cden.2019.02.014
dental.theclinics.com

urethane were the least used materials. This article will shed light on the characteristics of dental cements used in implant dentistry. It also provides selection criteria according to the material of the abutment and prosthesis.

CHARACTERISTICS OF AN IDEAL CEMENT

An ideal cement should have the following characteristics:

- Biocompatibility
- Adequate mechanical characteristics
- Promotion of tissue health
- Adequate marginal seal
- Dissolution resistance
- Radiopacity
- Excellent esthetics
- Cost effectiveness

An ideal cement is yet to be developed.[3–5] The clinicians' preference and clinical situation are the currently used selection criteria.[5]

DENTAL CEMENT MATERIALS

Several classification systems categorize cements based on characteristics such as composition and chemical bonding properties.[5] The classification of dental cements for cementing prostheses to natural abutments does not necessarily apply to implant-supported prostheses.[6] For instance, whereas (ZOE) is used for short-term cementation during provisionalization on teeth, ZOE provides sufficient retention for CRISP.[7] Because this article focuses on clinical applications, it is appropriate to classify dental cements as either provisional, semipermanent,[8] or permanent (**Table 1**).

PROVISIONAL CEMENTS

Provisional cements are highly soluble and show weak tensile strength.[8] This may be advantageous when completing a provisional CRISP or recementing a prosthesis that is associated with peri-implantitis.[9] Provisional cements allow for the retrievability of CRISP.[10,11] However, CRISP may lose retention when provisional cement is used. Both ZOE and eugenol-free ZnO (EF-ZnO) are considered provisional cements. According to Ma and Fenton's systematic review, 17.6% loss of retention of CRISP occurred when provisional cements were used.[4] The characteristics of ZOE and EF-ZnO are addressed in **Table 2**.

SEMIPERMANENT CEMENTS

Semipermanent cements provide sufficient retention to resist frequent decementation and allow retrievability. Zinc phosphate (ZnP) and GI are considered semipermanent

Table 1
Clinical classification of dental cements

Provisional	Semipermanent	Permanent
Zinc oxide eugenol	Zinc phosphate	Resin-modified glass ionomer
Eugenol-free zinc oxide	Glass ionomer	Zinc polycarboxylate
		Resin cement

Table 2
Provisional cements used to retain CRISP

Cement Type	Characteristics	Advantages	Disadvantages
ZOE	• Bactericidal[12] • Soluble[13] • Radiopaque[14] • Weak bond to titanium[15] • Lowest tensile strength[16–18] • High pH[19] • Excellent marginal seal[20]	• Significant reduction in periodontal pathogens[9] • No residual cement, hence low incidence of peri-implantitis • Excess cement is easily detected. • Easy removal of excess cement • Ideal for provisionalization • Biocompatible • Less bacterial microleakage	• Gap formation at the prosthesis-abutment interface • Frequent decementations
Eugenol-free zinc oxide	• Organic acid substitutes for eugenol[3,21] • Soluble • Low tensile strength[18,22] • Low inflammatory soft tissue parameters	• Hypoallergenic • Eliminate the negative effect of eugenol on resin polymerization if permanent cementation is considered[21] • Low incidence of peri-implantitis[7]	• Higher microleakage[2] • Low retention

cements when used with CRISP.[8,18] Semipermanent cements reduce the incidence of decementation when compared with provisional cements. When a cement's tensile strength is between provisional and permanent cements, it is classified as a semipermanent cement. A permanent cement, such as resin cement, can be made semipermanent by mixing it with petroleum jelly.[23] ZnP and GI offer a degree of retrievability when used with titanium or zirconia abutments.[6,18,24] Wittneben and Bragger's systematic review demonstrated a decementation rate of 0% for CRISP cemented with ZnP.[1] **Table 3** provides an overview of ZnP and GI characteristics.

PERMANENT CEMENTS

After careful evaluation of peri-implant tissue health, clinicians may wish to cement the prosthesis indefinitely. Permanent cements should have characteristics that prohibit the occurrence of any prosthetic complication. It must allow for long-term retention, peri-implant health and a desirable esthetic outcome. Resin-modified GI (RMGI), zinc PCB, and resin cements share properties of permanent cements. RMGI, PCB, and resin are used to retain permanent CRISPs. A systematic review by Chaar and colleagues[36] revealed a decementation rate up to 4% for CRISP retained with permanent cements **(Table 4)**.

SELECTION OF DENTAL CEMENTS

Selection of the proper dental cement for CRISP is largely based on retention and tensile strength of the material. However, esthetics become equally important when restoring anterior teeth. The retention and esthetics of CRISP are dependent on the interaction of the cement with the available abutment or prosthetic materials. Several studies assessed esthetics and retention of various abutment-prosthetic

Table 3
Commonly used semipermanent cements

Cement Type	Characteristics	Advantages	Disadvantages
ZnP	• Tensile strength is lower than GI, but higher than EF-ZnO[25] • Low viscosity • No adhesion to titanium or prosthesis[3,20] • Highest elastic modulus[3,20] • High solubility at setting time[3,26,27] • Least creep[28] • Highest radiopacity when compared with different luting agents[29] • Inexpensive	• Lower incidence of decementation than provisional cements • Flow easily for better mechanical retention[3,5,20] • Highly rigid, thus suitable for areas with high occlusal forces • Dimensionally stable, thus no stress generation on full ceramic prostheses • Easy detection of excess cement • Excess cement removal is the easiest compared with resin and GI cements[30,31] • Cost-effective	• Not recommended for short abutments or prostheses with increased prosthetic-abutment gab • Inadequate marginal seal[30,32]
GI	• Adequate mechanical strength, and adhesion to base metal alloys[3] • Critical manipulation during setting time[5,20] • High creep—deformation of the material with time[33] • High water sorption[3] • Low modulus of elasticity[33] • Radiopaque • retention increases over time due to continued polymerization[24,31,34] • Inexpensive	• Adequate retention • Some brands (GC Fuji Temp LT) can be detected radiographically[35]	• Inadequate moisture control during setting results in high microleakage[5] • Microcracks with excessive dryness during setting time[20] • Dimensional instability (not recommended for full lithium disilicate ceramic crown)[34] • Not recommended in areas subjected to high occlusal forces[33]

combinations in a quest to determine the best performing cement for each combination.

Esthetic Value

Shade selection

The combination of the prosthesis, cement, and abutment selection can change the overall appearance of the final outcome. Dede and colleagues[60] tested the effect of 3 different shades of resin cement (translucent, universal, and white opaque) on the visual perception of the final prosthesis. The study used discs to represent combinations of available abutments and cement shades when used with a lithium disilicate (LS_2) crown. The abutments tested were zirconium, gold-palladium, and titanium. The arrangement of discs is illustrated in **Fig. 1**. Of all the tested combinations, only the combination of zirconia or gold-palladium abutments with universal shade resin cement were esthetically acceptable.

Table 4
Commonly used permanent cements for CRISP

Cement Type	Characteristics	Advantages	Disadvantages
RMGI	• Less critical manipulation than conventional GI[37,38] • Increased tensile and flexural strength provided by the added resin[5,39] • Improved initial strength and less solubility compared with GI[5,34] • Highest water sorption[3,34,40,41] • Radiopacity is comparable with enamel[3,29,35] • Different shades are available	• Suitable for areas subjected to high occlusal forces • Indicated for metal, PFM, FPD, and high strength ceramics[34,42,43] • Less microleakage[3,32,41] • Excess cement can be detected radiographically • Excellent esthetics and retentive qualities[42,44]	• Dimensionally less stable (contraindicated with full ceramic prostheses)[3,43,45] • Excess cement removal can be difficult if not performed quickly.[3,5,20]
Zinc PCB	• Good retention[17,18] • High solubility and erosion in acidic medium[3,27,34,46] • Weak cohesive strength • Deformation under pressure[5,20] • Radiopaque at 0.5 mm thickness[29] • Corrosive behavior on titanium[47,48]	• Can be used in less than ideal retentive conditions, only when excellent prosthetic fit is present • Excess cement can be detected	• Loss of retention is anticipated with ill fitted prosthesis • Highest microleakage among dental cements[3,30] • Sandblasting of the abutment or the prostheses does not make a significant difference. • Not recommended for long span prosthesis • Not recommended with titanium abutments
Resin	• Insoluble and provide adhesion[3,20,49] • Highest retention[17,30,32,49–51] • High modulus of elasticity and flexural strength[3,52] • Strengthen all-ceramic prostheses[53,54] • Highly viscous • High water sorption, especially for unfilled resin[3,55,56] • High bonding affinity to titanium • radiolucent[29]	• Lowest microleakage[32,34] • Indicated for short abutments[57] • Excellent in posterior area[3,20] • Less fracture of all-ceramic prostheses • Excellent esthetics	• High incidence of peri-implantitis when excess cement is not removed[9] • High viscosity might prevent complete seating of the prosthesis, thus leading to marginal discrepancy or fracture of the veneering ceramic[17,58,59] • Removal of excess cement is not easy after setting of the cement • Excess cement is not detected radiographically

Color stability

Tertiary amines are components of self-cured and dual-cured resin cement, which activate the curing chemical reaction. However, they are also responsible for color instability within the resin.[61,62] Whether or not the gradual change in color in the

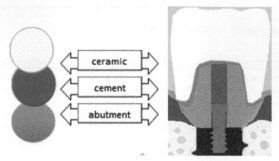

Fig. 1. Representation of the tested disc combinations to determine the best esthetic outcome.

composite cements affects the long-term esthetic outcome of the cemented prostheses is debatable.[63–66]

Retentiveness

Tensile strength of a cement determines the degree of retention. Researchers tested several cements with various abutment-prosthesis combinations. The retentiveness of titanium and zirconia abutments with several cements and prosthetic materials is reviewed below.

Zirconia abutments

Lithium disilicate Sellers and colleagues[24] investigated the retentiveness of 6 luting agents cementing LS_2 all-ceramic crowns to zirconia abutments. A thermocycling model was used to simulate the condition in the oral environment. The most retentive cement after thermocycling was resin cement (Multilink Hybrid Abutment). However, retention of 2 resin cements (Panavia 21 and RelyX Unicem) were significantly reduced after thermocycling.

Zirconia Rinke and colleagues[67] followed 42 anterior crowns cemented provisionally on prefabricated zirconia abutments for 7 years to assess survival and prosthetic complications rate. Only 4 decementations occurred over a period of 7 years. Rinke[68] recommended the use of provisional cement if sufficient retention is available. Otherwise, resin cement is preferred if excess cement removal can be achieved.

Titanium abutments

Cobalt-chromium In 2013, Mehl and colleagues[69] examined the retention of cobalt-chromium (Co-Cr) castings cemented to titanium abutments using several types of cements. The highest retention was obtained with resin cement. Polycarboxylate was the second most retentive cement followed by GI. Another study confirms that resin cement provides more retention for Co-Cr when compared with GI.[70]

Zirconia Schiessl and colleagues[71] investigated the retention of 2 prosthetic materials, Co-Cr and zirconia cemented to titanium abutments using PCB, ZnP, EF-ZnO, GI, and resin cements. In this study, PCB offered the most retention for Co-Cr. Retention of zirconia coping was noticed to be similar when ZnP, EF-ZnO, GI, or resin cements are used.

Gold The retention of gold copings cemented with resin cement was evaluated in relation to varying abutment heights.[72] In this study, a larger abutment surface area enhanced the amount of retention. Moreover, copings were successfully cemented to titanium abutments as short as 5 mm via resin cement.

Porcelain fused to metal Woelber and colleagues[73] conducted a retrospective study to evaluate the retention of porcelain fused to metal (PFM) prostheses cemented to titanium abutments using ZOE. The decementation rate was 8.77% over a mean period of 9.27 years. The investigators recommended ZOE as a viable option to retain PFM to titanium abutments. On the other hand, Rinke and colleagues[74] looked at prosthetic complications of 112 implant-supporting single PFM crowns retained by ZOE. Rinke did not recommend ZOE to retain PFM because of the high decementation rate. Furthermore, Worni and colleagues[75] tested the retention of several luting agents in combination with 2 different abutment heights. The outcome of this study suggested that the type of cement used was more influential than abutment height. Among the cement tested, PCB (Durelon, 3M ESPE) and resin cement (Improv, Alvelogro) provided the highest retention for PFM crowns supported by titanium abutments.

Based on these previously mentioned studies and other relatable articles, a proposed cement selection guideline based on the combination of the abutment and desired prosthesis is summarized in **Table 5**.

CEMENTATION TECHNIQUES

Proper cementation techniques ensure adequate retention of the prosthesis and decrease the incidence of potential complications. Every attempt should be made to minimize excess cement extrusion during seating of the prostheses. Thus, the prostheses should never be completely filled during cementation,[76] because this will most likely result in the expression of cement into the gingival tissue. Furthermore, the crown margins should be less than 2 mm apical to the gingival crest to allow for the detection and removal of excess cement.[77] Several methods (as mentioned later) have been advocated to cement prostheses supported by implants with the common goal of limiting excess cement,[78–82] and thus preventing cement-associated peri-implantitis.[7] **Fig. 2** shows a clinical case of cement-induced peri-implant mucositis.

Table 5					
Desired cements based on the abutment-prosthetic combination					
Type of Restoration	**PFM Crown**	**Zr Crown**	**All-Ceramic Crown**	**Gold Crown**	**Co-Cr Crown**
Gold/UCLA abutment	ZOE, universal shade resin cement	N/A	Universal shade resin cement	Calcium hydroxide temporary cement	N/A
Titanium abutment	PCB, resin cements	PCB, GI, resin cements	ZOE	Resin cement	PCB, GI, resin cements
Zirconia abutment	GI, resin cements	Resin cement	Translucent, universal shade resin, ZOE cements	N/A	N/A
All-ceramic abutment	N/A	Resin cement (Multilink)	Resin cement (Multilink)	N/A	N/A

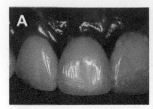 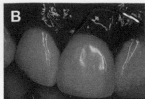 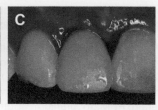

Fig. 2. Cement-induced peri-implant mucositis. (*A*) Cement-induced peri-implant mucositis. Note the mucosal inflammation around implant in site no. 8. (*B*) Excess cement was identified and removed. (*C*) Soft tissue healing at 2 weeks follow-up visit. Note the dissolution of mucosal inflammation.

Incomplete Coating of the Intaglio of the Prosthesis

One of the proposed techniques to minimize the excess cement in the peri-implant tissue is to coat only the coronal half of the intaglio of the prostheses.[78] Wolfart and colleagues[17] tested the retention of several luting agents using this method and they suggested that coating half of the intaglio surface of the prostheses was as effective as complete coating. This mode of cementation is thought to be beneficial in preventing incomplete seating of the prostheses.[78] However, it might result in a gap and bacterial leakage at the restorative-abutment interface.[83] Thus, clinicians may choose to coat only the apical half of the prostheses intaglio to address this issue (not the coronal).[17]

Extraoral Prosthetic Preseating Using Abutment Analog

The extra-oral preseating technique involves the use of a replica (abutment analog), on which the prosthesis is preseated. The cement is applied, and the prosthesis is seated on the abutment analog first. This ensures the elimination of excess cement before cementing the prosthesis intra-orally.[82,84–86] In 2016, Frisch and colleagues[7] investigated the clinical efficacy of this method with EF-ZnO. The results showed decementation in 6.19% of cases within the first 6 months. Jimenez and Vargas-Koudriavtsev[85] also investigated the use of EF-ZnOZ with this technique alone, or in combination with leaving the screw access channel open as a reservoir for excess cement. They did not recommend this technique with provisional cements, either alone or in combination with the open screw access channel. Santosa and colleagues[16] compared the retention attained by conventional cementation and abutment analog techniques using EF-ZnO and RMGI cements. No significant difference in retention was recorded, either for the EF-ZnO samples or for the RMGI samples when comparing the 2 cementation methods. However, extra-oral cementation did significantly minimize excess cement.

Creating a Vent Hole as a Cement Reservoir

Another method tested to reduce excess cement is to create a vent hole in the prostheses.[81,87] This provides a channel for cement escapement, thus limiting excess cement in peri-implant tissue. Some clinicians opt to leave screw access channel open as a reservoir for excess cement. Jimenez and Vargas-Koudriavtsev[85] measured the amount of excess EF-ZnO cement used in 3 different cementation protocols: creating a vent hole in the crown, leaving the screw channel open, or using a preseating technique. All 3 methods reduce excess cement. The investigators recommended a vent hole or open screw access channel because they both reduce the amount of excess cement while maintaining acceptable retention.

Extraoral Cementation (Screwmentation)

Another method used to limit excess cement in peri-implant tissue is screwmentation. This is achieved by cementing the prostheses extra-orally, wiping off any excess cement, then screwing the prostheses-abutment combination to the implant.[54,88] Screwmentation combines the advantages of screw-retention and cement-retention. It allows for retrievability of CRISP and eliminates the risk of excess cement.

Among the 4 previously mentioned methods, abutment analog provided the least amount of excess cement.[82] The Preseating technique is advisable when a luting agent with sufficient retention and difficult excess cement removal (eg, adhesive resin) is used, especially if the prosthesis margins are 3 mm below the gingival crest.[78]

CLINICAL CONSIDERATIONS

Multiple clinical situations are encountered when cementing the prosthesis to the implant. Removal of excess cement is of vast importance, and must be handled carefully and efficiently. Other considerations include permanent cementation after provisionalization, increasing the retention of CRISP and cantilever by abutment and prosthetic surface pretreatment. These prosthetic considerations are further discussed later.

Removal of Excess Cement

Excess cement should be removed immediately following cementation with scalers, dental floss, or probes. However, plastic or titanium instruments are preferred to avoid scratching the implant platform. A radiograph may confirm seating of the prosthesis and allow for large pieces of excess cement to be detected. However, all patients with a CRISP should routinely return for follow-up care and maintenance to monitor the condition of the peri-implant. The length of time that cement is present is directly correlated with the level of inflammation, suppuration, and periodontal destruction.[89]

Permanent Cementation After Provisionalization

Provisional cement residues on the abutment or the prosthetic intaglio surfaces can affect the adhesion of permanent cement, thus decreasing retention. ZOE, in particular, should be completely removed before permanently cementing the prosthesis with resin cement. Eugenol within ZOE inhibits polymerization of resin cement and prevents complete setting of the resin matrix.[90] The best way to completely remove all provisional cement residues is achieved with aluminum oxide air abrasion.[49]

Abutment and Prosthetic Surface Pretreatment

Loss of retention of CRISP is common and poses a risk of aspiration or swallowing of the prosthesis.[25] Increasing the retention of a prosthesis is possible for some dental cements by pretreating the prostheses intaglio or the abutment.[17] The most commonly used pretreatment method in the United States is sandblasting the prostheses with aluminum oxide. Al Hamad and colleagues[91] found that sandblasting the abutment improved the retention of ZnP, GI, and ZOE.

Cantilever Cement-Retained Implant-Supported Prostheses

Cantilever CRISP may be necessary in cases where placing additional implants is not feasible (lower incisor with lack of space). Sandblasting the abutment is advisable when the abutment height is less than 6 mm.[91] Kappel and colleagues[22] investigated the effect of sandblasting the abutment on the retention of different types of dental cements (EF-ZnO, ZnP, and GI) retaining cantilever CRISP. Sandblasting resulted in significantly higher retention for semipermanent cements (ZnP and GI) compared with samples without sandblasting. However, no significant difference in retention was recorded for EF-ZnO cements with or without sandblasting. Retention of cantilever CRISP with GI increases when sandblasting the abutment and the intaglio surface of the prosthesis is used,[92] whereas ZnP can be recommended for cantilever CRISP even without sandblasting.[20,22]

SUMMARY

Based on the information obtained from peer-reviewed articles, cements show different retention qualities for CRISP. These qualities might not be the same as those for cement-retained prostheses on teeth. However, the previously defined clinical guidelines for appropriate cement selection should be considered when planning the prosthesis. The use of provisional cement, such as ZOE, is widely accepted in implant dentistry. However, a more durable permanent cement such as RMGI is preferred. Although resin cement provides the highest retention, it is less popular because of the high incidence of peri-implantitis and the inability to retrieve the prosthesis in cases of complications. When selecting the cement, esthetics and retention should be considered when planning a case.

REFERENCES

1. Wittneben JG, Millen C, Bragger U. Clinical performance of screw- versus cement-retained fixed implant-supported reconstructions–a systematic review. Int J Oral Maxillofac Implants 2014;29(Suppl):84–98.
2. Tarica DY, Alvarado VM, Truong ST. Survey of United States dental schools on cementation protocols for implant crown restorations. J Prosthet Dent 2010; 103(2):68–79.
3. Rosenstiel SF, Land MF, Crispin BJ. Dental luting agents: a review of the current literature. J Prosthet Dent 1998;80(3):280–301.
4. Ma S, Fenton A. Screw- versus cement-retained implant prostheses: a systematic review of prosthodontic maintenance and complications. Int J Prosthodont 2015; 28(2):127–45.
5. Lad PP, Kamath M, Tarale K, et al. Practical clinical considerations of luting cements: a review. J Int Oral Health 2014;6(1):116–20.
6. Mansour A, Ercoli C, Graser G, et al. Comparative evaluation of casting retention using the ITI solid abutment with six cements. Clin Oral Implants Res 2002;13(4): 343–8.
7. Frisch E, Ratka-Kruger P, Weigl P, et al. Extraoral cementation technique to minimize cement-associated peri-implant marginal bone loss: can a thin layer of zinc oxide cement provide sufficient retention? Int J Prosthodont 2016;29(4):360–2.
8. Mehl C, Harder S, Wolfart M, et al. Retrievability of implant-retained crowns following cementation. Clin Oral Implants Res 2008;19(12):1304–11.
9. Korsch M, Marten SM, Walther W, et al. Impact of dental cement on the peri-implant biofilm-microbial comparison of two different cements in an in vivo observational study. Clin Implant Dent Relat Res 2018;20(5):806–13.
10. Schoenbaum TR, Chang YY, Klokkevold PR. Screw-access marking: a technique to simplify retrieval of cement-retained implant prostheses. Compend Contin Educ Dent 2013;34(3):230–6.
11. Merz BR, Hunenbart S, Belser UC. Mechanics of the implant-abutment connection: an 8-degree taper compared to a bull joint connection. Int J Oral Maxillofac Implants 2000;15(4):519–26.

12. Raval NC, Wadhwani CP, Jain S, et al. The interaction of implant luting cements and oral bacteria linked to peri-implant disease: an in vitro analysis of planktonic and biofilm growth–a preliminary study. Clin Implant Dent Relat Res 2015;17(6): 1029–35.

13. Weber HP, Kim DM, Ng MW, et al. Peri-implant soft-tissue health surrounding cement- and screw-retained implant restorations: a multi-center, 3-year prospective study. Clin Oral Implants Res 2006;17(4):375–9.

14. Wadhwani C, Hess T, Faber T, et al. A descriptive study of the radiographic density of implant restorative cements. J Prosthet Dent 2010;103(5):295–302.

15. Breeding LC, Dixon DL, Bogacki MT, et al. Use of luting agents with an implant system: part I. J Prosthet Dent 1992;68(5):737–41.

16. Santosa RE, Martin W, Morton D. Effects of a cementing technique in addition to luting agent on the uniaxial retention force of a single-tooth implant-supported restoration: an in vitro study. Int J Oral Maxillofac Implants 2010;25(6):1145–52.

17. Wolfart M, Wolfart S, Kern M. Retention forces and seating discrepancies of implant-retained castings after cementation. Int J Oral Maxillofac Implants 2006;21(4):519–25.

18. Akca K, Iplikcioglu H, Cehreli MC. Comparison of uniaxial resistance forces of cements used with implant-supported crowns. Int J Oral Maxillofac Implants 2002; 17(4):536–42.

19. Marvin JC, Gallegos SI, Parsaei S, et al. In vitro evaluation of cell compatibility of dental cements used with titanium implant components. J Prosthodont 2018; 28(2):e705–12.

20. Hill EE, Lott J. A clinically focused discussion of luting materials. Aust Dent J 2011;56(Suppl 1):67–76.

21. Wilson TG Jr. The positive relationship between excess cement and peri-implant disease: a prospective clinical endoscopic study. J Periodontol 2009;80(9): 1388–92.

22. Kappel S, Chepura T, Schmitter M, et al. Effects of cement, abutment surface pretreatment, and artificial aging on the force required to detach cantilever fixed dental prostheses from dental implants. Int J Prosthodont 2017;30(6):545–52.

23. Bresciano M, Schierano G, Manzella C, et al. Retention of luting agents on implant abutments of different height and taper. Clin Oral Implants Res 2005; 16(5):594–8.

24. Sellers K, Powers JM, Kiat-Amnuay S. Retentive strength of implant-supported CAD-CAM lithium disilicate crowns on zirconia custom abutments using 6 different cements. J Prosthet Dent 2017;117(2):247–52.

25. Schwarz S, Schroder C, Corcodel N, et al. Retrospective comparison of semipermanent and permanent cementation of implant-supported single crowns and FDPs with regard to the incidence of survival and complications. Clin Implant Dent Relat Res 2012;14(Suppl 1):e151–8.

26. Craig R, Powers J. Restorative dental materials. 11th edition. St Louis (MO): Mosby; 2002.

27. Baldissara P, Comin G, Martone F, et al. Comparative study of the marginal microleakage of six cements in fixed provisional crowns. J Prosthet Dent 1998;80(4): 417–22.

28. Wilson AD, Lewis BG. The flow properties of dental cements. J Biomed Mater Res 1980;14(4):383–91.

29. Pette GA, Ganeles J, Norkin FJ. Radiographic appearance of commonly used cements in implant dentistry. Int J Periodontics Restorative Dent 2013;33(1):61–8.

30. Pan YH, Ramp LC, Lin CK, et al. Comparison of 7 luting protocols and their effect on the retention and marginal leakage of a cement-retained dental implant restoration. Int J Oral Maxillofac Implants 2006;21(4):587–92.

31. Agar JR, Cameron SM, Hughbanks JC, et al. Cement removal from restorations luted to titanium abutments with simulated subgingival margins. J Prosthet Dent 1997;78(1):43–7.

32. White SN, Yu Z, Tom JF, et al. In vivo microleakage of luting cements for cast crowns. J Prosthet Dent 1994;71(4):333–8.

33. Cattani-Lorente MA, Godin C, Meyer JM. Early strength of glass ionomer cements. Dent Mater 1993;9(1):57–62.

34. Hill EE. Dental cements for definitive luting: a review and practical clinical considerations. Dent Clin North Am 2007;51(3):643–58, vi.

35. Cal E, Guneri P, Unal S, et al. Radiopacity of luting cements as a potential factor in peri-implantitis: an in vitro comparative study. Int J Periodontics Restorative Dent 2017;37(3):e163–9.

36. Chaar MS, Att W, Strub JR. Prosthetic outcome of cement-retained implant-supported fixed dental restorations: a systematic review. J Oral Rehabil 2011;38(9):697–711.

37. Cho E, Kopel H, White SN. Moisture susceptibility of resin-modified glass-ionomer materials. Quintessence Int 1995;26(5):351–8.

38. McComb D. Adhesive luting cements–classes, criteria, and usage. Compend Contin Educ Dent 1996;17(8):759–62, 64 passim; quiz 74.

39. White SN, Yu Z. Compressive and diametral tensile strengths of current adhesive luting agents. J Prosthet Dent 1993;69(6):568–72.

40. Kanchanavasita W, Anstice HM, Pearson GJ. Water sorption characteristics of resin-modified glass-ionomer cements. Biomaterials 1997;18(4):343–9.

41. Thonemann B, Federlin M, Schmalz G, et al. Resin-modified glass ionomers for luting posterior ceramic restorations. Dent Mater 1995;11(3):161–8.

42. Snyder MD, Lang BR, Razzoog ME. The efficacy of luting all-ceramic crowns with resin-modified glass ionomer cement. J Am Dent Assoc 2003;134(5):609–12 [quiz: 32–3].

43. Diaz-Arnold AM, Vargas MA, Haselton DR. Current status of luting agents for fixed prosthodontics. J Prosthet Dent 1999;81(2):135–41.

44. Ernst CP, Cohnen U, Stender E, et al. In vitro retentive strength of zirconium oxide ceramic crowns using different luting agents. J Prosthet Dent 2005;93(6):551–8.

45. Mount GJ. An atlas of glass-ionomer cements: a clinicians guide. 3rd edition. New York: Martin Duntiz; 2002.

46. Wilson AD, Nicholson JW. Acid-base cements: their biomedical and industrial applications. Cambridge: Cambridge University Press; 2005.

47. Wadhwani C, Chung KH. Bond strength and interactions of machined titanium-based alloy with dental cements. J Prosthet Dent 2015;114(5):660–5.

48. Schoenbaum T, Stevenson RG, Moshaverinia A. Single-unit cement-retained implant restorations: strategies, protocols, and techniques. Dentistry today 2017;36(6):64–8.

49. Ferrari M, Dalloca L, Kugel G, et al. An evaluation of the effect of the adhesive luting on microleakage of the IPS empress crowns. Pract Periodontics Aesthet Dent 1994;6(4):15–23 [quiz: 4].

50. Mojon P, Hawbolt EB, MacEntee MI, et al. Early bond strength of luting cements to a precious alloy. J Dent Res 1992;71(9):1633–9.

51. White SN, Furuichi R, Kyomen SM. Microleakage through dentin after crown cementation. J Endod 1995;21(1):9–12.

52. Ladha K, Verma M. Conventional and contemporary luting cements: an overview. J Indian Prosthodont Soc 2010;10(2):79–88.
53. Jensen ME, Sheth JJ, Tolliver D. Etched-porcelain resin-bonded full-veneer crowns: in vitro fracture resistance. Compendium 1989;10(6):336–8, 340-1, 344-7.
54. Roberts EE, Bailey CW, Ashcraft-Olmscheid DL, et al. Fracture resistance of titanium-based lithium disilicate and zirconia implant restorations. J Prosthodont 2018;27(7):644–50.
55. Giti R, Vojdani M, Abduo J, et al. The comparison of sorption and solubility behavior of four different resin luting cements in different storage media. J Dent (Shiraz) 2016;17(2):91–7.
56. Gerdolle DA, Mortier E, Jacquot B, et al. Water sorption and water solubility of current luting cements: an in vitro study. Quintessence Int 2008;39(3):e107–14.
57. Pegoraro TA, da Silva NR, Carvalho RM. Cements for use in esthetic dentistry. Dent Clin North Am 2007;51(2):453–71, x.
58. McAllister BS. The rationale for the vented-crown technique and its application in today's dental practice. Oper Dent 2008;33(2):116–20.
59. Linkevicius T, Vladimirovas E, Grybauskas S, et al. Veneer fracture in implant-supported metal-ceramic restorations. Part I: overall success rate and impact of occlusal guidance. Stomatologija 2008;10(4):133–9.
60. Dede DO, Armaganci A, Ceylan G, et al. Influence of abutment material and luting cements color on the final color of all ceramics. Acta Odontol Scand 2013; 71(6):1570–8.
61. Brauer GM, Dulik DM, Antonucci JM, et al. New amine accelerators for composite restorative resins. J Dent Res 1979;58(10):1994–2000.
62. De Souza G, Braga RR, Cesar PF, et al. Correlation between clinical performance and degree of conversion of resin cements: a literature review. J Appl Oral Sci 2015;23(4):358–68.
63. Berrong JM, Weed RM, Schwartz IS. Color stability of selected dual-cure composite resin cements. J Prosthodont 1993;2(1):24–7.
64. Prieto LT, Pimenta de Araujo CT, Araujo Pierote JJ, et al. Evaluation of degree of conversion and the effect of thermal aging on the color stability of resin cements and flowable composite. J Conserv Dent 2018;21(1):47–51.
65. Noie F, O'Keefe KL, Powers JM. Color stability of resin cements after accelerated aging. Int J Prosthodont 1995;8(1):51–5.
66. Mina NR, Baba NZ, Al-Harbi FA, et al. The influence of simulated aging on the color stability of composite resin cements. J Prosthet Dent 2019;121(2):306–10.
67. Rinke S, Lattke A, Eickholz P, et al. Practice-based clinical evaluation of zirconia abutments for anterior single-tooth restorations. Quintessence Int 2015;46(1): 19–29.
68. Rinke S. Anterior all-ceramic superstructures: chance or risk? Quintessence Int 2015;46(3):217–27.
69. Mehl C, Harder S, Steiner M, et al. Influence of cement film thickness on the retention of implant-retained crowns. J Prosthodont 2013;22(8):618–25.
70. Mehl C, Ali S, El Bahra S, et al. Is there a correlation between tensile strength and retrievability of cemented implant-retained crowns using artificial aging? Int J Prosthodont 2016;29(1):83–90.
71. Schiessl C, Schaefer L, Winter C, et al. Factors determining the retentiveness of luting agents used with metal- and ceramic-based implant components. Clin Oral Investig 2013;17(4):1179–90.

72. Menini M, Pera F, Migliorati M, et al. Adhesive strength of the luting technique for passively fitting screw-retained implant-supported prostheses: an in vitro evaluation. Int J Prosthodont 2015;28(1):37–9.

73. Woelber JP, Ratka-Krueger P, Vach K, et al. Decementation rates and the peri-implant tissue status of implant-supported fixed restorations retained via zinc oxide cement: a retrospective 10-23-year study. Clin Implant Dent Relat Res 2016; 18(5):917–25.

74. Rinke S, Roediger M, Eickholz P, et al. Technical and biological complications of single-molar implant restorations. Clin Oral Implants Res 2015;26(9):1024–30.

75. Worni A, Gholami H, Marchand L, et al. Retrievability of implant-supported crowns when using three different cements: a controlled clinical trial. Int J Prosthodont 2015;28(1):22–9.

76. Wadhwani C, Hess T, Pineyro A, et al. Cement application techniques in luting implant-supported crowns: a quantitative and qualitative survey. Int J Oral Maxillofac Implants 2012;27(4):859–64.

77. Wittneben JG, Joda T, Weber HP, et al. Screw retained vs. cement retained implant-supported fixed dental prosthesis. Periodontol 2000 2017;73(1):141–51.

78. Dumbrigue HB, Abanomi AA, Cheng LL. Techniques to minimize excess luting agent in cement-retained implant restorations. J Prosthet Dent 2002;87(1):112–4.

79. Wadhwani C, Pineyro A. Technique for controlling the cement for an implant crown. J Prosthet Dent 2009;102(1):57–8.

80. Present S, Levine RA. Techniques to control or avoid cement around implant-retained restorations. Compend Contin Educ Dent 2013;34(6):432–7.

81. Patel D, Invest JC, Tredwin CJ, et al. An analysis of the effect of a vent hole on excess cement expressed at the crown-abutment margin for cement-retained implant crowns. J Prosthodont 2009;18(1):54–9.

82. Chee WW, Duncan J, Afshar M, et al. Evaluation of the amount of excess cement around the margins of cement-retained dental implant restorations: the effect of the cement application method. J Prosthet Dent 2013;109(4):216–21.

83. Quirynen M, Bollen CM, Eyssen H, et al. Microbial penetration along the implant components of the Branemark system. An in vitro study. Clin Oral Implants Res 1994;5(4):239–44.

84. Frisch E, Ratka-Kruger P, Weigl P, et al. Minimizing excess cement in implant-supported fixed restorations using an extraoral replica technique: a prospective 1-year study. Int J Oral Maxillofac Implants 2015;30(6):1355–61.

85. Jimenez RA, Vargas-Koudriavtsev T. Effect of preseating, screw access opening, and vent holes on extrusion of excess cement at the crown-abutment margin and associated tensile force for cement-retained implant restorations. Int J Oral Maxillofac Implants 2016;31(4):807–12.

86. Jambhekar SS, Matani J, Sethi T, et al. Reduction of excess cement during cementation of implant-retained crowns: a clinical tip. J Dent Implants 2013; 3(2):168–71.

87. Wadhwani C, Pineyro A, Hess T, et al. Effect of implant abutment modification on the extrusion of excess cement at the crown-abutment margin for cement-retained implant restorations. Int J Oral Maxillofac Implants 2011;26(6):1241–6.

88. Chawla P, Saini S, Mehrotra A, et al. Combination implant crown: a crown with a difference. J Dent Herald 2014;1(4):14–7.

89. Korsch M, Robra BP, Walther W. Cement-associated signs of inflammation: retrospective analysis of the effect of excess cement on peri-implant tissue. Int J Prosthodont 2015;28(1):11–8.

90. Stark H. Does temporary cementing have an effect on the bond strength of definitively cemented crowns? Dtsch Zahnarztl Z 1991;46(11):774–6 [in German].

91. Al Hamad KQ, Al Rashdan BA, Abu-Sitta EH. The effects of height and surface roughness of abutments and the type of cement on bond strength of cement-retained implant restorations. Clin Oral Implants Res 2011;22(6):638–44.

92. Okuyama JY, de Brito RB Jr, Franca FM. Aluminum oxide sandblasting of hexagonal coping and abutment: influence on retention and marginal leakage using temporary cements. Implant Dent 2016;25(3):394–9.

Is Peri-Implantitis Curable?

Mohanad Al-Sabbagh, DDS, MS[a], Luciana M. Shaddox, DDS, MS, PhD[b],*

KEYWORDS

- Peri-implantitis • Peri-implant mucositis • Management of peri-implantitis
- Prevention of peri-implantitis

KEY POINTS

- Diagnosis of peri-implant mucositis and peri-implantitis is based on the combination of clinical and radiographic findings.
- Prevention of peri-implant mucositis and peri-implantitis remains the fundamental strategy for a long-term successful outcome of implants.
- Treatment of peri-implantitis is not standardized and several surgical techniques are available. However, none provides an evidence-based approach nor predictable therapeutic outcome. Peri-implantitis, like periodontitis, is manageable but not curable.

PERI-IMPLANTITIS: DEFINITION AND DIAGNOSIS

Peri-implant diseases were originally classified into 2 categories; peri-implant mucositis and peri-implantitis. Both diagnoses involve mucosal tissue inflammation around implants[1,2] with clinical signs that include redness, swelling, and bleeding on probing. Peri-implant mucositis is characterized by the marginal inflammation of mucosal tissues around the implant with no loss of supporting bone following initial bone remodeling, whereas peri-implantitis is characterized by inflammation of mucosal tissues around the implant including progressive loss of supporting bone beyond initial biological remodeling.[3]

The 2017 World Workshop on the classification of periodontitis and peri-implant diseases introduced a new classification scheme to further expand the definitions of peri-implant health, peri-implant mucositis, peri-implantitis, and peri-implant soft-tissue and hard-tissue deficiencies.[4–7] This expansion includes more stringent criteria for disease assessment to include patients with and without previous evaluation by the clinician. Based on these factors, a diagnostic tree can be used (**Fig. 1**):

Peri-implant health is characterized by absence of peri-implant signs of soft-tissue inflammation (redness, swelling, and profuse bleeding on probing) and absence of further additional bone loss following initial healing/bone remodeling (**Fig. 2**).

Disclosure: The authors have nothing to disclose.
[a] Division of Periodontology, Department of Oral Health Practice, University of Kentucky College of Dentistry, D-438 Chandler Medical Center, 800 Rose Street, Lexington, KY 40536-0927, USA; [b] Division of Periodontology, Department of Oral Health Practice, College of Dentistry, University of Kentucky, 800 Rose Street, Lexington, KY 40536, USA
* Corresponding author.
E-mail address: lshaddox@uky.edu

Dent Clin N Am 63 (2019) 547–566
https://doi.org/10.1016/j.cden.2019.02.003
0011-8532/19/© 2019 Elsevier Inc. All rights reserved.

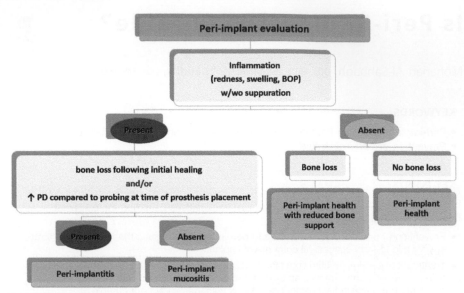

Fig. 1. Peri-implant evaluation flowchart.

Peri-implant mucositis is characterized by the presence of peri-implant signs of inflammation (redness, swelling, line or drop of bleeding, and/or suppuration within 30 seconds following probing), combined with no additional bone loss following initial healing (**Fig. 3**).

Peri-implantitis is based on following criteria:

1. Presence of peri-implant signs of inflammation
2. Radiographic evidence of progressive bone loss (≥2 mm) 1 year following delivery of implant prosthesis
3. Increasing probing depth compared with probing depth values collected after placement of the prosthetic reconstruction

In the absence of previous radiographs, a radiographic bone level of ≥3 mm along with bleeding on probing (BoP) and probing depths ≥6 mm along with bleeding indicates peri-implantitis as shown in **Fig. 4**.

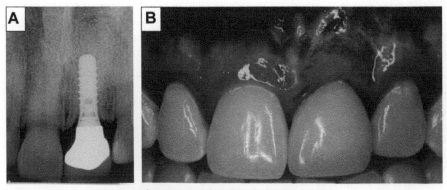

Fig. 2. Peri-implant health is demonstrated in site #9. (*A*) No evidence of radiographic bone loss around the implant. (*B*) Healthy mucosal tissue around the implant at 3-year follow-up.

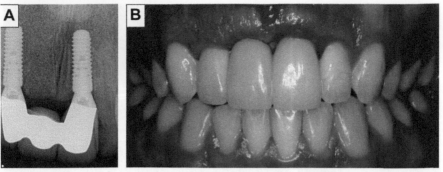

Fig. 3. Peri-implant mucositis around implant #9 at 2-year follow-up. (*A*) The radiographic bone level around implants #7 and #9 do not show additional bone loss following initial healing. (*B*) Marginal inflammation of mucosal tissue exists around implant #9.

Peri-implant soft-tissue and hard-tissue deficiencies may result from a multitude of factors including systemic and local diseases, medications, tissue healing, turnover, response to interventions, trauma, iatrogenic factors, malpositioned implants, biochemical factors, and tissue morphology and phenotype (**Fig. 5**). Furthermore, peri-implantitis can be further classified as mild, moderate, and severe according to probing depth, bone loss, and presence of bleeding and suppuration (**Fig. 6**).

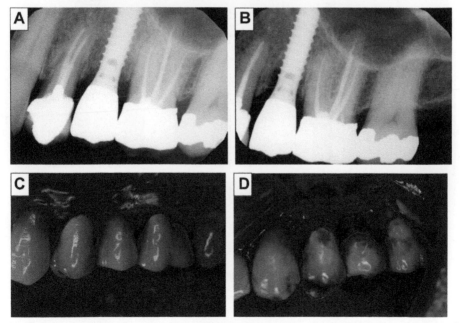

Fig. 4. Peri-implantitis of implant #13. (*A*) Radiographic bone level is normal at the time of implant loading (*B*) Radiographic crestal bone loss is present around the implant after 3 years of function. (*C*) Healthy mucosal tissue around implant at the time of implant loading. (*D*) After 3 years of function, circumferential bone loss around the implant as seen after the reflection of mucoperiosteal flap.

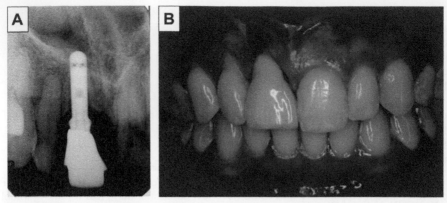

Fig. 5. Peri-implant soft-tissue and hard-tissue deficiencies in implant #8. (*A*) Bone deficiency around the implant is due to implant malposition (implant is more apically and facially positioned). (*B*) Mucosal deficiency is present on midfacial of the implant.

PREVALENCE AND RISK FACTORS

Joos-Jansaker et. al. reported that peri-implant mucositis is present in 48% of implants followed from 9 to 14 years.[8] However, this prevalence could be underreported because peri-implant mucositis is reversible. The prevalence of peri-implantitis is more difficult to assess because study methodologies, specifically in

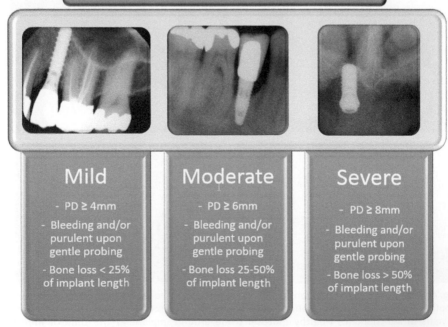

Fig. 6. Classification of peri-implant severity (*Data from* Froum SJ, Rosen, PS. A proposed classification for peri-implantitis. Int J Periodontics Restorative Dent 2012;32(5):533–40.)

terms of peri-implantitis criteria, vary greatly.[9] Peri-implantitis has been reported to range from 1.1% to 85% of implants and in 3% of nonsmokers to 53% of smokers with periodontitis history.[10] Prevalence of peri-implantitis also increases in patients without regular maintenance care (18% vs 9% in patients with regular maintenance).[11] Incidence of peri-implantitis also seems to increase with time: from 0.4% within 3 years after implant placement to 43.9% within 5 years after implant placement. According to a recent meta-analysis, the risk factors for peri-implant diseases include: smoking (odds ratio [OR] 1.7, 95% confidence interval [CI] 1.25–2.3), diabetes mellitus (OR 2.5, 95% CI 1.4–4.5), lack of prophylaxis, and a current or previous history of periodontal disease that has been shown to increase the incidence of peri-implant diseases.[11] Thus, these risk factors need to be taken into consideration when managing peri-implantitis.

PREVENTION AND MAINTENANCE

Peri-implantitis is known to be preceded by peri-mucositis; thus, preventive therapy aiming at the preservation and maintenance of mucosal health around an implant is essential. The "epithelial sealing" around implants is like that of teeth, and there is no evidence that structural differences affects the host response to bacterial challenge.[12–14] Therefore, the process of mucositis is very similar to that of gingivitis.[13] Additionally there is evidence to suggest that, like gingivitis, peri-implant mucositis is reversible when it is effectively treated.[12,13] Initial studies showing implant surface damage from the use of probe or common mechanical instruments, such as Cavitron tips and regular scalers,[15] deter practitioners from using basic prevention techniques, especially in the disruption of subgingival biofilm around implants. Subgingival biofilm disruption on a regular basis is essential to avoid initial inflammation (peri-mucositis). Instruments, such as titanium scalers, regular sonic and ultrasonic scalers with plastic tips, or piezoelectric scalers with carbon or plastic tips,[16] can be used around implant abutments and seem to be safe with regard to subgingival biofilm disruption.

There is a notable paucity of clinical trials addressing the efficacy of preventive measures, and most of these studies evaluated professional plaque control versus patient self-plaque control. There is a lack of a standard preventive measure with demonstrated efficacy to preserve peri-implant health.[17] It has been reported that the use of a triclosan/copolymer toothpaste significantly reduced plaque and gingivitis and BoP as well as microbiological variables compared with a routine fluoride dentifrice after 6 months of application.[18]

MANAGING PERIODONTITIS BEFORE IMPLANT PLACEMENT

Periodontitis should be treated before the placement of a dental implant. A systematic review revealed that significantly more patients developed peri-implantitis when a prior history of periodontitis-associated tooth loss was present (risk ratio, 9; 95% CI 3.94–20.57).[19] Moreover, significantly increased peri-implant marginal bone loss was observed in patients with periodontitis-associated tooth loss after 5 years, mean difference 0.5 mm (95% CI 0.06–0.94).[19] Regular maintenance care must be emphasized in patients with a history of periodontitis to avoid the initiation of peri-implant disease.

MANAGEMENT OF PERI-IMPLANT DISEASES

Once the diagnosis of peri-implant mucositis or peri-implantitis has been made, several nonsurgical and surgical treatment modalities are available.

Nonsurgical Approaches

Peri-implant mucositis

Treatment of peri-implant mucositis is essential for the prevention of peri-implantitis. Mechanical therapy (with or without adjunctive use of antiseptic rinses) is usually the initial treatment of choice for this condition. Graziani and colleagues[17] published a recent systematic review on the treatment of peri-implant mucositis. This publication concluded that only 6 parallel-arm randomized controlled trials (RCTs) evaluated the adjunctive effect of antimicrobial compounds (chlorhexidine [CHX], triclosan, essential oils, and tetracycline fibers) in the treatment of peri-implant mucositis. The results of these were as follows.

Chlorhexidine

- No adjunctive effect was noted with the use of CHX on these studies (with the exception of one study[20] that had low quality of evaluation methods[17])
- Irrigation of sulcus with CHX did not enhance clinical outcomes in terms of reducing periodontal parameters and periodontopathogens[21]
- BoP sites did not decrease with the application of CHX gel[22,23]

Essential oils

- Superior plaque control of mouth rinse essential oils (Listerine) occurred when compared with the control in the absence of mechanical therapy[24]

Triclosan

- Less BoP was noted after daily usage of triclosan/copolymer-containing toothpaste when compared with a sodium fluoride toothpaste[25]

Tetracycline fibers

- In a controlled case series study,[26] little effect was observed from the submucosal placement of tetracycline fibers

Peri-implantitis

Until recently, there was neither any standardized classification of peri-implantitis nor treatment approaches. In addition, the methods of decontamination of implant surfaces are still controversial. Most RCTs in the literature on this topic evaluate small sample sizes and are mostly of short duration.

Renvert and Polyzois[27] examined all recent case series and controlled trials that used mechanical debridement and an adjunctive therapy (local antimicrobial, laser, ultrasonic, or air-abrasive devices). No additional benefits were found with the use of different debridement approaches such as air abrasion,[28] ultrasonic scaling,[29–31] or Erbium:YAG lasers[32,33] in peri-implantitis lesions at 6 to 12 months after treatment. **Table 1** shows controlled studies evaluating different nonsurgical approaches in the treatment of peri-implantitis and their outcomes in terms of reduction of clinical parameters obtained from the different treatment modalities applied.

Air-abrasive devices

- A prospective clinical RCT comparing an air-abrasive device with mechanical debridement showed decreased BoP with the air-abrasive device.[28] Another comparative study, using laser therapy (Er:YAG) and an air-abrasive device (Perio-Flow) showed similar but limited clinical improvement between the 2 methods.[41]

Chlorohexidine

- An RCT[38] comparing mechanical therapy + matrix chips versus mechanical therapy + CHX chips (frequently placed) found both therapies to be effective

Table 1
Nonsurgical treatment studies, treatment approaches, and clinical parameter reductions

Studies	Treatment Approach	Time (mo)	PD/CAL Reduction	Other Parameters/Notes
Nonsurgical approach: mechanical				
Karring et al,[29] 2005	a. OHI + carbon-fiber tip and aerosol spray with HA b. OHI + carbon-fiber curette	6	Not significant from baseline	Reduction on PI and BoP (a only)
Renvert et al,[30] 2009	a. Titanium curette b. Ultrasonic system with specially designed tip	6	Not significant from baseline	Plaque index: mean difference from baseline to 6 mo (both groups) (P<.01) BoP: mean difference from baseline to 6 mo (both groups) (P = .026)
Sahm et al,[28] 2011	a. Air-abrasive device vs b. Mechanical debridement (carbon-fiber curettes)	6	a. PD: 0.6 mm CAL: 0.4 mm b. PD: 0.5 mm CAL: 0.5 mm	a. PI: 0.1 BoP: 43.5% R: 0.2 mm b. PI: 0.2 BoP: 11% R: 0.0 mm
Nonsurgical approach: local antimicrobials				
Buchter et al,[34] 2004	Removal of prosthetic restoration + abutment sterilized + CHX irrigation (0.2%) + scaling (plastic instruments) + a. 8.5% doxycycline hyclate b. No additional treatment	4	PD: a. 0.4 mm[a] b. 0.3 mm[a] CAL: a. 1.1 mm[a] b. 0.3 mm[a,b]	BI: a. 0.2[a] b. 0.1[b]
Renvert et al,[35] 2004	OHI + supra- and submucosal scaling + rubber cup polishing + submucosal administration of: a. 1 mg of Arestin b. 1 mL of 1% CHX gel	3	a. PD: 0.4 mm[a] b. PD: no change	a. PI: 24%[a]; BoP: 43%[a,b] b. PI: 23%; BoP: 15%

(continued on next page)

Table 1
(continued)

Studies	Treatment Approach	Time (mo)	PD/CAL Reduction	Other Parameters/Notes
Renvert et al,[36] 2006	OHI + supra- and submucosal scaling + rubber cup polishing + submucosal administration of a. 1 mg of Arestin b. 1 mL of 1% chlorhexidine gel	12	a. PD: 0.3 mm[a,b] b. PD: no change	a. PI: 23%[a], BoP: 17%[a,b] b. PI: 24%; BoP: 8% Microbiological improvements in both groups
Renvert et al,[37] 2008	a. Minocycline HCl microspheres (Arestin) b. 0.1% chlorhexidine gel	12	PD (deepest site): a. 0.6 mm[a] b. 0.5 mm[a] (significant differences between the groups were found for probing depths up to 6 mo but not at 12 mo)	PI: moderate improvements in both groups BoP (deepest site): a. 26%[a] b. 11%[a] No difference in mean total viable counts between groups
Machtei et al,[38] 2012	a. Mechanical therapy + matrix chips b. Mechanical therapy + chlorhexidine chips	6	PD: a. 1.59 mm[a] b. 2.19 mm[a] CAL: a. 1.56 mm[a] b. 2.21 mm[a]	BoP: a. 41%[a] b. 57.5%[a]
Schar et al,[39] 2013	a. Mechanical therapy + minocycline microspheres b. Mechanical therapy + photodynamic therapy	6	PD: a. 0.49 mm b. 0.36 mm CAL: a. 0.19 mm b. 0.16 mm	R: a. 0.3 mm b. 0.2 mm PI: a. 0.18 b. 0.13 Equally effective treatments
Bassetti et al,[40] 2014	a. Mechanical therapy + minocycline microspheres b. Mechanical therapy + photodynamic therapy	12	PD: a. 0.56 mm b. 0.11 mm CAL: a. 0.31 mm b. 0.08 mm	R: a. 0.27 mm b. 0.03 mm PI: a. 0.21 b. 0.1 Equally effective treatments

Nonsurgical approach: lasers and air-abrasive devices

Study	Months	Treatment	PD	CAL / Bone level	Other outcomes
Schwarz et al,[32] 2005	6	Hygiene program 2 wk before treatment a. Plastic curette + CHX irrigation (0.2%) + CHX gel b. Er:YAG laser	PD: a. 0.7 mm[a] b. 0.8 mm[a]	CAL: a. 0.6 mm[a] b. 0.7 mm[a]	PI: unchanged BoP: a. 22%[a] b. 52%[a]
Schwarz et al,[33] 2006	12	Hygiene program 2 wk before treatment a. Plastic curette + CHX irrigation (0.2%) + CHX gel b. Er:YAG laser Maintenance: supragingival cleaning and OHI (1,3,6 and 12 mo) Moderate disease: PD >4 mm + BoP + bone loss Advanced disease: PD >7 mm + BoP + bone loss	PD: a. 0.2 mm (moderate)[a]; 0.4 mm (advanced)[a] b. 0.5 mm (moderate); 0.4 mm (advanced)[a]	CAL: a. 0.1 mm (moderate); 0.3 mm (advanced) b. 0.3 mm (moderate); 0.2 mm (advanced)	PI: unchanged (higher at 12 mo) BI: a. 0.3 (moderate disease)[a]; 0.2 (advanced disease)[a] b. 0.4 (moderate)[a]; 0.2 (advanced)[a]
Renvert et al,[41] 2011	6	a. Perio-Flow monotherapy (n = 21 patients/45 implants) b. Er:YAG laser monotherapy (n = 21 patients/55 implants) OHI in both groups	PD: a. 0.9 mm b. 0.8 mm Bone level changes: a. −0.1 mm b. −0.3 mm		BoP: a. 65%[a] b. 60%[a] Clinical treatment results were limited and similar between the 2 approaches
Sahm et al,[28] 2011	6	a. Air-abrasive device b. Mechanical debridement (carbon-fiber curettes) + CHX	a. PD: 0.6 mm[a] b. PD: 0.5 mm[a]	CAL: 0.4 mm[a] CAL: 0.5 mm[a]	a. PI: 0.1 　BI: 43.5%[b] 　R: −0.2 mm b. PI: 0.2 　BI: 11% 　R: 0.0

Abbreviations: BI, bleeding index change; BoP, bleeding on probing (% reduction); CAL, clinical attachment level; CHX, chlorhexidine; HA, hydroxyapatite; OHI, oral hygiene instruction; PD, pocket depth; PI, plaque index change; R, recession change.

[a] Significant reduction from baseline.

[b] Significantly different from other treatment group.

Data from Renvert S, Polyzois IN. Clinical approaches to treat peri-implant mucositis and peri-implantitis. Periodontol 2000 2015;68(1):369–404.

in pocket depth reduction and clinical attachment level (CAL) gain, but with no significant difference between the 2 treatment modalities.

Local delivery A significant improvement in clinical parameters was observed in studies testing local application of antibiotics (minocycline microspheres[35–37] or doxycycline gel[34]) against mechanical debridement alone or debridement with CHX gel. The Doxy Gel study[34] was a single-blinded controlled study with 28 patients and 48 implants comparing CHX irrigation (0.2%) + implant scaling with plastic instruments + 8.5% doxycycline hyclate gel (Atridox) versus CHX and implant scaling alone. They found superiority of the adjunctive local-delivery antibiotic for bleeding index and probing CALs (0.2 mm difference). The minocycline microspheres (Arestin) study in 2008[37] showed that repeated treatment/applications (baseline, 30 days, and 90 days) showed superior significant differences in probing depths up to 6 months but not at 12 months.

Local delivery versus photodynamic therapy
- Two RCTs[39,40] comparing mechanical therapy + minocycline microspheres versus mechanical therapy and photodynamic therapy (PTD) found both treatments to be equally effective in reducing clinical parameters with no difference among the 2 modalities.

SURGICAL APPROACHES

Surgical approaches are regularly used in the treatment of peri-implantitis, especially in the more severe cases. Although the literature does not define the severity of peri-implantitis for which a recommendation for a surgical versus a nonsurgical approach should be given, studies have shown generally enhanced clinical results with surgical approaches for the treatment of peri-implantitis.

A systematic review conducted by Graziani and colleagues[17] to analyze differences in surgical approaches in the treatment of peri-implantitis showed broad range of variability in terms of quality of reporting, and methods indicate a trend toward low-quality studies. Additionally there was no standard control intervention in these studies. However, access flap, including debridement/degranulation of the lesion and decontamination of the implant surface, was included in all treatment arms. The results are summarized in **Table 2**.

The consensus of these studies revealed that the surgical treatments showed some improvements in clinical parameters. However, complete resolution of peri-implantitis was never reported and significant differences among different surgical modalities were rarely noted. Deppe and coworkers,[51] in a 4-arm controlled clinical trial, concluded that the use of CO_2 laser surface decontamination and soft-tissue resection around implants showed benefits in implant shoulder to bone height in the short term (4 months) compared with conventional open flap decontamination, but not in the long-term follow-up evaluation.[51] Romeo and colleagues[55,56] indicated a superiority of added implantoplasty in terms of clinical parameter reductions at both short and medium term.

In general, although reduction in clinical parameters can be achieved after surgical intervention in peri-implantitis, evidence-based determination of the efficacy of different surgical interventions cannot be concluded because of low sample sizes, marginal treatment differences, and the small overall number of clinical trials. Future studies including a control arm, a clear surgical design, proven methods for decontamination of the implant surface, and a composite outcome of disease resolution (absence of deep-probing pocket depths with bleeding and suppuration and no additional bone loss) are warranted.

Table 2
Surgical approach studies, treatment approaches, and clinical parameter reductions

Studies	Treatment Approach	Time (mo)	PD/CAL Reduction	Other Parameters/Notes
Surgical approaches				
Mercado et al,[42] 2018, prospective study	30 patients Surgical access and debridement + implant decontamination with 24% EDTA (2 min) + mixture of deproteinized bovine bone mineral with 10% collagen, EMD and doxycycline powder. Defects were covered with connective tissue grafts as needed	36	PD: 5.4 mm[a] Bone gain: 4.3 mm[a]	56.6% of the implants were considered successfully treated (PD < 5 mm, no further bone loss >10%, no BoP/suppuration, no recession >0.5 mm for anterior implants and >1.5 mm for posterior implants)
Heitz-Mayfield et al,[43] 2012, prospective study	All patients received OHI and nonsurgical treatment 4 wk before surgery. Access flap and implant surface debridement with amoxicillin (500 mg) and metronidazole (400 mg) for 7 d (36 implants in 24 patients)	12	PD: 2.4 mm[a]	PI: 34% BoP: 47% R: 1 mm
De Waal et al,[44] 2013	Resective surgical treatment combined with decontamination of the implant surface using 0.12% CHX +: a. 0.05% cetylpyridinium chloride (n = 15 pts/31 implants) b. placebo solution (n = 15 pts/48 implants)	12	PD: a. 2.3 mm b. 1.8 mm Marginal bone loss: a. −0.7 mm b. −0.3 mm Clinical improvements were observed in both groups; no difference between groups	PI: a. −30%; b. 11% BoP: a. 25%; b. 28% Significantly greater reduction of bacterial load on the implant surface on a group but no differences in other clinical parameters

(continued on next page)

Table 2
(continued)

Studies	Treatment Approach	Time (mo)	PD/CAL Reduction	Other Parameters/Notes
Roccuzzo et al,[45] 2011, comparative study	Access flap + granulation tissue removal by plastic curettes + implant cleaning (24% EDTA for 2 min + 1% chlorhexidine gel for 2 min + rinse with saline) + bovine-derived xenograft + connective tissue when necessary in TPS vs SLA implants	12	PD: TPS: 2.1 mm SLA: 3.4 mm[b] Complete defect fill occurred in 3/12 SLA vs 0/14 TPS implants	BoP: TPS: 34% SLA: 60.4%[b]
Khoury and Buchmann,[46] 2001, comparative study	Subgingival debridement and irrigation with CHX + systemic antibiotics a. CHX irrigation + citric acid + hydrogen peroxide + saline + bone blocks and particulate bone (n = 12 implants) b. as "a" + ePTF (expanded polytetrafluoroethylene) membrane (n = 20) c. as "a" + collagen membrane (n = 9)	36	PD: a. 5.1 mm[a] b. 5.4 mm[a] c. 2.61 mm[a] Probing bone levels: a. 3.2 mm[a] b. 4.4 mm[a] c. 2.3 mm[a]	58.6% of the barrier implant sites were compromised by early post-therapy complications All significant treatments but additional use of barriers did not improve overall outcomes 3 y following therapy
Schwarz et al,[47] 2006, comparative study	a. Granulation tissue removal + implant surface debridement by plastic curettes + saline irrigation + nanocrystalline hydroxyapatite (NHA) (Ostim) (n = 11 pts) b. As "a" + Bio-Oss and Bio-Gide (instead of HA)—nonsubmerged (n = 11 patients)	6	PD: a. 2.1 mm[a] b. 2.6 mm[a] CAL: a. 1.8 mm[a] b. 2.3 mm[a]	Postoperative wound healing: NHA compromised initial adhesion of the mucoperiosteal flaps in all patients Both groups showed decreased translucency within the intrabony component of the peri-implant bone defect

Study		Treatment		Results	Comments
Roos-Jansaker et al,[48] 2007, comparative study	12	Systemic antibiotic (amoxicillin, 375 mg, 3 times daily + metronidazole, 400 mg, twice daily)—10 d starting 1 d before surgery. a. Debridement of the granulation tissue + implant detoxification using hydrogen peroxide and irrigation with saline + bone substitute (Algipore) + resorbable membrane (Osseoquest) (n = 17 pts) b. as "a" but no membrane used. Nonsubmerged (n = 19 pts)		PD: a. 2.9 mm[a] b. 3.4 mm[a] Mean defect fills: a. 1.5 mm[a] b. 1.4 mm[a] No significant differences between the 2 groups	Additional use of a membrane was not supported by this study
Schwarz et al,[49] 2008, comparative study	24	a. Granulation tissue removal + implant debrided by plastic curettes + saline irrigation + nanocrystalline HA (Ostim) (n = 9 pts) b. As "a" but Bio-Oss and Bio-Gide (instead of HA). Nonsubmerged (n = 11 pts)		PD: a. 1.5 mm b. 2.4 mm CAL: a. 1.0 mm b. 2.0 mm (no statistics mentioned in paper)	BoP a. 36% b. 44% Both treatments showed efficacy over 24 mo but Bio-Oss + Bio-Gide performed better than HA
Schwarz et al,[50] 2009, comparative study	48	a. Granulation tissue removal + implant debrided by plastic curettes + saline irrigation + nanocrystalline HA (NHA) (Ostim) (n = 9 pts) b. As "a" but Bio-Oss and Bio-Gide used (instead of NHA). Nonsubmerged (n = 10 pts)		PD: a. 1.1 mm b. 2.5 mm CAL a. 0.6 mm b. 2.0 mm (no statistics mentioned in paper)	Application of Ostim resulted in clinical improvements over a period of 4 y but the performance is not as effective as Bio-Oss + Bio-Gide

(continued on next page)

Table 2
(continued)

Studies	Treatment Approach	Time (mo)	PD/CAL Reduction	Other Parameters/Notes
Laser treatment during surgery				
Deppe et al,[51] 2007, comparative study	a. Soft-tissue resection following CO_2 laser (22 implants) b. Soft-tissue resection following CO_2 laser + btricalcium phosphate/autogenous bone and PTF membrane (17 implants) c. Soft-tissue resection and decontamination (19 implants) d. Soft-tissue resection and decontamination + btricalcium phosphate/autogenous bone and PTF membrane (15 implants)	4 (second evaluation was performed after a variable period)	In the short term, CO_2 laser treatment had a beneficial effect on the distance from implant shoulder to the first bone contact	No difference between laser and conventional decontamination in the long term
Schwarz et al,[52] 2011; Schwarz et al,[53] 2012; Schwarz et al,[54] 2013	Nonsurgical therapy + subgingival application of CHX gel. In 2 wk: access flap, granulation tissue removal, implantoplasty. Remaining intrabony defects were randomly treated with: a. Er:YaG laser (9 pts) b. Plastic curettes + cotton pellets + sterile saline (12 pts) In both groups the defects were augmented with a natural bone mineral and covered by a collagen membrane	48	CAL: a. 1.2 mm b. 1.5 mm	BoP: a. 71.6% b. 85.2% The 48-mo clinical outcomes following this combined therapy was not influenced by initial defect configuration or the method of surface decontamination

Abbreviations: BI, bleeding index change; BoP, bleeding on probing (% reduction); CAL, clinical attachment level; CHX, chlorhexidine; HA, hydroxyapatite; OHI, oral hygiene instruction; PD, pocket depth; PI, plaque index change; R, recession change.
[a] Significant reduction from baseline.
[b] Significantly different from other treatment group.
Data from Renvert S, Polyzois IN. Clinical approaches to treat peri-implant mucositis and peri-implantitis. Periodontol 2000 2015;68(1):369–404.

IMPLANT SURFACE TREATMENT

There is a lack of clinical studies evaluating the effects of different implant surface treatments on healing after peri-implantitis therapy. Roccuzzo and colleagues[45] evaluated the treatment of peri-implantitis with mechanical instrumentation on surgical flap and implant decontamination with ethylenediaminetetraacetic acid (EDTA) and CHX gel and saline rinse, followed by placement of a xenograft and connective tissue on titanium plasma-sprayed (TPS) versus sandblasted acid-etched (SLA) surface implants. They observed that there was a complete defect fill in 3 of the 12 SLA implants versus none of the TPS implants. Additionally there was higher bleeding reduction on SLA implants compared with TPS implants.

Another recent retrospective study[57] in 50 patients who had received surgical treatment for peri-implantitis (oral hygiene instruction [OHI], professional supramucosal instrumentation, and surgical therapy: open flap, debridement, calculus removal, and osseous recontouring, when indicated) and supportive therapy at 4-month intervals showed that treatment was effective in resolving the inflammation by reduction in peri-implant pocket depth and BoP scores as well as crestal bone. Treatment outcome was significantly better at implants with nonmodified surfaces than at implants with modified surfaces (TiUnite, TiOblast, Osseospeed, TPS, and SLA).

A recent prospective study of 100 patients with advanced peri-implantitis were randomly assigned to surgical therapy aiming at pocket elimination, and pocket elimination with either systemic antibiotics, use of an antiseptic agent for implant surface decontamination, or both. Results showed that at 3 years after treatment there was a mean reduction in pocket depth of 2.7 mm and a reduction in bleeding/suppuration on probing of 40%, as well as stable peri-implant marginal bone levels (mean bone loss during follow-up of only 0.04 mm). Implant surface characteristics had a significant impact on 3-year outcomes in favor of implants with nonmodified surfaces, and systemic antibiotic benefits were limited to implants with modified surfaces (TiUnite, TiOblast, Osseospeed, Neoss Proactive, and SLA), up to the first year of follow-up.[58]

OUTCOME OF THERAPY

Tables 1 and **2** show means of clinical parameter reductions for surgical and nonsurgical peri-implantitis treatment approaches.[27] This table includes only studies limited to controlled trials or RCTs. Some comparative studies are also included in the table under surgical approaches because there is limited evidence from RCTs. Nonsurgical approaches show significant, albeit limited, reductions in pocket depth (average of 0.4 mm with mechanical therapy alone, 0.7 mm with lasers, and up to 0.8 mm with additional local delivery of antimicrobials) and CAL (ranging from 0.4 mm with mechanical therapy alone, 0.4 mm with lasers, and up to 0.9 mm with additional local delivery of antimicrobials). Compared with reductions in pocket depth (average 1–2 mm) and CAL (average 0.5–1 mm) obtained following nonsurgical and surgical treatment of periodontitis, these values are slightly lower. In vivo studies show that reosteointegration of previously contaminated implant surfaces is indeed possible.[59–61]

SUMMARY

The treatment of peri-implantitis remains controversial, and no standard of care has been defined to date. At present, the limited quantity and quality of RCTs preclude better or preferred treatment choices for the management of peri-implantitis.

Treatment of peri-implantitis, unlike periodontitis, is unpredictable, after either surgical or nonsurgical treatment. Currently there are no data indicating that severity of peri-implantitis lesions can be the basis for recommending nonsurgical or surgical therapy. However, surgical therapy may be required to provide proper access to implant surface decontamination. Although the evidence is limited, some animal studies have shown that reosteointegration of contaminated implant surfaces is possible.[59–61] However, the anatomy of the bone defect and its configuration might be the most important factors in predicting treatment outcomes following regenerative approaches.[27]

Is peri-implantitis curable? Similarly to periodontitis, we do not "cure" it, we manage it. Different treatment approaches, as summarized herein, do result in reduction of clinical parameters of disease and some bone fill in the attempt to maintain the implant for a longer period. However, evidence on the rate of recurrent or refractory peri-implant disease is still not sufficient for a definitive answer to this question.

Prevention is the best form of treatment of peri-implantitis. Thus, following implant placement, patients should be closely monitored with regular recalls to evaluate periodontal and implant health, and compliance with oral hygiene. Since peri-implant mucositis precedes peri-implantitis, and evidence shows it is reversible when effectively treated, this stage of marginal disease is the best time to diagnose the initial problem and reverse it before it becomes an unpredictable issue and challenging to treat.

REFERENCES

1. Mombelli A, Lang NP. The diagnosis and treatment of peri-implantitis. Periodontol 2000 1998;17:63–76.
2. Lindhe J, Meyle J, Group D of European Workshop on Periodontology. Peri-implant diseases: Consensus Report of the Sixth European Workshop on Periodontology. J Clin Periodontol 2008;35(8 Suppl):282–5.
3. Sanz M, Chapple IL, Working Group 4 of the VIII European Workshop on Periodontology. Clinical research on peri-implant diseases: consensus report of Working Group 4. J Clin Periodontol 2012;39(Suppl 12):202–6.
4. Berglundh T, Armitage G, Araujo MG, et al. Peri-implant diseases and conditions: consensus report of workgroup 4 of the 2017 World Workshop on the classification of periodontal and peri-implant diseases and conditions. J Periodontol 2018; 89(Suppl 1):S313–8.
5. Caton JG, Armitage G, Berglundh T, et al. A new classification scheme for periodontal and peri-implant diseases and conditions—introduction and key changes from the 1999 classification. J Clin Periodontol 2018;45(Suppl 20):S1–8.
6. Renvert S, Persson GR, Pirih FQ, et al. Peri-implant health, peri-implant mucositis, and peri-implantitis: case definitions and diagnostic considerations. J Periodontol 2018;89(Suppl 1):S304–12.
7. Hammerle CHF, Tarnow D. The etiology of hard- and soft-tissue deficiencies at dental implants: a narrative review. J Periodontol 2018;89(Suppl 1):S291–303.
8. Roos-Jansaker AM, Renvert H, Lindahl C, et al. Nine- to fourteen-year follow-up of implant treatment. Part III: factors associated with peri-implant lesions. J Clin Periodontol 2006;33(4):296–301.
9. Tomasi C, Derks J. Clinical research of peri-implant diseases—quality of reporting, case definitions and methods to study incidence, prevalence and risk factors of peri-implant diseases. J Clin Periodontol 2012;39(Suppl 12):207–23.
10. Rinke S, Ohl S, Ziebolz D, et al. Prevalence of periimplant disease in partially edentulous patients: a practice-based cross-sectional study. Clin Oral Implants Res 2011;22(8):826–33.

11. Dreyer H, Grischke J, Tiede C, et al. Epidemiology and risk factors of peri-implantitis: a systematic review. J Periodontal Res 2018;53(5):657–81.

12. Lang NP, Berglundh T, Working Group 4 of Seventh European Workshop on Periodontology. Periimplant diseases: where are we now?–Consensus of the Seventh European Workshop on Periodontology. J Clin Periodontol 2011;38(Suppl 11): 178–81.

13. Pontoriero R, Tonelli MP, Carnevale G, et al. Experimentally induced peri-implant mucositis. A clinical study in humans. Clin Oral Implants Res 1994;5(4):254–9.

14. Zitzmann NU, Berglundh T, Marinello CP, et al. Experimental peri-implant mucositis in man. J Clin Periodontol 2001;28(6):517–23.

15. Mengel R, Buns CE, Mengel C, et al. An in vitro study of the treatment of implant surfaces with different instruments. Int J Oral Maxillofac Implants 1998;13(1): 91–6.

16. Rapley JW, Swan RH, Hallmon WW, et al. The surface characteristics produced by various oral hygiene instruments and materials on titanium implant abutments. Int J Oral Maxillofac Implants 1990;5(1):47–52.

17. Graziani F, Figuero E, Herrera D. Systematic review of quality of reporting, outcome measurements and methods to study efficacy of preventive and therapeutic approaches to peri-implant diseases. J Clin Periodontol 2012;39(Suppl 12):224–44.

18. Sreenivasan PK, Vered Y, Zini A, et al. A 6-month study of the effects of 0.3% triclosan/copolymer dentifrice on dental implants. J Clin Periodontol 2011;38(1): 33–42.

19. Schou S, Holmstrup P, Worthington HV, et al. Outcome of implant therapy in patients with previous tooth loss due to periodontitis. Clin Oral Implants Res 2006; 17:104–23.

20. Felo A, Shibly O, Ciancio SG, et al. Effects of subgingival chlorhexidine irrigation on peri-implant maintenance. Am J Dent 1997;10(2):107–10.

21. Porras R, Anderson GB, Caffesse R, et al. Clinical response to 2 different therapeutic regimens to treat peri-implant mucositis. J Periodontol 2002;73(10): 1118–25.

22. Heitz-Mayfield LJ, Salvi GE, Botticelli D, et al. Anti-infective treatment of peri-implant mucositis: a randomised controlled clinical trial. Clin Oral Implants Res 2011;22(3):237–41.

23. Thone-Muhling M, Swierkot K, Nonnenmacher C, et al. Comparison of two full-mouth approaches in the treatment of peri-implant mucositis: a pilot study. Clin Oral Implants Res 2010;21(5):504–12.

24. Ciancio SG, Lauciello F, Shibly O, et al. The effect of an antiseptic mouthrinse on implant maintenance: plaque and peri-implant gingival tissues. J Periodontol 1995;66(11):962–5.

25. Ramberg P, Lindhe J, Botticelli D, et al. The effect of a triclosan dentifrice on mucositis in subjects with dental implants: a six-month clinical study. J Clin Dent 2009;20(3):103–7.

26. Schenk G, Flemmig TF, Betz T, et al. Controlled local delivery of tetracycline HCl in the treatment of periimplant mucosal hyperplasia and mucositis. A controlled case series. Clin Oral Implants Res 1997;8(5):427–33.

27. Renvert S, Polyzois IN. Clinical approaches to treat peri-implant mucositis and peri-implantitis. Periodontol 2000 2015;68(1):369–404.

28. Sahm N, Becker J, Santel T, et al. Non-surgical treatment of peri-implantitis using an air-abrasive device or mechanical debridement and local application of

chlorhexidine: a prospective, randomized, controlled clinical study. J Clin Periodontol 2011;38(9):872–8.

29. Karring ES, Stavropoulos A, Ellegaard B, et al. Treatment of peri-implantitis by the Vector system. Clin Oral Implants Res 2005;16(3):288–93.

30. Renvert S, Samuelsson E, Lindahl C, et al. Mechanical non-surgical treatment of peri-implantitis: a double-blind randomized longitudinal clinical study. I: clinical results. J Clin Periodontol 2009;36(7):604–9.

31. Persson GR, Samuelsson E, Lindahl C, et al. Mechanical non-surgical treatment of peri-implantitis: a single-blinded randomized longitudinal clinical study. II. Microbiological results. J Clin Periodontol 2010;37(6):563–73.

32. Schwarz F, Sculean A, Rothamel D, et al. Clinical evaluation of an Er:YAG laser for nonsurgical treatment of peri-implantitis: a pilot study. Clin Oral Implants Res 2005;16(1):44–52.

33. Schwarz F, Bieling K, Bonsmann M, et al. Nonsurgical treatment of moderate and advanced periimplantitis lesions: a controlled clinical study. Clin Oral Investig 2006;10(4):279–88.

34. Buchter A, Meyer U, Kruse-Lösler B, et al. Sustained release of doxycycline for the treatment of peri-implantitis: randomised controlled trial. Br J Oral Maxillofac Surg 2004;42(5):439–44.

35. Renvert S, Lessem J, Lindahl C, et al. Treatment of incipient peri-implant infections using topical minocycline microspheres versus topical chlorhexidine gel as an adjunct to mechanical debridement. J Int Acad Periodontol 2004;6(4 Suppl):154–9.

36. Renvert S, Lessem J, Dahlén G, et al. Topical minocycline microspheres versus topical chlorhexidine gel as an adjunct to mechanical debridement of incipient peri-implant infections: a randomized clinical trial. J Clin Periodontol 2006; 33(5):362–9.

37. Renvert S, Lessem J, Dahlén G, et al. Mechanical and repeated antimicrobial therapy using a local drug delivery system in the treatment of peri-implantitis: a randomized clinical trial. J Periodontol 2008;79(5):836–44.

38. Machtei EE, Frankenthal S, Levi G, et al. Treatment of peri-implantitis using multiple applications of chlorhexidine chips: a double-blind, randomized multi-centre clinical trial. J Clin Periodontol 2012;39(12):1198–205.

39. Schar D, Ramseier CA, Eick S, et al. Anti-infective therapy of peri-implantitis with adjunctive local drug delivery or photodynamic therapy: six-month outcomes of a prospective randomized clinical trial. Clin Oral Implants Res 2013;24(1):104–10.

40. Bassetti M, Schär D, Wicki B, et al. Anti-infective therapy of peri-implantitis with adjunctive local drug delivery or photodynamic therapy: 12-month outcomes of a randomized controlled clinical trial. Clin Oral Implants Res 2014;25(3):279–87.

41. Renvert S, Lindahl C, Roos Jansåker AM, et al. Treatment of peri-implantitis using an Er:YAG laser or an air-abrasive device: a randomized clinical trial. J Clin Periodontol 2011;38(1):65–73.

42. Mercado F, Hamlet S, Ivanovski S. Regenerative surgical therapy for peri-implantitis using deproteinized bovine bone mineral with 10% collagen, enamel matrix derivative and Doxycycline-A prospective 3-year cohort study. Clin Oral Implants Res 2018;29(6):583–91.

43. Heitz-Mayfield LJA, Salvi GE, Mombelli A, et al. Anti-infective surgical therapy of peri-implantitis. A 12-month prospective clinical study. Clin Oral Implants Res 2012;23(2):205–10.

44. de Waal YC, Raghoebar GM, Huddleston Slater JJ, et al. Implant decontamination during surgical peri-implantitis treatment: a randomized, double-blind, placebo-controlled trial. J Clin Periodontol 2013;40(2):186–95.

45. Roccuzzo M, Bonino F, Bonino L, et al. Surgical therapy of peri-implantitis lesions by means of a bovine-derived xenograft: comparative results of a prospective study on two different implant surfaces. J Clin Periodontol 2011;38(8):738–45.

46. Khoury F, Buchmann R. Surgical therapy of peri-implant disease: a 3-year follow-up study of cases treated with 3 different techniques of bone regeneration. J Periodontol 2001;72(11):1498–508.

47. Schwarz F, Bieling K, Latz T, et al. Healing of intrabony peri-implantitis defects following application of a nanocrystalline hydroxyapatite (Ostim) or a bovine-derived xenograft (Bio-Oss) in combination with a collagen membrane (Bio-Gide). A case series. J Clin Periodontol 2006;33(7):491–9.

48. Roos-Jansaker AM, Renvert H, Lindahl C, et al. Surgical treatment of peri-implantitis using a bone substitute with or without a resorbable membrane: a prospective cohort study. J Clin Periodontol 2007;34(7):625–32.

49. Schwarz F, Sculean A, Bieling K, et al. Two-year clinical results following treatment of peri-implantitis lesions using a nanocrystalline hydroxyapatite or a natural bone mineral in combination with a collagen membrane. J Clin Periodontol 2008;35(1): 80–7.

50. Schwarz F, Sahm N, Bieling K, et al. Surgical regenerative treatment of peri-implantitis lesions using a nanocrystalline hydroxyapatite or a natural bone mineral in combination with a collagen membrane: a four-year clinical follow-up report. J Clin Periodontol 2009;36(9):807–14.

51. Deppe H, Horch HH, Neff A. Conventional versus CO_2 laser-assisted treatment of peri-implant defects with the concomitant use of pure-phase beta-tricalcium phosphate: a 5-year clinical report. Int J Oral Maxillofac Implants 2007;22(1): 79–86.

52. Schwarz F, Sahm N, Iglhaut G, et al. Impact of the method of surface debridement and decontamination on the clinical outcome following combined surgical therapy of peri-implantitis: a randomized controlled clinical study. J Clin Periodontol 2011;38(3):276–84.

53. Schwarz F, John G, Mainusch S, et al. Combined surgical therapy of peri-implantitis evaluating two methods of surface debridement and decontamination. A two-year clinical follow up report. J Clin Periodontol 2012;39(8):789–97.

54. Schwarz F, Hegewald A, John G, et al. Four-year follow-up of combined surgical therapy of advanced peri-implantitis evaluating two methods of surface decontamination. J Clin Periodontol 2013;40(10):962–7.

55. Romeo E, Ghisolfi M, Murgolo N, et al. Therapy of peri-implantitis with resective surgery. A 3-year clinical trial on rough screw-shaped oral implants. Part I: clinical outcome. Clin Oral Implants Res 2005;16(1):9–18.

56. Romeo E, Lops D, Chiapasco M, et al. Therapy of peri-implantitis with resective surgery. A 3-year clinical trial on rough screw-shaped oral implants. Part II: radiographic outcome. Clin Oral Implants Res 2007;18(2):179–87.

57. Berglundh T, Wennstrom JL, Lindhe J. Long-term outcome of surgical treatment of peri-implantitis. A 2-11-year retrospective study. Clin Oral Implants Res 2018; 29(4):404–10.

58. Carcuac O, Derks J, Abrahamsson I, et al. Surgical treatment of peri-implantitis: 3-year results from a randomized controlled clinical trial. J Clin Periodontol 2017; 44(12):1294–303.

59. Alhag M, Renvert S, Polyzois I, et al. Re-osseointegration on rough implant surfaces previously coated with bacterial biofilm: an experimental study in the dog. Clin Oral Implants Res 2008;19(2):182–7.

60. Kolonidis SG, Renvert S, Hämmerle CH, et al. Osseointegration on implant surfaces previously contaminated with plaque. An experimental study in the dog. Clin Oral Implants Res 2003;14(4):373–80.

61. Mohamed S, Polyzois I, Renvert S, et al. Effect of surface contamination on osseointegration of dental implants surrounded by circumferential bone defects. Clin Oral Implants Res 2010;21(5):513–9.

Does Peri-Implant Mucosa Have a Prognostic Value?

Mohanad Al-Sabbagh, DDS, MS[a],*, Pinelopi Xenoudi, DDS, MS[b],
Fatimah Al-Shaikhli, BDS, DMD[c], Walied Eldomiaty, BDS[c],
Ahmed Hanafy, BDS, MSc, PhD[d]

KEYWORDS

- Peri-implant mucosa • Soft-tissue augmentation • Keratinized mucosa
- Mucosal biotype • Aesthetic outcome • Implant health

KEY POINTS

- The effect of peri-implant mucosa thickness and keratinization on the long-term health of implants remains controversial.
- Peri-implant mucosa characteristics have an effect on the aesthetic outcome of implants.
- Implant placement position and macrostructure design play an important role in the final soft-tissue status.
- The surgical technique and timing of soft-tissue augmentation are determined according to peri-implant soft-tissue condition, objective of the procedure, and desired final aesthetic outcome.

INTRODUCTION

Teeth and implants have comparable surrounding soft-tissue configurations including elements of connective tissue and epithelium. However, they have several structural differences.[1] The junctional epithelium around teeth attaches to the enamel surface via desmosomes and internal basal lamina along the length of the junctional epithelium, whereas in implants the junctional epithelium attach to implant surface via hemi-desmosomes.[2] Peri-implant tissues lack cementum and periodontal ligament (with direct contact between alveolar bone and implant surface), and have less

Disclosure: The authors have nothing to disclose.
[a] Division of Periodontology, Department of Oral Health Practice, University of Kentucky College of Dentistry, D-438 Chandler Medical Center, 800 Rose Street, Lexington, KY 40536-0927, USA; [b] Division of Periodontology, Department of Orofacial Sciences, University of California, San Francisco, School of Dentistry, 707 Parnassus Ave, San Francisco, CA 94143, USA; [c] Division of Periodontology, Department of Oral Health Practice, College of Dentistry, University of Kentucky, 800 Rose Street, Lexington, KY 40536-7001, USA; [d] Department of Periodontology, School of Dental Medicine, British University in Egypt, Suez Desert Road, P.O. Box 43, El Sherouk City, Cairo 11837, Egypt
* Corresponding author.
E-mail address: malsa2@email.uky.edu

vascular supply and fewer fibroblasts with parallel rather than perpendicular orientation of supracrestal connective tissue[3,4] (**Table 1**).

The transmucosal attachment around implants is formed after adaptation of the mucosal wound edges to the transmucosal part of the implant. Therefore, following surgical intervention the soft-tissue attachment around the implant develops whereby the development of the periodontium around teeth takes place simultaneously and remains structurally continuous with the surrounding tissues.[5]

There has always been debate surrounding the significance of soft tissue at implant sites on aesthetic outcome and long-term stability of dental implants. The objective of this article is to discuss the controversy of this importance and illustrate suggested surgical techniques and timings for soft-tissue augmentation around implants.

FACTORS INFLUENCING THE PERI-IMPLANT MUCOSAL BARRIER
Supracrestal Attached Tissues Around Implant "Biological Width"

The term supracrestal attached tissues, previously known as "biological width,"[6] refers to the vertical dimension extending from the coronal portion of the junctional epithelium to the apical aspect of the connective tissue attachment.[4] The supracrestal attached tissues provide a biological protective seal around the implant or tooth against any external or biological impingement.[7] Gargiulo and Arrocha[8] and Vacek and colleagues[9] studied the supracrestal attached tissue dimensions in natural dentition in humans. The former study reported that the supracrestal attached tissues' "biological width" consists of a gingival sulcus (average 0.69 mm), an epithelial attachment (average 0.97 mm), and a connective tissue attachment (average 1.07 mm). The latter study confirmed the results of the earlier study, reporting average values of epithelial attachment as 1.14 mm and connective tissue attachment as 0.77 mm. The authors of both studies concluded that the most consistent value between individuals was the dimension of the connective tissue attachment.

In peri-implant mucosa, early studies have shown that the supracrestal attached tissues' "biological width" around dental implants consists of a sulcular epithelium width ranging between 1.5 and 2 mm and connective tissue width ranging between 1 and 2 mm.[10–12] Therefore, dental implants have longer supracrestal attached tissues (2.5–4 mm) in comparison with natural tooth (2–3 mm).[13]

It is important to mention that there are several factors that may influence the dimension of the supracrestal attached tissues around an implant, such as different designs and surface characteristics of different commercially available implant systems, and various placement and surgical protocols. Many studies noted similar mucosal attachment formation around various titanium implant systems[7,14] and around intentionally

Table 1		
Comparison between tooth and implant surrounding tissue		
Clinical Characteristics	**Tooth**	**Implant**
Connection	Cementum, bone, PDL	Osseointegration Ankylosis
Junctional epithelium	Desmosome Internal basal lamina	Hemidesmosome
Connective tissue	Perpendicular fibers	Parallel/oblique fibers
Vascularity	More	Less
Probing depth	≤3 mm	3–4 mm

submerged and intentionally nonsubmerged implants.[15,16] The peri-implant junctional epithelium was significantly longer in initially submerged implants to which an abutment was connected later than in intentionally nonsubmerged implants.[16]

Regarding the design of macrostructure topography, the use of 1-piece or 2-piece implants has been the most relevant factor in determining the vertical dimension of the supracrestal attached tissues.[17] There is an absence of a gap (implant-abutment interface) at crestal bone level when 1-piece (tissue level) dental implants are used, whereas 2-piece (bone level) dental implants have a gap at this region.[18] Herman and colleagues[19] revealed that 1-piece implants showed soft-tissue dimension relatively smaller than that of 2-piece implants, and the supracrestal attached tissues of the 1-piece implant more closely resembled that of the natural dentition.

Hermann and colleagues[19–21] also demonstrated that in 2-part implant systems, bone remodeling occurred 2 mm apical to the micro gap, regardless of the positioning of the implant relative to the bone crest (ie, depth of placement). The investigators postulated that the microbial contamination (or leakage) from the micro gap after the abutment connection could be the cause of the greater apical extension of epithelial attachment in submerged 2-part implants.

Platform switching has been developed to overcome crestal bone loss resulting from the re-establishment of supracrestal attached tissues apical to the implant-abutment interface, where there is a horizontal mismatch between the diameter of the implant and the abutment. The rationale for this development is that the internal repositioning of the implant-abutment interface would shift the inflammatory cell infiltrate (formed at this interface) away from the crestal bone. This results in re-establishment of the supracrestal attached tissues in a predominantly horizontal rather than vertical dimension.[22] Furthermore, it would minimize the vertical bone resorption that occurs as a result of physiologic remodeling associated with biological width formation. In addition, it has been postulated that platform shifting has a biomechanical advantage by moving stress concentration from the outer edges of the implant.[23]

PAPILLA HEIGHT

Papilla height next to dental implants is one of the most significant factors that can affect the aesthetic outcome around an implant. Clinical studies were conducted to evaluate the presence or absence of the papilla between implants and teeth.[24] The presence of the papilla between an implant and adjacent tooth was demonstrated to depend on the vertical position of the periodontal attachment of the neighboring tooth. In cases with a vertical distance between the contact point and the bone crest of 5 mm, complete papilla fill is anticipated. When the distance was greater than 5 mm, the presence of the papilla was reduced to a frequency of 50%. In a clinical study, the mean papilla height between 2 adjacent implants was 3.4 mm, which is 1.5 mm less than between an implant and a natural tooth.[25] Compared with natural teeth, the papilla at implant sites are reported to be significantly shorter.[26]

In addition to the vertical position, the horizontal distance between the implant and the adjacent tooth needs to be considered. It was suggested that a minimal distance of 1.5 mm would be necessary to compensate for remodeling processes following establishment of the biological width.[27,28] Tarnow and colleagues[29] evaluated the horizontal distance of bone between 2 adjacent implants and the respective presence of the papilla. When the measurement of interimplant distance was ≤3 mm, the amount of crestal bone loss was 1.04 mm, whereas 0.45 mm of bone loss was noted with an interimplant distance of greater than 3 mm. These findings indicate the need for a minimum distance of 3 mm between 2 adjacent implants for the presence of a normal papilla. These distances may have to be reconsidered in the future following the introduction of dental implants with platform-shifting modifications.[30–32] Such implants have been shown to result in less peri-implant bone loss compared with the standard types of implant.[33]

MUCOSAL PHENOTYPE

Mucosal thickness of soft tissue around implants is of clinical importance because of the influence on the aesthetic outcome and implant health. In addition, it may partly compensate for missing bone on the buccal side of dental implants.[34,35]

At implant restorations, the gingival phenotype has been described as one of the key elements that lead to a successful treatment outcome.[36] In particular, papilla between immediate single-tooth implant and adjacent teeth was significantly correlated with a thick-flat phenotype.[37] According to Evans and Chen,[38] mucosal recession increases in patients with thin gingiva immediately after single-implant restorations. Implant sites with thin mucosa were vulnerable to angular bone defects, and implants with thick mucosa have shown a stability in crestal bone dimension.[39] In addition, patients with thick-flat mucosa had the ability of retaining the implant papilla height,[37] resisting recession,[40,41] concealing titanium,[42] and an overall better aesthetic outcome[43] that is more amenable to various implant positions.[38,42] Therefore, thick soft-tissue phenotype around dental implants is more favorable to thin phenotype.

The critical soft-tissue thickness on the buccal aspect of implants has been demonstrated to be 2 mm.[42,44] In cases where the buccal soft-tissue volume is <2 mm, when the choice of the soft-tissue augmentation material can significantly influence the aesthetic outcome at the implant site, the results of all-ceramic restorations were superior than metal-ceramic restorations.[31,45,46] In another study, the presence of >1 mm of thick mucosa around dental implants had lower gingival recession than <1 mm of thin mucosa.[47]

KERATINIZED MUCOSA

The influence of keratinized mucosa (KM) dimension around implants on the maintenance of soft and hard tissue is a controversial topic,[47] as is the need to augment the keratinized tissue around implants in patients with lack of width or reduced width.[48] Preserving healthy peri-implant tissue around a dental implant might be related to presence of an adequate amount of attached mucosal tissue.[49] According to a study conducted by Adibrad and colleagues[50] in 2009, a significant association exists between a limited zone of keratinized mucosa around dental implants and increased plaque accumulation, mucosal inflammation, bleeding on probing, recession, alveolar bone loss, and probing depth.

The response of the peri-implant mucosa to plaque formation was investigated in human and animal studies.[51,52] It was observed that plaque formation and soft-tissue response develop in a similar manner around teeth and dental implants. However, with increasing duration of plaque accumulation, the peri-implant mucosa showed less efficiency in encapsulating the inflammatory lesion.[53] Thus, the rate of tissue destruction in peri-implant mucositis is higher than that in periodontal lesions.[54] As a result, having an adequate amount of peri-implant soft tissue that firmly attaches to underlying bone has been suggested as a key factor for long-term success of dental implants.[55]

The existence of an adequate band of KM around dental implants might be imperative for plaque control and plaque-associated mucosal lesions because the potential for plaque control was better for implants with KM for the same patients.[56] Warror and colleagues[57] reported that tissue breakdown and early loss of attachments is more likely to arise from plaque accumulation in an area with inadequate amount of KM around a dental implant. A higher rate of plaque accumulation and peri-implantitis was expected after placing an implant in an area with no KM implants in comparison with implants placed in an area with KM.[58,59] This finding is in agreement with other studies that support the significance of KM around dental implants in controlling plaque and maintaining overall health of peri-implant tissues[60–63] (**Fig. 1**).

Langer and Langer,[64] Landi and Sabatucci,[65] and Lee and colleagues[66] concluded that a minimum width of 2 mm of KM was needed to maintain peri-implant tissue because it decreased plaque accumulation, bleeding around the implant, and mucosal recession. Zigdon and Machtei[47] reported that the width of KM around implants might be critical in the early identification and diagnosis of mucosal recession.[67,68] These investigators suggested that patients with less than 2 mm of KM have a significantly higher plaque accumulation associated with peri-implantitis over a period of 3 years.

On the other hand, different systematic reviews dispute that an adequate width of KM around dental implants is critical for the health of the peri-implant mucosa, improved aesthetic outcome, and higher survival rates of dental implants.[69–71] In their systematic review, Wennstrom and Derks[71] reported that there is no strong evidence with regard to risks/benefits of absence/presence of KM at dental implants. They also stated that proper plaque control is more important than the presence of KM around implants. Another study revealed that the width of keratinized band had no critical impact on the health condition of peri-implant tissue or plaque control.[49]

Although a conclusion cannot be reached on the influence of KM on long-term survival of dental implants, the preservation and/or reconstruction of KM around dental implants may be needed to facilitate restorative procedures, improve aesthetics, and control plaque formation (**Table 2**).[72,73]

TIMING OF PERI-IMPLANT SOFT-TISSUE AUGMENTATION

At present there is not enough evidence in the literature to allow formulation of a guideline for the most suitable timing and technique for performing soft-tissue augmentation around implants. Soft-tissue management of dental implant sites may be completed before placement, after placement, before prosthetic loading, or even after the prosthetic loading of a dental implant.[58] In a study by Stimmelmayr and colleagues[78] on 70 implants, the amount of shrinkage of free gingival graft (FGG) at the time of implant placement was greater compared with FGG placed at the second-stage surgery.

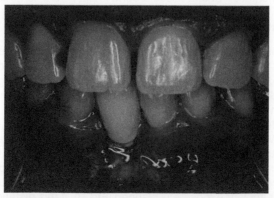

Fig. 1. Implant in site #25 with mucosal recession and no keratinized mucosa. Note the plaque accumulation around the implant-abutment interface.

Table 2
Systematic reviews evaluating the influence of peri-implant keratinized mucosa (KM)

Authors, Year	Objective of Research	No. of Studies Included	Conclusion
Lin et al,[74] 2013	Examination of KM effect on peri-implant health parameters	11	Lack of adequate KM around dental implants is associated with more plaque accumulation, tissue inflammation, mucosal recession, and attachment loss
Gobbato et al,[75] 2013	Effect of KM width on clinical parameters of soft-tissue health and stability around dental implants	8	Predictive value of KM width was limited, although reduced KM width was associated with inflammation and poor oral hygiene
Brito et al,[76] 2014	Importance of KM around dental implants to maintain proper health of peri-implant tissue	7	Adequate zone of KM may be necessary for better peri-implant tissue health, but more randomized controlled trials are needed to support this claim
Pranskunas et al,[77] 2016	Influence of peri-implant soft-tissue condition and plaque accumulation on peri-implantitis	8	• Insufficient KM does not necessarily mediate adverse effects on the hygiene management and soft-tissue health condition • The risk of increase in gingival index, plaque index, pocket depth, and bleeding on probing/modified bleeding index is present • Presence of an appropriate amount of keratinized gingiva is required

Timing of the most effective surgical techniques with clinical outcomes and drawbacks in the augmentation of soft tissue around implants are summarized in **Table 3**.

SURGICAL TECHNIQUES

Several techniques have been proposed to obtain an adequate amount of KM around 2-stage implants. If the amount of KM is minimal, FGG is suggested at the time of implant exposure. Apically positioned flap (using mid-crestal or lingually positioned incision) or laterally positioned flap was also proposed to reconstruct an adequate zone of KM around implants.[64,79]

Barone and colleagues[80] proposed a surgical protocol for soft-tissue reconstruction around implants. When the baseline width of KM is minimal (<2 mm), an FGG is placed before fixture installation (**Fig. 2**). At the time of fixture installation, the distance between the bone crest and the mucogingival junction is measured and the type of second surgical procedure is scheduled. If the distance is ≤3 mm, the use of an apically positioned flap for implant exposure is planned (**Fig. 3**). If this distance is >0 mm, circular gingivectomy is scheduled. Barone and colleagues[80] used FGG to augment soft